Infectious
CONNECTIONS

How Short-term Foodborne Infections Can Lead to Long-term Health Problems

T0273419

BEATRICE TRUM HUNTER

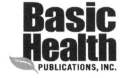

Basic
Health
PUBLICATIONS, INC.

Basic Health Publications, Inc.
28812 Top of the World Drive
Laguna Beach, CA 92651
949-715-7327 • www.basichealthpub.com

Library of Congress Cataloging-in-Publication Data

Hunter, Beatrice Trum.
  Infectious connections : how short-term foodborne infections can lead to long-term health problems / by Beatrice Trum Hunter.
      p. cm.
   Includes bibliographical references and index.
   ISBN 978-1-59120-244-8
   1. Food—Toxicology—Health aspects. 2. Food contamination—Health aspects. 3. Food--Microbiology. I. Title.
   RA1258.H86   2009
   615.9'54—dc22

                                                        2009024676

Editor: Cheryl Hirsch
Typesetting/Book design: Gary A. Rosenberg
Cover design: Mike Stromberg

Printed in the United States of America

10   9   8   7   6   5   4   3   2   1

To Norman Goldfind
with appreciation of his efforts
to afford authors the opportunity
to enlighten readers.

Contents

Part Four
Reducing Your Risk of Foodborne Illness

PART ONE

Foodborne Diseases and Infectious Connections

CHAPTER 1

Introduction

By the early twentieth century, it was understood that most known killer diseases were caused by infectious pathogens, not from "bad blood" or "bad air" (miasma). Diseases such as smallpox, bubonic plague, yellow fever, tuberculosis, diphtheria, and whooping cough were held in check by improved sanitation, vaccines, surveillance, and antibiotics.

Although there was success in controlling these scourges, since then newly emerged infectious diseases have appeared. Some examples are acquired immune deficiency syndrome (AIDS), Legionnaires' disease, hepatitis C, antibiotic-resistant tuberculosis, and methicillin-resistant *Staphylococcus aureus* (MRSA). In addition, new foodborne infections are emerging, and other foodborne infections, long with us, have become more virulent. This book will focus on the main foodborne infections, and how the short-term illnesses that they produce may lead to long-term chronic health disorders. Also, foodborne infections may compound the problems of other health conditions already present.

We have come to recognize that many chronic health disorders, including some forms of heart disease, arthritis, and cancer, may have infectious connections. Diseases long ascribed to genetics or environmental factors actually may be linked to infections. Opposite is a list of some infectious agents and the diseases they can induce. Among them are many foodborne infections.

KOCH'S FOUR POSTULATES TO PROVE INFECTIVITY

By 1905 Robert Koch, the distinguished German bacteriologist (1843–1910), was well known for isolating and identifying the bacteria that causes anthrax (1876), tuberculosis (1882), and cholera (1883). With all this experience behind him, by 1905 Koch set out four postulates that must be proved before it can be accepted that particular bacteria cause

Infectious Agent	Disease Induced or Suspected
Borrelia burgdorferi	Chronic Lyme arthritis
Borna disease virus	Schizophrenia*
Chlamydia pneumoniae	Alzheimer's disease*, atherosclerosis, bronchitis, heart disease, periodontitis, pneumonia
Coxsackie B virus	Obsessive-compulsive disorder*, type 1 diabetes (once known as juvenile diabetes or insulin-dependent diabetes)
Clostridia	Gallstones
Cytomegalovirus (CMV)	Heart disease
Epstein-Barr virus	Burkitt's lymphoma, multiple sclerosis (MS)
Eubacteria	Gallstones
Hepatitis B and C viruses	Chronic liver disease
Herpesvirus	Kaposi's sarcoma, heart disease
Human papilloma virus	Cervical cancer, prostate cancer*
Influenza vaccines	Guillain-Barré syndrome
Listeria monocytogenes	Blood infections, encephalitis, meningitis, spontaneous abortion (miscarriage)
Mycobacterium tuberculosis	Crohn's disease
Various infective organisms, including *Streptococcus*	Tourette's syndrome
West Nile virus	Paralysis, post-polio syndrome

* Organism is suspected of causing this condition.

particular disease. According to these four postulates—still recognized as valid—a microbe must be:

• Found in a person or animal with the disease

• Isolated or grown in culture

• Injected into a healthy experimental animal to produce the disease

• Recovered from the experimentally diseased animal, and shown to be the same pathogen as the original one

Applying Koch's four postulates, some infectious connections with chronic health problems are established firmly; others, tentative and circumstantial. Additional ones, as yet, may be unrecognized and unidentified. This book will discuss some infectious connections that are well recognized, such as *Helicobacter pylori* with stomach ulcers and *Campylobacter jejuni* with Guillain-Barré syndrome. Also, this book will discuss many other foodborne infections that likely are associated with various health disorders of various systems and organs of the body.

FOODBORNE DISEASES IN THE TWENTY-FIRST CENTURY

The incidence of foodborne illness in the United States keeps increasing. The Atlanta-based Centers for Disease Control and Prevention (CDC), a branch of the U.S. Public Health Service, estimates that about 76 million cases of foodborne illness occur annually in the United States, resulting in 325,000 hospitalizations and 5,000 deaths. Some researchers suggest that these figures are gross underestimations. Many cases go unreported. Gastrointestinal (GI) distress that resembles stomach flu (often called gastroenteritis) is the most common initial symptom. Yet, unless the GI distress is severe, few individuals seek medical help, and many are not hospitalized. Some cases are misdiagnosed. Deaths may be ascribed to other health conditions (to AIDS for example), with foodborne illness being an accessory to, and increasing the gravity of, the main illness.

The incidence of foodborne diseases could be lowered dramatically through various means discussed in this book. The end result would be far fewer cases of short-term gastroenteritis, and perhaps more important, far fewer cases of long-term chronic diseases associated with foodborne infections.

GLOBALIZATION INCREASES RISK OF FOODBORNE DISEASES

In an article titled "Infectious Diseases of the Twenty-First Century," Jesús Kumate, at Hospital de Especialidades in Mexico City, wrote about global factors that contribute to infectious diseases. Among them are "the industrialization of food, national and international commerce, and the combination in some places of economic deterioration, an increase in poverty, and less available potable water." Kumate continued, "Important factors leading to continued foodborne disease in the next century [twenty-first century] will be the growing need for convenience foods prepared on an industrial scale or consumed in the street, and the globalization of the economy which increases contact between people, vectors, and object carriers of pathogenic microbes."
—*Archives of Medical Research*, Summer 1997

CHAPTER 2

Foodborne Infections and Chronic Diseases

A growing body of medical evidence links many chronic diseases, directly or indirectly, to pathogenic organisms that contaminate food (and sometimes water used in growing or in processing food). In many instances, the pathogens function as "environmental triggers." That is, how the body responds to the pathogen, or to any toxin that the pathogen produces, varies depending on one's immune system, genes, intestinal permeability, and other factors unique to one's own internal environment.

A complex interaction between the pathogen and the immune system can lead to autoimmune reactions, and result in tissue damage in organ systems. One's individual genetic makeup also plays a role. Specific genes can increase the risks. At times, the pathogen or its toxin may interrupt the intestinal integrity of the individual, and permit entry of substances normally excluded. Or, the pathogen may disrupt nutrient transport in the individual. This may result in nutritional deficiencies and in turn, lead to immunological impairment or autoimmune disease. (The immune system, the digestive system, and nutritional impact of infection will be discussed shortly.)

There are three possible outcomes of foodborne illness. The person (1) makes a full recovery, (2) dies, or (3) suffers a long-term consequence that can lead to debilitating illness or death.

A mild reaction to a pathogen can range from a simple stomach upset, headache, muscle aches, and fever to abdominal cramps, vomiting, and diarrhea. The symptoms are transient, with no lasting health problems.

Death is an infrequent outcome, other than with a few notable exceptions. For example, botulism (see Chapter 17) can lead to rapid death due to the neurotoxic effects of the virulent toxin produced by *Clostridium bot-*

ulinum. Or, fish poisoning from the virulent tetrodotoxin produced by puffer fish (also known as blowfish or swellfish) can cause death within hours after ingestion of the toxin. What is not as well recognized is that death can follow an invasion of certain bacterial organisms such as *Listeria monocytogenes* (see Chapter 8) or certain strains of *Salmonella* (see Chapter 3) into the bloodstream, as a direct result of the interaction between the bacteria and the individual. Such cases do occur, and they are dramatic as well as tragic.

In more common episodes, infectious bacteria initially cause acute gastrointestinal distress, and then invade the bloodstream. The bacteria establish themselves at various sites within the body and then begin to cause problems. For example, *Salmonella* can infect heart valves and later lead to bacterial endocarditis. Or, it can infect the walls of the larger blood vessels, and later lead to endarteritis, a condition found in people with some degree of atherosclerosis. The minor change in the blood vessel wall (caused by the atherosclerosis) allows the *Salmonella* to gain entry and become established. Or, *Salmonella* may go from the bloodstream into bone, and later lead to osteomyelitis. These three different health problems result in distinctly different clinical conditions, and have different outcomes. However, all three result in chronic health problems, which, if untreated, can be fatal.

If *Listeria monocytogenes* invades the bloodstream and infects specific target organisms such as a pregnant woman's placenta, it can lead to spontaneous abortion (miscarriage). Or, the pathogen can invade the central nervous system, and lead to meningitis. Even if the person recovers fully from meningitis following the *L. monocytogenes* infection, some persistent brain damage can be inflicted.

Campylobacter jejuni (see Chapter 5), the most common cause of acute bacterial gastroenteritis in the United States, is associated with the chronic health disorder, Guillain-Barré syndrome. Unlike *L. monocytogenes*, which gets into the bloodstream and infects other sites in the body, *C. jejuni* bacteria remain in the intestines of the person with Guillain-Barré syndrome and cause nerve damage. The body's immune response to the infecting *C. jejuni* bacteria is to generate antibodies to the outer surface of the bacteria. These antibodies then attack the tissue that normally acts as insulation around some of the nerves. Gradually, the unprotected nerves cease to function, and the body becomes paralyzed.

These cited chronic health problems serve as illustrations of infectious connections with foodborne illnesses. Now, we will discuss the effects of foodborne illnesses on various systems and organs of the body.

FOODBORNE INFECTIONS AND THE IMMUNE SYSTEM

The immune system is composed of sets and subsets of cells with different functions that communicate through a complex system of chemical signals. The cells interact specifically with other cells of the immune system or affect other organs of the body, to thwart disease-causing organisms from entering and proliferating within the body. The skin and the mucous membrane linings of the gastrointestinal, respiratory, and genitourinary tracts provide the first line of defense against the invasion of infectious organisms.

The immune system in the gastrointestinal tract needs to cope with an enormous load of substances (foods) foreign to the body. The system functions in its own distinctive ways, even though it is related to the larger systemic immune system. The complexities of the intestine's immune system are recognized, both in humans and in other living organisms. For example, 90 percent of all immunoglobulin-secreting cells (antibodies) of rodents are in their small intestines. Similarly, a large percentage of the human immune system is located in the intestinal tract. The integrity and optimal functioning of the immune system in humans, as well as in other creatures, are vital for health and survival.

An antigen is a substance that, when introduced into the body, causes the body to produce antibodies to fight the foreign substance and create immunity to it. Antigens can be toxins, bacteria, or viruses in blood cells. They are foreign to the body. T cells are immune cells that activate other cells to destroy pathogens. Several foodborne pathogens have been identified as antigens in tissues of Crohn's disease patients: *L. monocytogenes, E. coli,* and some species of *Streptococcus,* as we'll see shortly.

FOODBORNE INFECTIONS AND THE DIGESTIVE SYSTEM

Numerous foodborne pathogens include bacteria, viruses, one-celled protozoa, helminthes (worms), fungi, and toxins produced by microbes. These pathogens can induce gastrointestinal illness and may be factors in chronic diseases. The digestive system is the port of entry for all the foodborne pathogens discussed in this book. As just mentioned, a large portion of the immune system is located in the digestive system.

Leaky Gut Syndrome

A condition exists that has been termed leaky gut syndrome. Leaky gut syndrome (also called increased intestinal permeability) is a condition that results from damage to the intestinal lining, making it less able to protect the internal environment against entry of inappropriate substances, such as food and toxins, into the bloodstream. Foodborne infections may alter the permeability of the gut. This triggers an autoimmune reaction, which can lead to autoimmune disorders such as hypersensitivity or allergic reactions, Crohn's disease, and other inflammatory bowel conditions.

Inflammatory Bowel Disease

Inflammatory bowel disease (IBD) is a collective term for Crohn's disease and ulcerative colitis. Both conditions are chronic inflammatory diseases in the gastrointestinal tract. The two conditions can be difficult to differentiate because often the symptoms are similar.

Although the cause of IBD and its mechanism(s) for flare-ups and remissions are unknown, transmissible infectious agents, including foodborne pathogens, are suspected. In studies, species of *E. coli, Pseudomonas, Mycobacterium,* and *Enterococcus faecalis* have all been identified, at times, in affected tissue of some people with IBD, but not in the healthy controls.

Mycobacterium paratuberculosis may be associated with Crohn's disease. This pathogen causes diseases in ruminant animals. Infected cows shed *M. paratuberculosis,* and the viable organism has been identified in pasteurized milk. It is thought that a susceptible human newborn infant could become infected with this organism by ingesting commercial dairy products, and lead to chronic low-grade inflammation. Over time, the severity of the immune system's response could increase, and ultimately would produce the pathologic features of Crohn's disease.

Crohn's disease was recognized in 1913 by a Scottish surgeon, Thomas Kennedy Dalziel (1861–1924). The disorder is in the small intestine and involves malfunctioning of the autoimmune system, especially of T4 cells, a type of T cell, and causes inflammation in the intestinal tract. The disease is debilitating and chronic.

Dalziel recognized similarities between Crohn's disease and a mycobacterial infection in livestock, termed Johne's disease. The pathogen was isolated in 1895 by Heinrich Johne, a bacteriologist and veterinarian, and L. Frothingham, a pathologist, who had been investigating a serious intestinal infection in a cow from Germany.

Both Crohn's disease in humans, and Johne's disease in livestock and in other animals, share some common features. Both are associated with mycobacterial infections. Both are diseases centered in the ileum, the final section of the small intestine. Both begin early in life with long incubation periods. Both have very similar symptoms and immune responses in their hosts. Whether Johne's disease is transmissible from animals to humans (a feature known as zoonotic) is unclear.

Mycobacteria are among the most damaging bacteria to health. *Mycobacterium tuberculosis* is responsible for many deaths through the respiratory illness of tuberculosis. Another species, *M. leprae,* causes leprosy. *M. avium paratuberculosis* (MAP) has emerged as a widespread pathogen among livestock herds and causes a severe intestinal disease. MAP is linked, too, with Crohn's disease as well as an opportunistic infection in immunosuppressed individuals. This pathogen has an unusual ability to withstand heat and can survive pasteurization. This feature makes the pathogen worrisome as a potential contaminant in the food supply of items, such as meat and dairy products as well as in drinking water.

Shiga toxin-producing *E. coli* infection, like other foodborne infections, usually begins with acute gastroenteritis. However, this group of pathogens produces potent toxins that may go into the bloodstream and attack small blood vessels or other vital organs, such as the kidney, pancreas, and brain.

The major foodborne viruses linked to chronic health problems are hepatitis A and E (see Chapter 13). Both are transmitted orally in contaminated food or water, and lead to acute hepatitis (liver inflammation).

SOME DISEASES WITH POSSIBLE VIRAL ORIGINS

In the National Institute of Allergy and Infectious Diseases' 1992 *Report of the Task Force on Microbiology and Infectious Diseases,* the following diseases were cited as having viral infectious origins:

- Alzheimer's disease
- Atherosclerosis
- Certain leukemias and lymphomas
- Cervical cancer
- Connective tissue diseases
- Diabetes mellitus
- Kawasaki syndrome
- Multiple sclerosis
- Sjögren's syndrome

FOODBORNE INFECTIONS AND NUTRITIONAL STATUS

Malabsorption and Nutrient Loss

Repeated diarrheal episodes caused by foodborne illness or by other infections can lead to malabsorption and loss of nutrients, fluids, and electrolytes. To some degree, malabsorption results in malnutrition and weight loss. Even the nutrient stress from short-duration diarrhea can cause subtle changes in the efficient functioning of the immune system. Chronic diarrhea may compromise the nutritional status so gravely that the immune system's functioning may be impaired. For example, *C. jejuni* has been found to cause such severe and prolonged diarrhea and malabsorption of nutrients in infants that they fail to thrive.

Other foodborne pathogens that cause malabsorption and nutrient loss in the intestine include Enterobacteriaceae, rotaviruses (see Chapter 10), amoebas, *Cryptosporidia* (see Chapter 15), and *Giardia lamblia* (beaver fever). Deaths due to diarrheal illness in immune-suppressed individuals, and in persons with acquired immune deficiency syndrome (AIDS) are estimated at nearly 80 percent. Even with treatment, AIDS patients may develop additional health problems. For example, *Cryptosporidia* are host-adapted, which in AIDS patients may lead to pulmonary or tracheal cryptosporidiosis, accompanied by coughing and frequent low-grade fever. In such cases, there is no effective treatment. In AIDS patients with cryptosporidiosis, the intestinal infection is chronic.

FOODBORNE INFECTIONS AND JOINT DISEASES

Two types of arthritis, septic and aseptic, may be triggered by foodborne infections, as well as by other pathogens.

Septic Arthritis

Septic arthritis is a common health problem in which the infective organism is present in the joints. The problem arises from the ready accessibility of blood to the synovial space. Synovial fluid is secreted and found in joint cavities, bursae (pad-like sacs that reduce friction between joints), and tendon sheaths. Generally, the risk factors in septic arthritis are similar to those for sepsis, a condition in which microbes or their toxins infect blood or tissue. Even with medical treatment judged successful, there may be permanent joint damage.

Aseptic Arthritis

Aseptic arthritis is known more commonly as reactive arthritis (ReA). Formerly, ReA was known as Reiter's syndrome, named to honor the German physician Hans Conrad Reiter (1881–1969). He had written about the syndrome, and in the early 1940s, he was given public recognition. However, in the 1990s, his war record was publicized, and it was revealed that he had voluntarily served as a senior Nazi official during the Hitler regime. As a result, many medical journals and textbooks have dropped the term Reiter's syndrome, and use ReA.

Unlike septic arthritis, with ReA, pathogenic organisms are not active in the joints. Antigen components of the infective organisms are there, but they are not viable.

ReA, as well as ankylosing spondylitis, is linked to the HLA-B27 gene. (See the inset below.) ReA affects the joints, eye, urethra, and skin. Ankylosing spondylitis is a rheumatic disease that causes arthritis in the spine and sacroiliac joints, and also can cause inflammation in the eyes and heart valves. Individuals who suffer an infection in the small intestine, and who also carry the HLA-B27 gene, are eighteen times more at risk of

GENES AND ARTHRITIS: MOLECULAR MIMICRY

Genes may play a role in arthritis. Individuals who carry the gene responsible for producing the human leukocyte antigen HLA-B27 are more susceptible to arthritis than individuals who do not carry this gene. The molecular structure of antigens from particular foodborne bacteria linked to arthritis mimics the HLA antigen. This molecular mimicry could be a mechanism linking foodborne bacteria and arthritis.

Microbes can disguise themselves with proteins that mimic those of their hosts, as a way of evading detection by the immune system of the host. Such molecular mimicry, advantageous to the microbe, harms the host by causing the immune system's protectors to mistakenly attack the body's own tissue. This is the basis for the development of autoimmune diseases. Molecular mimicry has been identified as a factor in disparate disorders, such as eye disease, chronic arthritis from Lyme's disease, and heart disease from *Chlamydia*.

developing ReA than individuals who have the intestinal infection but lack the gene; those with ankylosing spondylitis, and who also carry the gene, are 126 times more at risk.

Some common infectious foodborne agents that can trigger ReA include certain strains of *Salmonella*, especially *S*. Typhimurium and *S*. Enteriditis. Of some 2,000 *Salmonella* serotypes (types of a microorganism determined by their characteristic sets of antigens), twenty-two have been reported to trigger ReA.

It is difficult to connect ReA with a prior *Salmonella* infection. By the time ReA symptoms appear, detection of the offending pathogen in the stool is unlikely. It is thought that in cases of ReA, a faulty interleukin-1 and lymphocyte response in the body to the initial infection fail to eliminate the pathogen efficiently. Then, the *Salmonella* is transported to bones. From there, it may continue to joints, where it can become established and perpetuate joint inflammation.

Juvenile ReA, generally regarded as an immune system disorder, also may be caused by microbial infection, as demonstrated by indirect evidence. The offending pathogen, *Mycoplasma pneumoniae*, is a common cause of atypical pneumonia. In a nearly two-decade Canadian study, diagnosed cases of juvenile ReA peaked in the same year as *M. pneumoniae* infections. This evidence, however, does not prove cause and effect.

Other foodborne pathogens also can induce ReA. All pathogens that can induce ReA share some similar characteristics. They can cause infections on mucosal surfaces. They all have lipopolysaccharides (lipids and sugars) on their outer membranes. Additionally, all the organisms are capable of penetrating cells within human bodies.

Other foodborne infections that can trigger ReA include: *C. jejuni*, *Shigella dysenteriae*, *Shigella flexneri*, *E. coli*, and *Klebsiella pneumoniae*. This last-named microbe is associated especially with ankylosing spondylitis. Additional *Salmonella* strains are involved with ReA, but less frequently. They include *S*. Montevideo, *S*. Agona, *S*. Saintpaul, and *S*. Java.

Salmonella, Shigella, and Yersinia can lead to arthritis of the large joints, such as the knees. The antibodies produced to combat the infectious bacteria then attack their own tissue in the autoimmune process.

Following a 1985 outbreak of gastroenteritis caused by *S*. Typhimurium-contaminated milk in the Chicago area, a physical examination of the people made ill showed a 2.3 percent incidence of ReA among them. One patient, who carried the HLA-B27 gene, was the most seriously affected. A year after the outbreak, twenty out of twenty-nine individuals reported persistent symptoms of ReA. Six people had worsened, with a tendency toward arthropathy. Arthropathy is chronic and progressive degeneration of the stress-bearing portion of joints.

A subsequent U.S. outbreak in the mid-1990s of milkborne salmonellosis made nearly 200,000 people ill. After the episode, investigators found ReA in about 2.3 percent of the people made ill—a strikingly similar incidence as the 1985 outbreak. In this episode, however, due to the large numbers of people made ill, more than 4,500 individuals developed ReA.

Symptoms of ReA may last for less than a year in some individuals. In others, it may last longer, with multiple episodes of arthritis accompanied by debilitating symptoms. Some individuals develop rheumatoid arthritis (RA).

For decades, numerous microbial pathogens have been linked to RA. Impaired functioning of the immune system may be involved, in addition to the infection. Abnormal thio-reactive immunoglobulin A (IgA) is present in RA. Much of the serum IgA is complexed with alpha-1 antitrypsin, a major antiprotease. Similarly, high levels of abnormal IgA are found in ankylosing spondylitis patients. Many of these individuals also have elevated levels of IgA directed against the infective agent, *K. pneumoniae*. The reactivity of T lymphocytes from RA patients is increased by another infective agent, *Mycobacterium paratuberculosis,* which cross-reacts with human cartilage. Also, the HLA-DR4 gene is associated with the immune response to *M. paratuberculosis.* All these factors may offer clues to the pathogenesis of RA. The ability of the mycobacteria to persist and degrade very slowly in phagocyte cells (cells that ingest microorganisms or foreign particles) would account for the chronic condition that results from an immunologic or inflammatory stimulus.

FOODBORNE INFECTIONS AND THE CARDIOVASCULAR SYSTEM

Inflammatory Heart Disorders

Several foodborne pathogens have been linked, directly or indirectly, to inflammatory heart disease. One disorder is endocarditis, associated with bacteria or viruses. Endocarditis is marked by infection of the heart valves. The acute form has both a rapid onset and progression. Sometimes the infection is caused by a virulent bacterium, *Staphylococcus aureus,* which can invade other tissues as well. The subacute form has an insidious onset, and a protracted progression. It is caused by various bacteria, usually alpha-hemolytic streptococci.

Another inflammatory heart disorder is myocarditis. This disorder also is associated, either directly or indirectly, with bacteria or viruses. Myocarditis is an inflammation of the myocardium, the middle and thickest layer of the heart wall. It is composed of cardiac muscles. Damage to the cardiac muscles or the heart valves may be permanent.

If *Salmonella* bacteria reach the walls of some of the larger blood vessels, the infection can lead to endarteritis, an inflammation of the innermost coat of an artery. This disorder often occurs in people who have some degree of atherosclerosis such that the minor damage to the blood vessel wall allows the *Salmonella* to gain entry.

If *Salmonella* goes from the bloodstream into bone, it can result in an inflammation known as osteomyelitis.

Atherosclerosis

The process of atherogenesis is complex and involves numerous factors. Recently, *E. coli* and *S.* Typhimurium have been implicated in atherosclerosis, as well as in ReA and IBD.

Macrophages are phagocyte cells in the blood vessel walls that ingest pathogens. In the progression of atherosclerosis, endotoxins from degrading bacteria in macrophages can act in tandem with cytokines (inflammatory factors) induced by endotoxins from endothelial and smooth muscle cells.

All these examples of inflammatory conditions in the cardiovascular system linked to foodborne pathogens lead to very different clinical conditions. They have different outcomes. However, all of them can result in prolonged illnesses.

FOODBORNE INFECTIONS AND NEUROMUSCULAR DISORDERS
Meningitis

Meningitis is an inflammation of the meninges, membranes that cover the brain and spinal cord. Some cases of meningitis result from foodborne infections. Nearly half of all cases of *L. monocytogene* infections reported to the CDC between 1980 and 1982 took the form of meningitis. If untreated, the fatality rate of this disorder can be as high as 90 percent. Treatment with antibiotics has become ineffective due to the development of antibiotic resistance. *Listeria*-induced meningitis can begin with a low-grade fever and personality changes. As inflammation progresses, it is indistinguishable from other forms of bacterial meningitis. Identification is based on symptoms and laboratory tests, especially by analyzing the cerebral spinal fluid. *L. monocytogenes* is the pathogen responsible for inducing many cases of meningitis in adults.

Listeriosis is a foodborne infection, mainly from contaminated soft cheeses, unpasteurized milk, and undercooked chicken, fish, and meats. In April 2009, an outbreak of *Listeria* was reported in several New England states from contaminated salad sprouts. The Food and Drug Administration (FDA) considers the pathogen a grave health threat, and adopted a zero-tolerance level for *Listeria* in ready-to-eat foods.

Cerebral Palsy

Inflammatory infections may be linked to cerebral palsy, a form of brain damage that impairs movements. Traditionally, this disorder was attributed to difficult birthing that temporarily deprived oxygen to the fetus. Asphyxia may be the cause of cerebral palsy, but newer evidence shows that the brain damage also may result from another type of assault on the unborn child, such as inflammatory infection. Karin B. Nelson, a pediatric neurologist at the National Institute of Neurological Disorders and Stroke (NINDS) in Bethesda, Maryland, led a team of researchers who found that cytokines were abundant in newborn infants who later were diagnosed with cerebral palsy. An infection in the placenta, or in the pregnant woman, might cause the fetus's immune system to produce cytokines to combat the infection. The researchers stored blood taken from infants immediately after birth. They compared thirty-one infants who displayed cerebral palsy symptoms several months after birth with a control group of sixty-five infants without signs of cerebral palsy. They tested the stored blood for dozens of immune-system compounds and found that all the stricken children harbored greater concentrations of five types of cytokines than any of the controls. According to the researchers, the cytokine production might indicate a subtle attack on the fetus from a long-present maternal infection, transmitted via her placenta to the developing fetus.

The study also showed that the infants with cerebral palsy were much more likely than the control group to have excess amounts of several proteins that regulate blood clotting, as well as an anticoagulant associated with systemic lupus erythematosus (see next paragraph). Thus, in addition to finding an inflammatory connection with cerebral palsy, in some fetuses there also was an autoimmune reaction.

Myasthenia Gravis and Lupus

Autoantibodies are formed to combat an antigen of an individual's own tissues. A body of medical evidence demonstrates the role of autoantibodies. They are associated with the acetylcholine receptor in the pathology of myasthenia gravis, a debilitating disorder of muscular weakness. The antigenic determinants are shared between the acetylcholine receptor and surface proteins of certain strains of *E. coli*, a frequent food contaminant, as well as other pathogens, such as *Proteus vulgaris* and *K. pneumoniae*.

The onset of systemic lupus erythematosus, an autoimmune disease involving connective tissue, also may be linked to foodborne pathogens. In mouse studies, the onset of lupus was hastened by prolonged polyclonal stimulation of the animals' B cells with bacteria that form toxins in the intestines.

Neurologic Dysfunction

People who live near the ocean are familiar with red tide, periods when waters are closed to fishing due to toxins. A number of other toxins, too, may contaminate seafoods, and affect the neuromuscular system. Amnesic shellfish poisoning is one, caused by domoic acid, a naturally occurring toxin produced by microscopic algae. A small amount of ingested domoic acid has an excitatory effect; a large amount, a neurotoxic effect. At first, there are gastrointestinal symptoms, followed by neurologic dysfunction. In chronic cases, people may have signs of confusion or disorientation, and may lack speech or responsiveness. Individuals may suffer deep pain due to blocked receptors in the spinal cord. The autonomic nervous system is dysfunctional, which results in seizures, abnormal eye movements, and loss of visual-spatial recall, grimacing postures, loss of reflexes, and coma. The elderly are especially at risk.

FOODBORNE INFECTIONS AND THYROID DISEASE

Graves' Disease

Graves' disease, named in honor of its identification by an Irish physician, Robert J. Graves (1797–1853), is exophthalmic goiter, known as hyperthyroidism. It is caused by an excessive production of thyroid hormones. Signs and symptoms include enlarged thyroid glands, protrusion of the eyeballs, rapid heartbeat, and nervous excitability. George Herbert Walker Bush, his wife, Barbara Bush, and their dog, all suffer from Graves' disease.

The hormone system, the immune system, and genes may all be factors. So, apparently, is a foodborne infection. *Yersinia enterocolitica* (see Chapter 12) is found in patients with Graves' disease significantly more frequently than in controls. The finding suggests that the pathogen may trigger autoimmune thyroid disorders, especially Graves' disease.

Other evidence suggests molecular mimicry is at work. (See insert on page 11). Receptor autoantibodies mimic the biological effects of thyroid-stimulating hormones. Thyroid-stimulating binding sites, present in *Y. enterocolitica*, are recognized by immunogloblins of people with Graves' disease.

FOODBORNE INFECTIONS AND KIDNEY DISEASE

Hemolytic Uremic Syndrome

Hemorrhagic colitis, caused by *E. coli* O157:H7, an especially virulent strain of the bacterium, frequently leads to hemolytic uremic syndrome (HUS) both in children and adults (see Chapter 4). HUS is characterized by acute kidney failure, thrombocytopenia (a decrease in the number of platelets in circulating blood), and microangiopathic hemolytic anemia (a disease of the small blood vessels). Shiga toxin, produced by certain types of infectious microbes, may be involved. Diarrheal episodes of HUS may follow infection caused by common gram-negative foodborne pathogens, such as *Shigella*, *Salmonella*, *Campylobacter*, and *Escherichia*.

Thrombotic Thrombocytopenic Purpura

Thrombotic thrombocytopenic purpura (TTP) was described first in 1925. TTP shows similar symptoms as HUS, as well as fever and neurological symptoms. Several intestinal bacterial pathogens and endotoxins can cause TTP. *E. coli* O157:H7, already noted as an especially virulent strain, is associated with TTP as well as HUS. TTP has a high mortality rate.

IgA Glomerulonephritis

Another kidney disorder, IgA glomerulonephritis, is an inflammatory disorder that is thought to be immune-complex mediated. This condition may be caused by any prolonged stimulation of the IgA-producing lymphoid tissue, as, for example, a foodborne infection in the intestines. Or, it may result from the formation of IgA immune complex in response to an influx of food antigens when intestinal integrity is compromised, such as with leaky gut syndrome, mentioned earlier. Genetics, too, may play a role. Some individuals produce high levels of IgA; others do not. Any large load of antigenic material entering the general circulation, such as foodborne pathogens, can lead to IgA glomerulonephritis.

Kidney Stones

In 1997, Finnish researchers found that nanobacteria (organisms smaller even than many viruses) may cause kidney stones. The researchers found that the nanobacteria can live in urine and surround themselves with a mineralized coating, on which additional proteins and minerals can accumulate. In examining the kidney stones from thirty people, all showed traces of nanobacteria in their cores. This develops kidney-stone formation. DNA studies suggested that the nanobacteria are related to small, slow-growing, rod-shaped bacteria lacking in rigid cell walls. The bacteria are known to cause blood poisoning in humans, and abortions in animals.

Researchers have detected nanobacterial proteins in human kidneys, and also have grown them from blood samples. But blood may not be the primary target of these nanobacteria. Injected experimentally into animals, nanobacteria move quickly to the kidneys, and then into the urine.

The medical symptoms of nanobacteria may extend beyond kidney-stone formation. In a variety of human diseases, including atherosclerosis, arthritis, cancers, and dementias, unexplained calcium precipitation occurs in many body tissues. Also, people who frequently receive blood transfusions in dialysis often develop dangerous levels of calcium deposits. In a Turkish study, nanobacteria were found in 80 percent of all patients undergoing dialysis. Researchers suggest that the possible association of nanobacteria and many diseases with pathological extraskeletal calcification should be investigated.

FOODBORNE INFECTIONS AND GALLBLADDER DISEASE

Gallstones

A microbial infection may be associated with the development of gallstones. Studies led by Philip B. Hylemon of the Medical College of Virginia in Richmond showed that gallstone patients have from 100 to 1,000 times higher levels of *Clostridia* and eubacteria in their intestines than do people without gallbladder dysfunction. These bacteria produce deoxycholic acid, which induces the liver to secrete bile that is especially high in cholesterol. This development is a key risk factor for gallstone development.

FOODBORNE INFECTIONS AND MENTAL DISORDERS

Obsessive-Compulsive Disorder

Infectious microbes have been recognized to cause mental disorders. An example is syphilitic dementia, a form of dementia caused by the bacterium *Treponema pallidum* that results in personality changes and psychosis.

In recent years, it was suggested that some cases of infection were associated with cases of childhood obsessive-compulsive disorder (OCD). Susan E. Swedo at the National Institute of Mental Health in Bethesda noted a strong resemblance of OCD to Sydenham's chorea (formerly known as St. Vitus Dance). This is a nervous disorder, also occurring in children, and characterized by rapid, jerky, involuntary movements of the body. Like rheumatic heart disease, Sydenham's chorea can be a complication of an untreated streptococcal infection. Streptococcal antibodies enter the brain and attack the basal ganglia region, causing clumsiness, arm flapping, and senseless obsessive-compulsive movements and fixed ideas. Swedo wondered if some cases of childhood OCD are a milder version of Sydenham's chorea.

By the early 1990s, the two disorders appeared to be connected. A new syndrome known as pediatric autoimmune neuropsychiatric disorder associated with streptococcus (PANDAS) gained recognition. Some children with OCD improved when given intravenous immunoglobulin, or underwent plasma exchange to remove the antibodies from their blood.

An Odd Assortment of Psychological Symptoms

Ciguatera fish poisoning presents a weird assortment of symptoms in individuals who are infected. They suffer from a reversal in hot and cold discrimination, and a distorted sense that their teeth are loose when in reality they are not. Also, individuals may experience formication, a sensation of ants crawling over the body.

Ciguatera fish poisoning is caused by a dinoflagellate, *Gambierdiscus toxicus*. Fish such as barracuda, grouper, and red snapper, especially in the Caribbean area and in the Pacific Islands, may become infected with the dinoflagellate, but continue to thrive. However, people who eat the infected fish suffer gastrointestinal, cardiovascular, and neurological symptoms. The infected fish looks, smells, and tastes normal. The toxin is not destroyed by cooking, freezing, smoking, drying, water-soaking, or marinating the fish. Drinking alcohol worsens the symptoms inflicted by the toxin. Physical exercise in hot weather or sexual activity can intensify the symptoms. Even six months after recovery from this disorder, eating finfish or shellfish that are contaminated with the toxin can cause a recurrence of the bizarre symptoms described above. If the individual has had ciguatera poisoning in the past, subsequent encounters with the toxin can result in far more severe illness. Frequently, after thousands of dollars in medical tests, this disorder has been misdiagnosed as brain tumor, multiple sclerosis, chronic fatigue syndrome, or other disorders unrelated to ciguatera poisoning. If ciguatera poisoning is diagnosed properly, mannitol, a polyol sugar, may be administered for relief.

It has been discovered that the toxin in ciguatera infection opens the channels that allow sodium to pass in and out of cells, resulting in a disruption of the cells' permeability and electrical activity. These channels are widespread in nerve and muscle tissue. Derailing their formation interferes with their normal neurological, biochemical, and muscular functions.

Schizophrenia

Epidemiologic studies indicate that infectious agents may be linked to some cases of schizophrenia. In acute human infections of the foodborne pathogen *Toxoplasma gondii* (see Chapter 7), psychotic symptoms can be produced that are similar to those displayed by people with schizophrenia.

In animal studies, infection with *T. gondii* can alter neurotransmitter function and behavior. Studies have found that exposure to cats in childhood is a risk factor for later development of schizophrenia. Other studies have reported the presence of *T. gondii* antibodies in people with schizophrenia and other severe psychiatric disorders.

FOODBORNE INFECTIONS AND CANCERS

Tumor Development and Growth

The connections between infections and cancers have been given credence with the evidence that certain neoplasms (new and abnormal growths) develop when an organism is immunosuppressed. This was a recognized feature in organ transplantation. Then, it was illustrated dramatically by the global HIV (human immunodeficiency virus) epidemic, which linked infections with cancer. Additionally, other diseases, formerly regarded as noninfectious, came to be recognized as being associated with infections (for example, peptic ulcers or some forms of arthritis).

Proto-oncogenes are genes that are normal but have the potential to become oncogenic (tumor-inducing). In human studies, the expression of proto-oncogenes was greater in patients with systemic lupus erythematosus than in normal controls. Substances produced by bacteria are capable of mitosis (cell division) in humans for both T cells and B cells. This development activates tumor-inducing genes (the proto-oncogenes).

Cervical and Prostate Cancers

The old idea that infectious microbes might cause cancer or predispose an organism to malignancy had been dismissed by many people. However, the idea has been strengthened by newer knowledge based on findings in microbiology, molecular genetics, epidemiology, and cancer biology. For example, epidemiologists linked human papilloma virus infections to cervical cancer, and possibly to prostate cancer, too. They also linked a sexually transmitted infection to Kaposi's sarcoma, and are credited with initiating a search that led to the discovery of a new human herpesvirus (KSHV), which may be needed in order for the Kaposi's sarcoma to develop.

SUSPECTED INFECTION-INDUCED CHRONIC DISEASES

Some of the suspected infection-induced chronic diseases are from foodborne infections. According to David A. Relman, associate professor of medicine, microbiology, and immunology at Stanford University in Palo Alto, California, the ever-increasing list of infection-induced chronic diseases now includes:

- Arthritis (RA)

- Cirrhosis

- Kawasaki disease, a condition that causes inflammation in the walls of small- and medium-sized arteries throughout the body, including the coronary arteries, which supply blood to the heart

- Sarcoidosis, a degenerative disease characterized by the development and growth of a tumor-like mass of inflammatory cells involving almost any organ or tissue

- Systemic lupus erythematosus

- Tropical sprue, a malabsorption disease characterized by the impaired absorption of fats, vitamins, and minerals

Relman noted that, to date, less than one-half of one percent of all existing bacterial species have been identified. Bacterial infections represent only a portion of infections. Viruses, parasites, protozoa, helminthes, fungi, and toxins produced from these organisms need to be considered in the total number of infectious organisms. Others would add to Relman's list, as this book will demonstrate. They include infectious connections with heart diseases, atherosclerosis, Alzheimer's disease, autoimmune diseases, multiple sclerosis, gastroenteritis, gastric ulcers, some major psychiatric diseases, Hashimoto's thyroiditis, cerebral palsy, polycystic ovary disease, periodontitis, eating disorders, obesity, and some cancers.

As recently as 2006, Siobhán M. O'Connor from the CDC noted: "Evidence now confirms that noncommunicable chronic diseases can stem from infectious agents. Furthermore, at least thirteen of thirty-nine recently described infectious agents induce chronic syndromes. Infectious agents likely determine more cancers, immuno-mediated syndromes, neuro-developmental disorders, and other chronic conditions than currently appreciated."

PART TWO
"The Big Four"

CHAPTER 3

Salmonella: Ubiquitous Bacterium

Alice and Ken were anticipating the holidays. There would be four generations of family members for the Christmas dinner. The children were coming with the grandchildren, and Ken would bring his eighty-nine-year-old mother, Nellie, from her assisted-living residence for part of the day's celebration.

Alice and Ken lived in rural New England. Ken's recreational pleasure was his vegetable garden. In December, he was able to cut some kale, still growing in a well-protected area. Alice took pleasure raising a flock of hens. Her "girls" produced wonderful fresh eggs. Alice promised Ken that she would make hollandaise sauce to accompany his kale. With an abundance of eggs, Alice also planned to make her traditional eggnog for the adults, and soft custard for the children and for her pregnant daughter, Lois, who was abstaining from alcoholic beverages. Alice figured that she would still have an ample supply of eggs to make French toast for the group the following morning.

The Christmas celebration was enjoyed by all. However, as the adults were ready for bedtime, the telephone rang. Sandra, the head nurse at Sunhaven, reported that Nellie was experiencing stomach cramps and felt nauseous. She was in too much discomfort to remember clearly what she had eaten that day. Could Alice and Ken help?

Sandra winced when she heard about the homemade hollandaise sauce and the homemade eggnog. She knew that a number of nursing homes and hospitals in the New England area were experiencing foodborne outbreaks of infections from eggs. Fortunately, so far, Sunhaven had escaped the outbreaks.

During the night, Alice and Ken were awakened by activity in the hallway and bathrooms. Several of the family members were not well. Lois and the small children had bouts of diarrhea and were vomiting. By day-

break, the entire group suffered from gastroenteritis. The beautiful holiday turned into a disaster, and it was far from over. The thought of French toast appealed to no one.

Salmonella Enteritidis bacteria were identified in Nellie's stools in a laboratory test ordered by Sunhaven. Nellie would be isolated and bedridden for weeks. Even after she recovered and was asymptomatic, she was a carrier. It was thought that she infected other residents. One was a frail ninety-four-year-old woman with several chronic health conditions. The salmonellosis was a tipping point, and she succumbed.

Lois and the two youngest children required medical attention. One of these children had to be hospitalized. Alice and Ken's eldest son developed pancreatitis. Ken and Alice recovered. Ken went back to work. However, like his mother, Ken was an asymptomatic carrier, and probably infected four coworkers at the office. They all had short bouts. Alice recovered, yet could not be convinced that her fresh, clean, Grade A shell eggs could have been responsible for the disaster, but the eggs were responsible.

Salmonella is a zoonotic infection, one that can be transmitted from animals to humans. *Salmonella* has long been with us. As one Food and Drug Administration (FDA) official remarked, "*Salmonella* in its hundreds of configurations . . . has been with man since time immemorial . . . perhaps since man himself arose from the primeval slime." *Salmonellae* commonly are present in the intestinal tract of warm-blooded animals, including both domestic and wild ones.

In recent decades, salmonellosis has increased as a problem due to

A BACTERIUM'S NAME HONORS THE WRONG MAN

In 1894, Dr. Theobald Smith (1859–1934), a researcher in the USDA's Bureau of Animal Industry, was the first to identify a certain bacterium as a separate genus. Smith identified the bacterium, which was causing hog cholera. However, when his findings were published, the name of his administrator appeared first, before his own in the article. Such deference was customary. His administrator was Dr. Daniel E. Salmon. Thus, the bacterium honored his name as *Salmonella*, and Smith's pioneering efforts were unheralded. —*Bergey's Manual of Systematic Bacteriology, 1984*

many factors, including agricultural and lifestyle changes. The growth of intensive farming has resulted in increased animal infections, including salmonellosis. Changes in feed and in feeding practices have resulted in increased salmonellosis. The addition of antibiotics and the mineral, selenium, to animal feed has had a profound impact on the rise of salmonellosis. The closing of local abattoirs has led to longer journeys of livestock to large slaughterhouses and to greater transfer of feces between animals. Changes in methods of slaughtering and processing animal foods, and in national and international distribution systems of food and feed, have increased the risks of foodborne infections such as salmonellosis.

Other factors are food preparation and storage practices in food service establishments and homes, and environmental contamination from animal wastes. The improper cooling of food; lapses of a day or more between preparation and serving food; inadequate cooking or heat processing; cross-contamination; and eating contaminated raw or undercooked ingredients—all add to the problem of salmonellosis.

Changes in lifestyle contribute to salmonellosis. The increased eating away from home, bringing home more ready-to-serve foods that have been prepared elsewhere, and greater consumption of raw fruits, vegetables, and sprouts are additional factors. Some of these features in changed agricultural practices and lifestyle will be discussed in detail in this chapter.

SALMONELLA IS WIDESPREAD

Currently, salmonellosis, caused by *Salmonella* bacteria, is the leading cause of foodborne disease in the United States, followed by *Escherichia coli*, *Shigella*, and *Campylobacter*. They are known as "The Big Four." *Salmonella* is a worldwide problem, and is the most frequently reported foodborne disease in many countries.

Of more than 2,400 serotypes of *Salmonella* identified to date, fewer than 200 are known to cause illnesses in humans. The bacterium is ubiquitous in all basic food groups. Contamination has occurred in foods from animal sources such as livestock, poultry, and eggs; from produce such as vegetables, fruits, fruit juices, salads, and sprouted seeds; from dairy products such as milk and cheeses; from grains processed into ready-to-eat cereals; and from tree nuts (pistachios) and ground nuts (peanuts). A Centers for Disease Control and Prevention (CDC) report, issued in April 2009, noted a rise in the incidence of *Salmonella*.

Outbreaks of salmonellosis occur in many environments: in home kitchens; in cafeterias and restaurants; in schools and camps; in institutions such as hospitals and nursing homes; at military bases; at recreation halls and senior citizen centers; and at social gatherings, such as receptions, banquets, firemen's benefit barbecues, picnics, and church christenings.

Estimates of the number of Americans infected with salmonellosis vary widely from year to year. In recent years, CDC figures for the annual number of reported cases have ranged from 1.2 to 1.4 million. However, the CDC estimated that for every case reported, 100 cases go unreported. Annual hospitalized salmonellosis cases reported to the CDC have ranged from 15,000 to 18,000 persons; 5,000 with bloodstream infections; and from 400 to 600 deaths. Annually, salmonellosis causes the subsequent development of chronic diseases in some 120,000 persons. The economic costs, too, are staggering. They are estimated to be billions of dollars, resulting from investigations, diagnoses, and treatments.

HOW *SALMONELLAE* INVADE HUMAN CELLS

Bacteria have evolved numerous ingenious techniques for invading the human body. Of all the pathogens, some strains of *Salmonellae* have been especially intriguing to microbiologists. How do these bacteria manage to penetrate the cells that line the human intestine?

Salmonellae achieve this invasion with the cooperation of target cells. *Salmonellae* that survive the acid in the human stomach migrate to the intestines, where they attach themselves to intestinal cells. The *Salmonellae* are equipped with a molecular syringe to inject their own proteins into the intestinal cell. They make a hole in the cell and dock with it. The *Salmonellae* adhere firmly to the human cells and then begin to build a type of scaffolding that permits them, like Trojan horses, to enter the cells. To do this, the *Salmonellae* hijack human proteins to make the cells do things they ordinarily would never do. Once inside the cells, the *Salmonellae* replicate themselves, and then escape back into the intestine and induce diarrhea. Sometimes, the *Salmonellae* migrate into other parts of the body and cause more serious illnesses, such as typhoid fever.

SIGNS AND SYMPTOMS OF SALMONELLOSIS

There are two types of food poisoning symptoms with salmonellosis. One is self-limiting, and the other is more severe and leads to complications.

In the self-limiting type, the incubation period may be from six to forty-eight hours, but sometimes from five to seventy-two hours, and occasionally, as long as seven days. After the incubation period, acute gastroenteritis begins as early as twelve to thirty-six hours, but usually after two to five days. The symptoms include diarrhea, abdominal cramps, vomiting, mild fever, malaise, prostration, and loss of appetite. The active state passes fairly rapidly, within a week. However, the carrier state, when the patient continues to shed the bacteria and infect others, may last for three months.

Another type of salmonellosis is characterized by high fever. This symptom should be taken seriously because the infection can be life threatening. The illness may be more severe in infants and in the elderly, with deaths more likely in these two especially vulnerable groups than in other age groups. The high fever infection usually is caused by S. Typhi, associated with typhoid fever, which will be discussed later in this chapter.

HEALTH PROBLEMS CONNECTED WITH SALMONELLOSIS

Health complications can result from salmonellosis. In persons with underlying diseases such as cancer, salmonellosis can lead to septicemia (blood poisoning). Certain strains of *Salmonella*, especially S. Dublin, S. Typhimurium and S. Choleraesuis, cause septicemia.

Salmonellae become systemic by invading the bloodstream and many body organs, where they trigger severe and sometimes fatal inflammations. Nontyphoid salmonellosis is usually a killer only when it invades the bloodstream and colonizes in the brain or other organs. The intestine attempts to prevent this from happening by discharging the bacteria through diarrhea and vomit. Although this is unpleasant, the individual should realize that these are immune responses to ingested pathogens. By flushing out the *Salmonellae* that permeate the protective mucosa coating, the action prevents the pathogens from attaching themselves to the intestinal walls.

There are serious focal and septic forms of salmonellosis that occur as part of septicemia. Some may be isolated abscesses. Frequently, the gastrointestinal tract is involved, including the appendix and the gallbladder. The *Salmonellae* can localize and cause necrosis (death of cells) in almost any part of the body (for example, lungs, genitourinary tract, soft tissues, central nervous system, upper respiratory tract, joints, bones, or heart valves). *Salmonellae* tend to localize in abnormal tissues, such as in tumors. Salmonellosis can result in a range of health disorders, including pericarditis, pancreatitis, and neurological and neuromuscular diseases such as reactive arthritis, ankylosing spondylitis, and osteomyelitis, and cause damage to the mucous membrane of the small intestine and colon. Salmonellosis can lead to malabsorption and loss of nutrients, allergies, and some illnesses in malnourished individuals.

Salmonellosis is associated strongly with recipients of organ transplantations who are on antirejection therapy. Such individuals are at risk of certain illnesses, including meningitis, urinary tract infections, abscesses of soft tissues, septic arthritis, osteomyelitis, and vascular infections, including infections of vascular grafts. Recurrence of nontyphoidal salmonellosis occurs in up to 35 percent of renal transplant recipients.

About 10 percent of the American population carries the gene HLA-B27. About 2 to 3 percent of those people, if infected with salmonellosis, will develop reactive arthritis.

A small number of people infected with *Salmonella*—about one person in ten thousand—will experience septic arthritis, a painful condition in which the bacteria invade the joints.

Of the numerous strains of *Salmonella* that infect humans, the two most prevalent ones are *Salmonella* Typhimurium and *Salmonella* Enteritidis (formerly known as *Salmonella typhimurium* and *Salmonella enteritidis*). Both strains will be discussed shortly. *Salmonella* Typhi (formerly known as *Salmonella typhosa*) also also will be discussed shortly. Although this strain is less common, it is far more virulent. It is the strain that causes typhoid fever, which can be fatal.

Of all the strains of *Salmonella* that infect humans, only a relatively few cause most of the reported cases of salmonellosis outbreaks. Some strains that cause no symptoms in animals can make people ill, and vice versa.

An infective dose of *Salmonella* bacteria (or other infective organisms) is the amount needed to cause disease. Studies of healthy people have shown that large doses of *Salmonellae* are needed for them to contract salmonellosis. However, infection with some strains can occur with as few as one to ten *Salmonella* cells. Groups who are especially vulnerable are infants, pregnant women, the elderly, alcoholics, and people with impaired immune systems.

SOURCES OF SALMONELLA INFECTIONS

Salmonella bacteria are common in the intestinal tracts of farm animals and are shed in the waste of livestock and poultry. *Salmonella* is the only pathogen tested by the federal government at meat plants because it serves as an indicator of the safety of the country's supply of food from animal sources.

Any raw food of animal origin may carry *Salmonella*. The bacteria can survive if these foods are not cooked thoroughly. The bacteria also can contaminate other foods that come in contact with the raw animal food, either directly, or by way of dirty hands or dirty equipment.

There are numerous reservoirs for *Salmonella* bacteria. They have been detected in: barbecued chicken (undercooked or unevenly cooked); bakery items (containing eggs and/or milk); carmine dyes from cochineal insects (used as food coloring and in laboratory dyes); cockroaches; coconuts; companion animals (dogs, cats, hamsters, etc.); eggs (liquid, frozen, and dried); fleas; houseflies; fish (fresh and smoked); headcheese; livestock; meat scraps; milk (fresh and dried); nutritional supplements (bone meal, desiccated glandulars such as dried liver powder, stomach, and whole lung); peppermint sticks; pet chews, feed, meals, and feed mixes; poultry and poultry meals; processed foods containing eggs (cake mixes, noodles, etc.); processing machinery; snakes; turkeys (frozen); turtles; and well water.

The pervasiveness of salmonellosis is reflected by numerous recalls of foods, food products, and food ingredients. These are some recent recalls: beef (chopped and formed); brewer's yeast; buttermilk pancake mix; cheese from Canada in Lunchmate product; chicken nuggets (imported); chocolate/fiber nutritional beverage powder; chorizo sausage; coleslaw packaged by Dole; cooked beef rounds; cooked chicken breasts and wraps; Danish cheese; doughnut mix; Easter chocolate bunnies; fermented sausage; flame-broiled beef steaks; freshly cooked ham; frozen pasteurized egg products; frozen shrimp from India; frozen uncooked cheese ravioli; ground chicken; ground pork; live lobsters from Honduras; masala (spice) from India; meal-in-one strawberry powder mix; meat; mortadella cheese (vacuum-packaged, ready-to-eat); nondairy creamer; noodles; peanuts from Georgia; pet food from China, pistachios from California; Polish sausage; pork sausage (ready-to-eat); prosciutto ham; salami; shark cartilage powder; shellfish from New Zealand; smoked sausage; vanilla nutritional beverage powder; peanut butter; almonds; and vegetable sprouts.

No doubt, such recalls have averted numerous salmonellosis out-

COMPANION ANIMALS AS SOURCES OF HUMAN SALMONELLOSIS

A study published in *Pediatrics* (Jan 1999) found that young children are more likely to be infected with *Salmonella* from handling companion animals than from eating *Salmonella*-contaminated foods.

Many salmonellosis outbreaks have occurred with companion animals, including cats, dogs, pet turtles, hamsters, lizards, iguanas, snakes, Easter chicks, and pet ducklings, as well as from environmental sources such as petting zoos. *Salmonella*-contaminated pet treats of beef and seafood origin have resulted in salmonellosis outbreaks in the United States in 2004 and 2005.

At times, the companion animals are more exotic. In 1994, a ten-month-old girl was hospitalized for severe symptoms due to salmonellosis. The family owned a breeding herd of eighty apparently healthy African pygmy hedgehogs. Tests showed that three of the animals were infected with *Salmonella*. The infant had not had direct contact with the hedgehogs, but the animals were handled frequently by a family member who may have transmitted the infection to the infant. Although the African pygmy hedgehog is an unusual pet, these animals are being bred in the United States, and ownership of them is increasing.

There are other unusual pets that may be infected with *Salmonella*. In Australia, orphaned kangaroos and wallaby infants have been found to be zoonotic sources of *Salmonella* transmissible to humans.

Often, children care for pet fish, and clean the tanks. There have been recent *Salmonella* outbreaks in North America, Europe, and Australia associated with pet fish and aquariums. Microbiologist Diana Lightfoot, a *Salmonella* specialist at the University of Melbourne, Australia, cautioned that in cleaning a fish tank, the water, pebbles, and other items, as well as the fish, may be contaminated with *Salmonella*. In Quebec, Canada, health workers developed posters and brochures, distributed in pet shops, with tips for safe handling of aquariums. Among the tips, pet fish owners were advised to avoid washing aquarium accessories in the kitchen or bathroom sinks, or in the bathtub. Lacking options, the fish owners were advised to clean and disinfect thoroughly with a bleach solution all the surfaces used, and rinse these surfaces before further use.

breaks. Nevertheless, many outbreaks still occur. This fact is evident by the listing of outbreaks in the Main Sources for this chapter.

In one year alone, salmonellosis outbreaks were reported with the following: baby foods; cheese; chicken; eggnog; green bananas; ham; ice cream; macaroni salad; meat loaf; Mexican food; milk; pork and beans; potato salad; roast duck; roast pork; salad; shellfish; turkey; and twenty-four reported salmonellosis outbreaks of unknown causes. Remember, for every reported outbreak, many more are unreported. The CDC suggests that *most* salmonellosis outbreaks are not reported.

Feeding Farm Animals Routinely with Antibiotics

Until the routine use of antibiotics with farm animals, animal husbandry relied on high standards of cleanliness to prevent infectious diseases in animals, and the isolation of sick animals. These practices became more challenging as tens of thousands of livestock were reared intensively in feedlots, and thousands of poultry also were reared intensively indoors. There was a false sense of assurance that antibiotics could substitute for high standards of sanitation.

The purpose was economic. Animals were given antibiotics routinely to increase weight more rapidly and get them to market earlier, and thus increase profits. The antibiotics were not being used judiciously to treat individually infected animals in order to prevent outbreaks. At the same time, antibiotics were being misused with humans, to treat conditions for which they are ineffective. The sale of antibiotics soared, and their use with farm animals has been greater than with humans. The two abuses of antibiotics—overuse and misuse with farm animals and humans—have led to major health problems.

In 1983, Michael Osterholm, a state epidemiologist in Minnesota, led a team of investigators who traced a salmonellosis outbreak in humans eating beef, back to beef cattle given antibiotics routinely. This was the first time that a clear and direct link was established between human illness and the use of antibiotics in animal feeds.

The outbreak of salmonellosis occurred with eleven people who were ill. All were infected with *S. enterica* serotype Newport, a bacterial strain not usually found in the northern region of the United States. Another odd fact was that most of the affected people had taken amoxicillin, a widely used penicillin derivative, one or two days before they became ill. Their stool samples showed that they were infected with the same strain of *S*. Newport that was resistant to common antibiotics such as penicillin and tetracycline. After painstaking research, the epidemiologists were able to pinpoint the specific farm and the chain of movement of the beef to a particular slaughterhouse, a meat processor, all the way to supermarkets in the Minneapolis-St. Paul area. Most of the salmonellosis sufferers had purchased their beef in stores selling the beef in question. The accumulated evidence showed that the beef cattle from a specific farm became 'biological factories' of drug-resistant *S*. Newport after being fed routinely low doses of antibiotics.

Osterholm and his CDC colleagues concluded that the fatality rate for people infected with drug-resistant *Salmonella* was twenty-one times greater than for people ill from salmonellosis that was not antibiotic resistant. Also, they concluded that food animals usually were the source of the drug-resistant bacteria that infect people. Based on a review of CDC's records of all outbreaks of drug-resistant salmonellosis between 1971 and 1983, the team found that 69 percent of the strains of drug-resistant *Salmonella* that made people sick were traced to food animals. Osterholm concluded that the investigation "represents bad news for the meat industry and for humans if indiscriminate antibiotic use continues." Despite repetitious demands for a federal ban on the use of penicillin and tetracycline in animal feed that followed the clear and direct linkage between foodborne salmonellosis and the use of antibiotics in animal feeds, the practice continued. In recent years, antibiotic resistance has loomed as an ever increasing and major public health problem. Multidrug resistance continues to increase. The number of effective antibiotics keeps dwindling in numbers, and with fewer and fewer effective ones in reserve.

In Denmark, the routine supplementation of an antibiotic, avoparcin, in animal feed, was discontinued with broiler chickens in 1998, and with pigs the following year. This decision had a remarkable outcome. There was a precipitous drop in the incidence of salmonellosis in these farm animals only four months after discontinuation of routine supplementation of the feed with the antibiotic. Avoparcin had been recognized for its ability to increase shedding of *Salmonella* in animal feces.

The Selenium/Antibiotic/*Salmonella* Connections

Selenium is a trace element that is essential for farm animals as well as for humans and crops. Some sections of the United States are selenium-deficient, and other sections have such excessively high amounts of selenium in their soils that they would be toxic for growing crops and for grazing animals. In order to provide adequate selenium in low-selenium areas, in 1987, the FDA published its first feed additive regulation permitting the addition of 0.3 parts per million (ppm) of selenium in animal feed. By the early 1990s, many livestock raisers were using far more selenium in their animal feed in a practice known as "extra label"—using amounts beyond the approved limit. The FDA legalized this practice by *tripling* the amount of selenium allowed to be added to animal feeds.

In response, the Microbiology and Analytical Chemistry section of the American Council of Independent Laboratories recommended that the FDA regulate selenium as an animal *drug* rather than as a feed additive because of selenium's potential toxicity and narrow margin of safety. Too much selenium intake by humans and other creatures leads to selenosis, (selenium poisoning) a chronic health disorder that, among other effects, damages the liver and skin. The group recommended, that in order to protect the public from risk, "meat and poultry derived from animals fed selenium-supplemented feed should be analyzed."

The increased levels of selenium in animal feed overlapped with the practice already noted: the addition of antibiotics to animal feed. The two introductions were a double whammy.

As farm animals were given feed with selenium, and at the same time, antibiotics were administered routinely, salmonellosis emerged as an even greater problem. Salmonellosis, long present, began to increase both in frequency and severity of complications, due to the elimination of com-

THE SELENIUM-*SALMONELLA* CONNECTION KNOWN EARLY

The selenium-*Salmonella* connection was known long before the problem surfaced in the 1990s. As early as 1936, Einar Leifson developed a specific liquid-enrichment medium containing sodium selenite (a selenium salt) to isolate and grow various pathogenic strains of *Salmonella*. Leifson found that the selenium salt was extremely useful as an enrichment medium. Even a few *Salmonella* organisms, such as the strain *S.* Typhimurium, present in feces, grew easily and would multiply a million times within twenty-four hours of incubation.

petitive flora in the intestines of animals, destroyed by the antibiotics. The addition of selenium increased the problem.

Selenium promotes the growth of *Salmonella.* The continuous intake of selenium in the feed resulted in a bioaccumulation of selenium in food animals. This concentration can result in an amount sufficient to act as a culturing agent for *Salmonella* in food animals and in the eventual transmission of the infection to humans via the meat and poultry derived from animals fed selenium-containing feed. At the same time, the antibiotics administered to the animals fostered the infection by destroying the beneficial organisms present, as well as the targeted pathogenic organisms in the intestinal tracts of the animals.

SALMONELLA TYPHIMURIUM

Salmonella Typhimurium (formally called *Salmonella enterica* serotype Typhimurium) currently accounts for the largest number of *Salmonella* infections in the United States.

S. Typhimurium was isolated in 1984 in the United Kingdom. It was identified a year later from an ill person, and found to be multidrug resistant (MDR) to antibiotics.

By the mid-1990s, *S.* Typhimurium DT104 emerged as a strain most frequently reported to the CDC in people infected by *Salmonella* in the United States, and the strain most frequently reported to the U.S. Department of Agriculture (USDA) in farm animals infected by *Salmonella.*

LARGE-SCALE S. TYPHIMURIUM OUTBREAKS

S. Typhimurium-Contaminated Milk

A large-scale outbreak of *S.* Typhimurium involved milk. Hillfarm Dairy in Melrose Park, Illinois, used to process about 1.5 million pounds of milk each day. The dairy was the sole supplier of milk to 217 supermarkets operated by the Jewel Food Stores chain in Illinois, and in neighboring states. The dairy was owned by the Jewel Company and had been in operation since 1968.

In 1985, a multistate outbreak of *S.* Typhimurium-contaminated milk from Hillfarm Dairy was so large and so devastating that it caused the dairy to close down. At least 16,284 persons were known victims. Most of them were from Illinois, but some were from Indiana, Iowa, Michigan, Minnesota, and Wisconsin. The outbreak directly caused two deaths, and was a contributing factor in the deaths of four or possibly five more people.

One of the characteristics of the *S.* Typhimurium infection was its resistance to several common antibiotics. Bernard Turnick, director of the Illinois State Department of Health, reported that the antibiotic resistance of *S.* Typhimurium "is an added dimension in this case, and is an issue we ought to be addressing because of the potential health problems."

At the time, the outbreak triggered one of the most intensive investigations ever conducted with a milkborne epidemic. What made the outbreak so frightening was the fact that so many people were made ill from drinking one of the most closely regulated products in the food supply. For years, milk had an enviable record of being one of the nation's safest foods, due to pasteurization.

After extensive examination of the Hillfarm Dairy, a large team of

CONTROLLING *S.* TYPHIMURIUM ON FARMS

Low doses of sodium chlorate are useful against *S.* Typhimurium and *E. coli* O157:H7 in the intestinal tracts of cows and pigs. This was the finding of researchers led by microbiologist David J. Nisbet at the USDA's Food and Feed Safety Research Unit at College Station, Texas.

Both pathogens contain an enzyme that converts the chlorate to chlorite and kills both *S.* Typhimurium and *E. coli* O157:H7. Beneficial bacteria in the intestinal tracts of these animals lack the enzyme, so they are not affected by the sodium chlorate.

The gut and lymph tissues of meat animals and chickens are major reservoirs for *S.* Typhimurium and *E. coli* O157:H7. Both of these pathogens can live both anaerobically (without air) or aerobically (with air). This characteristic makes them different from most gut bacteria, which are solely anaerobic.

In laboratory studies, Nisbet and his colleagues found that sodium chlorate produced a 150-fold reduction in the number of *S.* Typhimurium cells in the intestines of pigs. Sodium chlorate may offer a practical approach to reduce on-farm concentrations of these pathogens. Fewer bacterial pathogens in the guts of the animals can reduce significantly the potential for carcass contamination during food processing.

The Nisbet team's study was advanced by another group at College Sta-

investigators concluded that the most likely source of the outbreak was a stainless steel cross-connection pipe. On one side, it was linked to piping that carried unpasteurized low-fat milk; on the other side, pasteurized skim milk. Valves at each end of the pipe were intended to prevent unpasteurized milk from mixing with pasteurized milk. However, testing of the pipe arrangement showed that small amounts of milk could collect in the cross-connection and remain there long enough for bacteria to multiply. When the processing system for producing unpasteurized low-fat milk was activated, the pasteurized skim milk was pumped at high speed. It created a tremendous suction vacuum, and a potentially contaminated product in the cross-connection could be sucked into the line for pasteurized skim milk during blending. This was a possible explanation for some, but not all, of the causes of the outbreak.

tion led by microbiologist Robin Anderson. Sodium chlorate, added to the feed or water for livestock, two days prior to their slaughter, was extremely effective in reducing *Salmonella* and *E. coli* O157:H7 in the animals' intestinal tracts. The pathogens were reduced a thousandfold in more than a hundred swine and sheep tested.

Allen Byrd, a microbiologist colleague of Anderson's, tested the sodium chlorate in market-age birds: 200 turkeys and 2,000 broiler chickens, forty-eight hours before their slaughter. The *Salmonella* rate fell dramatically from 35 percent to 0 in the turkeys, and from 37 percent to 2 percent in the broiler chickens.

Additional studies by another colleague, Leon Kubena, an animal scientist, showed that the compound had good activity in preventing molting hens from shedding *Salmonella* in their feces.

Lactose (milk sugar) reduced the number *of S.* Typhimurium bacteria in infected chickens. Mannose, a natural sugar produced by a Mediterranean plant, was equally effective but more costly.

John R. DeLoach, a biochemist, led a research team at the USDA's Veterinary Toxicology Research Unit at College Station to find ways of reducing *S.* Typhimurium. The treated birds had 99.9 percent fewer bacteria than the control birds that had been infected with the pathogen, but given no lactose in their drinking water.

—*Agricultural Research*, Mar 2001

Another technical feature may have contributed to the contamination. The plant had "reclaimed" milk that for various reasons was unsuitable for delivery to stores, and was not supposed to leave the dairy plant. The milk was salvaged for use with products such as ice cream. Although all reclaimed milk was supposed to be repasteurized, investigators found that some reclaimed milk could bypass the pasteurization units and get into the cross-connection pipe, where it would remain until it was drawn into the pasteurized skim milk piping during the blending for low-fat milk.

Yet another potential contamination source was the plant's Clean-in-Place system for cleaning and sanitizing the equipment, piping, and critical areas of the dairy operations. There was one exception, discovered by the investigators: a T-shaped pipe connection leading from the pasteurized skim-milk tank to the skim-milk transfer line. Tests showed that small amounts of milk could collect in the T-connection long enough for *S.* Typhimurium to multiply. The T-connection had threaded caps. Plant employees admitted that they were unaware of the need to remove the end caps of the valve, and manually clean the caps.

The investigators' efforts were cited as "the most comprehensive dairy investigation ever undertaken." In releasing the final report on the outbreak, the Illinois Inspector General, Jeremy D. Margolis, remarked that "This wasn't sabotage, this wasn't a superbug, this wasn't a failure of the pasteurization process. It was a unique microbiological engineering phenomenon."

Increase in Outbreaks of *S.* Typhimurium DT104

The prevalence of *S.* Typhimurium DT104 isolates increased from less than 1 percent of salmonellosis in the 1980s to 34 percent by 1996. The incidence keeps rising. *S.* Typhimurium DT104 has emerged as the major strain in reported salmonellosis outbreaks.

By 2004, 58 percent of *Salmonella* strains were resistant to one or more antibiotics. These MDR strains accounted for 74 percent of all resistant isolates. Fifty percent of resistant drug isolates were *S.* Typhimurium DT104.

By 2005, the incidence of MDR *S.* Typhimurium infections, especially with DT104, increased substantially. This finding is similar in many other countries, too. An international survey, conducted among countries with available surveillance data, and covering a period from 1992 to 2001, showed that overall, the incidence of MDR *S.* Typhimurium DT104 increased continually. The infection affected primarily industrialized countries in North America and Europe. The survey suggested that MDR

S. Typhimurium constitutes an increasing public health problem in many parts of the world.

The Largest *S.* Typhimurium Outbreak—to Date

A multistate outbreak of the typhimurium strain of *Salmonella* occurred from late 2008 to early 2009. It was one of the largest foodborne outbreaks, to date, that has occurred in the United States. Contaminated peanut butter and peanut paste were responsible for causing illnesses in nearly 20,000 people, with at least nine deaths in forty-three states and Canada. The CDC estimated that for every identified case, there were probably an additional thirty unreported cases. The source of the contaminated peanut products was traced to a single facility, the Peanut Corporation of America (PCA) in Blakely, Georgia. PCA's King Nut peanut butter and peanut paste had been distributed in bulk packaging to food service industries, private label food companies, and other institutions, but not sold directly to consumers in retail stores. Both King Nut peanut butter and peanut paste had been used as ingredients in more than 200 different types of food products, including cookies, crackers, cereals, candies, ice creams, and pet foods. The large outbreak led to a worldwide recall of pails of peanut butter and peanut paste shipped to schools, nursing homes, military bases, and other institutions.

Earlier outbreaks associated with contaminated peanut butter had occurred with other strains of *Salmonella,* in Australia in 1996, and in the United States in 2004 and 2007. However, these earlier outbreaks had affected fewer people.

The large 2008 to 2009 outbreak reflected many common features of foodborne contamination, and the inadequacies of food safety surveillance. Official inspection has been stretched at all levels of government. Federal inspection by the FDA of food plants has been as infrequent as once in a decade. This was the case with the PCA plant. The state of Georgia, typical of many states, has a staff of only sixty-six inspectors responsible to supervise some 16,000 food-handling facilities. Georgia state officials claim that budgetary constraints, and attention to outbreaks of other foodborne illnesses diminished the ability to inspect the PCA plant. Like other states, Georgia contracted with the FDA to monitor food plants. The FDA's own science board had determined in 2007 that the FDA lacked the capacity to ensure a safe food supply, due to a greatly expanded number of food plants as well as imported foods.

After the outbreak was traced to the PCA plant, officials stonewalled. They refused to provide FDA inspectors with plant records. The inspectors were able to obtain the records only by invoking a recently acquired power under bioterrorism legislation. The records showed that PCA's tests had identified *Salmonella* contamination of its peanuts a dozen times since 2007, yet the company deliberately shipped its contaminated peanut butter and peanut paste. There was further stonewalling. At a congressional hearing, a PCA official refused to testify. All the features of the PCA case point to the inadequacies of food safety measures, and the need for strengthening the system for better consumer protection. As an aftermath, in April 2009, the Texas Department of State Health Services fined a Texas plant owned by PCA $14.6 million.

The Salmonella-Contaminated Pistachio Recall

Even as the peanut episode was exiting the stage, the spotlight turned on pistachios. The new scare began on March 24, 2009, when Kraft Foods notified the FDA that repeatedly, shipments of pistachios from Setton Pistachios of Terra Bella, the second largest pistachio company in the country, were contaminated with several strains of *Salmonella*. Kraft Foods had destroyed the contaminated nuts or had refused to accept them. A joint inspection by the FDA and the California Department of Public Health revealed troubling gaps of sanitation in the plant. Setton employees often used the same transport bins, conveyors, and packing machines for both raw and roasted pistachios, potentially contaminating the roasted nuts.

The FDA promptly issued a public advisory not to eat pistachios. Setton agreed to destroy the entire 2008 crop. Although no illnesses had been reported, the FDA action represented a new, tougher stance of the agency. At present, the FDA lacks the power to recall food unless there has been an outbreak of illness. David Acheson, associate commissioner of foods at the FDA, said, "We're going to try to stop people from getting sick in the first place, as opposed to waiting until we have illness and death before we take action."

SALMONELLA ENTERITIDIS

In the past, most eggborne *Salmonella* infections were due to cracked and dirty eggs and "leakers" contaminated by feces that would penetrate the shells. In the late 1980s, widespread outbreaks of eggborne salmonellosis

CAN PATHOGENIC *S.* TYPHIMURIUM BE USEFUL?

Vion Pharmaceuticals, located in New Haven, Connecticut, has been researching potential medical uses of genetically engineered *S.* Typhimurium. The modified strain can grow within tumors, but not elsewhere in the body, and slow the tumor's growth. The mechanism is uncertain. The hypothesis is that the bacteria compete for the same nutrients as the tumor for its growth in the cell. The bacteria induce apoptosis (death of the cells) of the tumor by its starvation.

—*Modern Drug Discovery,* Jan/Feb 1999

Vion Pharmaceuticals also is attempting to use genetically engineered *S.* Typhimurium bacteria to attack melanoma, a virulent form of skin cancer. In experiments with mice, the researchers inactivated the bacteria's ability to cause foodborne illness in the animals. The mice treated with the modified pathogen lived twice as long as the untreated mice with melanoma.

—*Nature Biotechnology,* 1999

occurred in the northeast, and spread to other regions of the United States. The infection was from *Salmonella enteritidis,* later renamed *Salmonella enterica* serotype Enteritidis.

FACTORS CONTRIBUTING TO RISE IN *S.* ENTERITIDIS

From the mid-1970s to the late 1980s, there was a sevenfold increase of *S.* Enteritidis in the Northeast from eggborne infections. For every reported case, it was estimated that there were ten unreported cases. Why the Northeast? The arrangement of the hen and egg production was distinctive. Unlike eggs, chicks were not shipped far from their hatcheries. Thus, when the disease spread, it traveled slowly and locally.

Investigators expected to find the usual suspects: contaminated feed, or feces from the poultry, or from invading rodents or wild birds. Yet none of these suspects were present. What puzzled the investigators was that the infection was traced to clean, intact Grade A shell eggs that had been washed and sanitized, free of feces, and had passed inspection.

Ultimately, investigators found that *S.* Enteritidis could be transmitted through the chicken's reproductive organs of ovary and oviduct, contaminating the egg content of yolk and white even before the eggshell formed.

The *S.* Enteritidis could migrate to the reproductive tract from an infected cloaca (the combined opening of a hen's reproductive and excretory tracts). Obviously, any program that focused on washing, sanitizing, and grading eggs was ineffective in controlling a hitherto unrecognized means of infection.

The CDC estimated that about one in ten thousand intact shell eggs was infected with *S.* Enteritidis. This sounds like a low risk, except that when eggs are pooled for mass feeding in restaurants or institutions, a single contaminated egg can lead to massive outbreaks. Food preparers at such places were encouraged to use previously pasteurized eggs.

By the 2000s, the outbreaks from *S.* Enteritidis-contaminated eggs declined somewhat, but still continued as a problem. Currently, it causes some 1.3 million reported cases annually, including 15,000 hospitalizations, and accounts for some 500 deaths.

S. Enteritidis-Contaminated Poultry

Changes in poultry production, as the process moved from the individual farm to mass industrial facilities, contributed to the rise of *S.* Enteritidis-contaminated poultry. Defeathering machines pressed the birds so hard that feces could spurt from the cloaca and drop onto the feathers. "Mechanical fingers" that removed the feathers inadvertently pressed the bacteria onto the skin, where *Salmonellae* could attach themselves in the empty feather follicles. High-speed disemboweling equipment could rip the intestines, and spatter fecal matter onto the carcasses.

Also, there were changes in egg production. For one, there was the invention of the shell-breaking machine. In large restaurants and food processing plants, hundreds, or even thousands of shell eggs are hand-broken daily. This labor-intensive activity could be replaced by an automated machine, which would be especially useful for large egg producers who also process eggs and convert them into powdered, liquefied, or frozen egg products used by bakers, restaurateurs, and institutional food servers.

With shell-breaking machinery, the eggs were placed in a cylinder that contained perforated baskets. The machine was spun at high speed to break the shells and strain the edible portion through the baskets. Such machines could crack about 20,000 eggs per hour. However, the large machine could spread *Salmonella* from contaminated eggs to other eggs.

The shell-breaking machine was approved for use in egg-processing

SALMONELLA ENTERITIDIS:
FROM MILD TO VIRULENT

Among various strains of *S.* Enteritidis, their genomes appear to be virtually identical. Yet they may behave differently within hens. This feature was discovered by a team of researchers, led by veterinarian officer Jean Guard-Bouldin at the USDA's Egg Safety and Quality Research Unit in Athens, Georgia. Using a technique known as whole-genome mutational mapping, the rresearchers were able to identify differences among the genomes of various strains of *S.* Enteritidis.

The researchers studied how *S.* Enteritidis evolved from being an innocuous bacterium, to becoming a virulent one. Under favorable conditions, this bacterium reproduces rapidly—every twenty minutes. The researchers speculated that about thirty-six years ago, a large-scale DNA exchange occurred between strains of *S.* Enteritidis in conjunction with the emergence of egg contamination. However, evolution of the bacterium, from mild to virulent, may have begun hundreds of years ago, probably setting the stage for the problem.

The strain that emerged recently has the ability to contaminate the internal contents of eggs. An additional problem emerged. The hybrid strain carries incompatible viruses within its genome. As a result, the hybrid strain splits very rapidly into two lineages, each around one virus. Except for the different virus, the two strains have identical genomes. Both of the newly split lineages contributed to the beginning of the pandemic of *S.* Enteritidis-contaminated eggs. Both continued to evolve by accumulating small changes in their genomes. Eventually, they survived on the farms. They began to vary in their ability to contaminate eggs. According to Jean Guard-Bouldin, their developments "challenge our ability to understand their association with chickens." She continued, "The information about the differences between genomes could help streamline the process of finding out how human disease organisms evolve to become more virulent . . . If we can understand how *Salmonella* [Enteritidis] evolved to become pathogenic, perhaps we can apply the same principles to other foodborne pathogens and begin to study foodborne illness the way influenza is being managed—with equal importance on the small, as well as the large, genetic changes."

—Agricultural Research, April 2009

facilities regulated by the USDA's Food Safety and Inspection Service (FSIS). However, another USDA branch, the Agricultural Marketing Service, in charge of eggs, received complaints, and had FSIS rescind its approval. Egg producers lobbied the FDA. The United Egg Producers, fearing for the reputation of the industry, declared that the machine was "a health hazard." The egg industry lobbyists succeeded in having six states ban use of the machine, and attempted, through an act of Congress, to put the company manufacturing the egg-shelling machine out of business.

CONTROLLING *SALMONELLA* IN POULTRY AND EGGS

Because of the frequent association of *Salmonella* with poultry and eggs, numerous types of controls have been suggested or instituted. The best controls are sanitation in the environments of producing, processing, and cooking these foods. *Salmonella* is destroyed if all portions of food are heated to 145°F.

Other techniques include microwaving, radiating, vaccinating, scalding, and pasteurizing. Use of chemical compounds include a trisodium phosphate (TSP) solution near the end of processing operations, and poultry dips such as peroxide catalyzed chemical (PC) plus agitation by ultrasound. Attempts were made to supplement broiler feed with organic acids, such as lactic, fumaric, citric, or formic/propionic, but these acids were ineffective. Also, it was suggested that formaldehyde be added to poultry feed. (Formaldehyde is an acknowledged carcinogen.)

Often eggs are processed into liquid, dried, and frozen forms, and used by bakers, and manufacturers of candies, pastas, mayonnaises, and salad dressings. Gluconic acid (the acid form of glucose) is added to liquid eggs to delay the growth of *Salmonella* in liquid eggs.

In an attempt to lower *Salmonella* in young chicks, researchers at the USDA's Poultry Microbiological Safety Research Center in Athens, Georgia, attempted to devise a control. *Salmonella* bacteria cannot digest certain naturally occurring sugars found in wheat, onions, and garlic. The researchers combined these sugars with various benign bacteria, and added the mix to chicken feed. The supplement crowded out *Salmonella* in the intestines of young chicks. The sugars—fructooligosaccharides (FOS)—made the chicks' intestines inhospitable to *Salmonella*. As an added bonus, FOS could replace antibiotics added to poultry feed to promote growth.

Official Advisories

Health officials have cautioned the public regarding eggborne salmonellosis. These are some of the specifics of the advice:

- Do not eat raw or lightly cooked eggs. Cook scrambled eggs for one minute at 250°F; poached eggs, five minutes in boiling water; "sunny-side up" eggs, seven minutes at 250°F, or four minutes at 250°F in a covered pan; "fried over easy" eggs, three minutes at 250°F for one side, and another minute after turning the egg to the other side; and boiled eggs, cook for seven minutes in water that boils continuously. (Some egg lovers have lampooned these directions, and suggested that eggs cooked this long would be the consistency of hockey pucks.)

- Do not eat food dishes likely to contain raw or lightly cooked eggs, such as homemade versions of mayonnaise, eggnog, and ice cream containing eggs. The commercial counterparts are considered safe because pasteurized eggs are used in such products. Lightly cooked eggs may be present in dishes such as French toast, omelettes, scrambled eggs in which the whites are still runny, Caesar salad, tiramisu (an Italian dessert containing raw eggs and mascarpone cheese), meringues, éclairs, soft custards, and sauces such as hollandaise and béarnaise.

- Discard eggs if shells inadvertently drop into the bowl while eggs are being cracked. Do not lick egg-containing, uncooked, cookie or cake dough from the bowl, or allow children to engage in this practice.

- Avoid the temptation to use inexpensive but riskier eggs with cracked shells, or "leakers." Check the soundness of the shells by opening the egg carton before purchasing it. Promptly refrigerate shell eggs and all products made with eggs.

S. Enteritidis-Contaminated Ice Cream

In 1994, a large outbreak of *S.* Enteritidis occurred with ice cream, produced by Schwan's Sales Enterprises in Minnesota. The product not only affected a large number of people within the state of Minnesota, but also 87 percent of the ice cream was shipped nationwide and distributed in the forty-eight contiguous states, affecting an even larger number of people. Nearly 30,000 people in Minnesota became ill with *S.* Enteritidis gastroenteritis, and countless numbers elsewhere. As many as 25,000 people brought a class action lawsuit against Schwan's. It was one of the largest class-action foodborne poisoning cases ever brought to court in U.S. history.

Investigators of the outbreak found that the cause of the contamination was due to the ice cream being hauled in a tanker that previously carried raw egg products. After processing, the ice cream had not been given any heat treatment. As a result of this outbreak, stricter regulations and practices were instituted.

Martin Blaser, at Vanderbilt University's School of Medicine in Nashville, Tennessee, termed salmonellosis "a disease of civilization." In an editorial in the *New England Journal of Medicine,* Blaser added:

> *Modern food production is often so complex that many points at which contamination could occur are simply not recognized. Thus, in the outbreak of salmonellosis, the use of tanker trailers to ship both pasteurized and nonpasteurized products represents a classic cross-connection that was not identified until the investigation was undertaken . . . This*

S. ENTERITIDIS WEAKENED BY YOGURT AND CALCIUM

Fermented milk products, as well as calcium present in milk, stimulate gastric acid secretion in the stomach that helps destroy pathogens. This fact suggested to Bovee-Oudenhoven and colleagues at the Netherland Institute for Dairy Research in BA Ede, that these substances might help lessen the severity of S. Enteritidis and other foodborne infections.

In rat experiments, the researchers found that both yogurt and calcium contained in milk increased the animals' resistance to salmonellosis. One day after researchers intentionally infected yogurt-fed rats orally with S. Enteritidis, significantly fewer of these pathogens were found in the rats' feces than in the rats orally infected but given no yogurt. Also, the number of *Salmonella* organisms declined rapidly in the feces excreted by rats given high-calcium milk. The rats fed low-calcium milk continued to excrete large numbers of *Salmonella.*

The protective effect of yogurt may be due to the slower gastric emptying rate of fermented milk—half that of regular milk. The slower emptying subjects the ingested pathogens to prolonged exposure of gastric acid that destroys them.

outbreak underscores the fact that to minimize risk from unrecognized hazards, pasteurization—one of the most powerful tools against bacterial pathogens—should be undertaken at the latest possible step in food production.

SALMONELLA SAINTPAUL

In 2008, the United States experienced its largest foodborne disease outbreak in a decade. The contaminant was *Salmonella* Saintpaul, short for *Salmonella enterica* serovar Saintpaul, an uncommon serotype. At the beginning of the outbreak, certain types of raw tomatoes were the prime suspects. As the epidemiologic studies were conducted, after the infections grew and spread, raw jalapeño peppers, and perhaps raw serrano peppers, were suspect as likely vehicles. Other raw produce, such as cilantro, parsley, and products made with these ingredients in raw salsa and guacamole (consisting of raw ingredients such as avocado, Roma tomatoes, red onions, serrano peppers, and cilantro), were also suspected as vehicles.

The outbreak began in May 2008 in New Mexico, and expanded rapidly to forty-three states, the District of Columbia, and Canada. Three months later, in August 2008, a total of 1,442 people had been reported to be infected with the outbreak strain, of which at least 280 persons required hospitalization. The infection may have contributed to two deaths.

Traceback investigations failed to identify a single packer, distributor, or growing area of tomatoes. The FDA finally traced the likely source of the contaminated jalapeño peppers to one farm in Tamaulipas, Mexico, where serrano peppers and Roma tomatoes also were grown. At another farm in Tamaulipas, the outbreak strain of *Salmonella* was identified from a sample of serrano peppers and from a sample of water from a holding pond at the farm used for irrigation. This farm also grew jalapeño peppers, but did not grow tomatoes. Both farms shipped produce through a common packing facility in Mexico that exports to the United States.

The CDC reported that, often, official response capacity to such large and complex outbreaks is strained, and can cause delays in identifying cases during investigations. The interim report, issued by the CDC three months after the initial outbreak, attests to this feature. Although a well-established traceback system for produce and other foods has been set-up under the Hazard Analysis and Critical Control Point (HACCP) program, the long delay may have resulted from a political decision. According to an editorial in the *New York Times* (July 24, 2008), "Four years ago, the Bush administration and food-industry leaders watered down regulations on tracing food supplies from farms to consumers that were supposed to be part of the nation's bioterrorism preparedness law. The effort they said would be too cumbersome and too costly." To learn about the HACCP program, see page 209.)

This decision may have been penny-wise and pound-foolish. The weakening of the traceback system, in this instance, resulted in the needless action of many tomato farmers to plow under their crops, resulting in estimated losses of hundreds of millions of dollars. This economic loss was accompanied by the sufferings of persons infected, and the hospitalizations and death of some, inflicted by this large outbreak.

The *New York Times* editorial concluded that "Congress could relieve consumers and food producers alike with a comprehensive food-safety bill that would require a system for tracing food, better oversight of food-safety plans by producers, and more authority to the FDA to investigate and recall tainted products."

SALMONELLA TYPHI

Salmonella Typhi bacteria cause typhus fever (typhoid). Although this *Salmonella* serotype, formally known as *Salmonella enterica* serovar Typhi, is more common in developing countries, it does occur, albeit infrequently, in developed countries. In the United States, generally a few hundred cases are reported annually, with some fatalities. Often outbreaks are traced to food handlers who are asymptomatic carriers, and practice poor personal hygiene. The potential for large outbreaks exist, especially in restaurants or institutions, when hands of preparers are in contact with raw foods that are eaten uncooked.

A FOODBORNE PATHOGEN LONG WITH US

S. Typhi bacteria enter the body through contaminated food or water, penetrate the small intestine, and invade the bloodstream, where they cause blood poisoning and carry infection into other parts of the body. Early symptoms of the infection begin with headache, general aches, restlessness, coughing, nosebleeds, bloody diarrhea or constipation, and fever. A week or two later, a rash appears on the torso. If the patient manages to survive, the fever begins to decline after about four weeks. But complications may arise, including heart failure, and ulceration or perforation of the intestinal wall. Then, typhoid generally is fatal.

About 30 percent of people infected with typhoid remain as carriers. They continue to excrete the organism in their stools or urine for weeks or months. About 5 percent are long-term carriers, who keep shedding *S.* Typhi bacteria for years, even though they are asymptomatic. They harbor the bacteria in their gallbladders and bile ducts.

The Infamous Mary Mallon

Mary Mallon (1868–1938), the first typhoid carrier identified in the United States, was asymptomatic. During her lifetime, she prepared food in many different locations, and by the end of her working career, directly infected at least fifty-one people, three of whom died; and infected, indirectly, countless more people.

In 1906, a banker, his family of three, and a staff of seven servants, rented a summerhouse in Oyster Bay, Long Island. Six of them were stricken with typhoid fever. George Soper, a sanitary engineer, investigated the outbreak, and suspected Mary Mallon as the source of the infection. She had begun to cook for the household before the outbreak, and left soon after Soper began his investigation. Soper found that several other typhoid outbreaks had occurred at six out of the seven households where Mary Mallon had previously been employed as a cook. Soper was able to trace her to an affluent family on Park Avenue in New York City. He learned that the laundress had recently been struck with typhoid, and the sole child of the family was also ill with typhoid. The child died shortly after Soper contacted the family.

Soper attempted to persuade Mary Mallon to stop cooking for others, but she was unconvinced that she was ill. Soper requested that the New York City Health Department take her into custody, in order to protect the public health. The police seized her and took her by ambulance to the Health Department's Detention Hospital. There, Mary Mallon's bowel movements were examined three times weekly for six months. Most of the time, the investigators could identify *S.* Typhi bacteria in her stools. By summer, there were five consecutive negative tests, followed by one positive one. Mary Mallon was kept in the isolation ward. Physicians thought that her gallbladder was the locus of the infection, and recommended that the organ be removed. Mary Mallon refused to consent to the surgery, convinced that she was well.

The authorities transferred Mary Mallon to Riverside Hospital, a so-called "typhus house" located on North Brother Island in the East River of New York City. After being in custody for about two years, Mary Mallon hired a lawyer, and in 1909 brought suit in the New York Supreme Court under habeas corpus proceedings. The doctor who had supervised her testified that she still harbored S. Typhi bacteria, and that she was "a public menace to the community." The judge dismissed the case, but the publicity generated by the trial circulated worldwide and Mary Mallon was dubbed "Typhoid Mary."

Mary Mallon was released in 1910, with her promise that she would not cook for other people. She was to report to the Health Department every three months. For a while, she reported dutifully, and then she disappeared. She had tried other occupations, but none paid as well as cooking. So, she resumed cooking, under assumed names.

In January and February of 1915, twenty-five staff members—mostly nurses and attendants—at the Sloane Hospital for Women in Manhattan, were stricken with typhoid fever. Two of them died. A Mrs. Brown (a.k.a. Mary Mallon) had begun cooking in the hospital three months before the first case was reported. Mary Mallon disappeared from the hospital, but she was traced to a private home on Long Island. She was arrested and returned to Riverside Hospital, and kept in confinement there for twenty-three years until her death.

Although Mary Mallon was the first identified asymptomatic carrier of S. Typhi, such carriers are still with us. Some may be food preparers in institutions, restaurants, and food-processing plants.

Early Typhoid Outbreaks

Typhoid outbreaks occurred frequently in New York City in the late 1880s, as scores of immigrants settled in squalid, crowded slums. In January 1892, some 200 Russian Jews, who fled pogroms and famine, settled in the Lower East Side of Manhattan. A month later, an epidemic typhoid outbreak occurred among them. Infected persons were sent to the same "typhus house" on North Brothers Island where Mary Mallon was housed. For three months, some 1,200 people—1,150 of whom actually were healthy—were placed in unsanitary, badly equipped, and poorly monitored tents and pavilions. More than 100 people died.

The prevalent anti-Semitism and general anti-foreign sentiments used the typhoid outbreak to demand immigration restrictions on Jews (and

Italians). Congressional hearings foundered because the medical experts were unable to describe the etiology and transmission of this infectious disease. Also, the issue became political, involving state's rights versus federal centralization of quarantine control.

More Recent *S.* Typhi Outbreaks

An outbreak occurred in Skagit County, in Washington State, in 1990, following a family gathering of 293 people from five different states. From the group, seventeen became ill from food, traced to a food handler who was a typhoid carrier.

Another outbreak occurred at a resort hotel in New York State in 1992, resulting in typhoid fever in forty-three hotel guests and one hotel staff member. Two persons required surgery for perforated bowels, and a secondary case occurred in a child of one of the hotel guests. The outbreak was the largest *S.* Typhi outbreak in the United States since 1981. Investigators identified many poor food-preparation practices in the hotel. Orange juice was a suspected food, with several opportunities for fecal contamination during the preparation and serving of the juice.

GARLIC EXTRACT KILLS *S.* TYPHI

In 1858, the famous French bacteriologist Louis Pasteur (1822–1895) reported on the antibacterial activity of garlic. In 1944, researchers isolated allicin, the active agent, from garlic. An extract of allicin inhibits the growth of *S.* Typhi as well as other foodborne pathogens. Boiled garlic is less effective because allicin is denatured by high heat.

CHAPTER 4

E. coli: From Mild to Deadly Strains

Although a year had passed, the sense of loss and the grieving remained with both parents. The counseling had not helped. Ann and Tim looked at the picture of their daughter, Robin, on the mantle. Tim had taken the picture last year on Robin's fourth birthday. She was blowing out the candles on her birthday cake, surrounded by her four preschool friends at the local restaurant. The picture showed a beautiful, vibrant child. Now, she was dead.

Tim and Ann had taken the five young children to a popular chain restaurant, where the children enjoyed hamburgers, french fries, and soft drinks. When Robin opened her birthday presents, Tim was too busy taking photographs to eat. Nor did Ann eat. She was busy serving the food and picking up the paper wrappings and ribbons. It was a happy scene.

By the next morning, Robin was not well. She had stomach cramps and a low fever. Later, she began to have a series of loose bowel movements. On the second day, Ann became alarmed when she noticed that the stools were bloody and the toilet bowl water was red. Tim phoned the parents of the other children, and learned that, like Robin, the children were ill with similar symptoms.

All five children required hospitalization. Robin was given an antibiotic, and it seemed to make her worse. After six days, two of the children were discharged from the hospital, but Robin and two others remained. Robin had high fever and her kidneys were failing. She required dialysis. The second child had seizures. The third child was confused, did not seem to comprehend, and had difficulty expressing herself.

After four months in the hospital, Robin was showing signs of rapid deterioration. All her vital organs functioned poorly. The two other children had progressed and were discharged. Although they were recovering, they were not as robust as previously.

In the sixth month after the original infection, all of Robin's systems failed and she died. Laboratory analysis of the stools of all five of the children had identified the infection. It was a rapidly emerging strain of E. coli *and was extremely virulent. Investigators thought that the pathogen most likely was present in the hamburgers eaten by the children at the restaurant, and probably the meat was undercooked.*

*E*scherichia coli are bacteria usually found in domestic as well as wild animals. Usually *E. coli* coexists with numerous competitive organisms in the intestinal tract, held in check by beneficial microflora.

"THE RENEGADE *E. COLI*"

This scenario changed with the emergence of a new strain. In 1982, following outbreaks of a distinctive pattern of bloody diarrhea in persons living in Oregon and Michigan, investigators identified a newly emerged bacterial strain, *E. coli* O157:H7. Subsequently, this strain, and a few related ones, developed into a major health problem throughout the United States, elsewhere in North America, the European continent, and beyond.

E. coli O157:H7 has been dubbed "the renegade *E. coli.*" It does not act like other *E. coli* strains. It is hardier, more difficult to detect, more virulent, and can be deadly. The 1982 investigation showed that fewer than ten bacteria of *E. coli* O157:H7 could be an infective dose.

According to Kristine L. MacDonald and Michael T. Osterholm, "the emergence of *E. coli* O157:H7 as an important foodborne pathogen represents an example of the changing epidemiology of foodborne disease in this country."

Why *E. coli* O157:H7 Is Virulent

Although most *E. coli* strains live peacefully in the intestine, the virulent strain *E. coli* O157:H7 incorporates toxin-producing genes. This strain is the best known for this characteristic, but it is only one in a family of *E. coli* strains that produce shiga-like toxins. To date, more than a hundred different strains of toxin-producing *E. coli* have been identified. In addition to O157:H7, the strains of O261:H11, O111:NM, and O113:H21 appear to be isolated from patients more frequently than other strains.

The most common and most studied member of this group of enterohemorrhagic *E. coli* is O157:H7. Infections carried by this strain are being recognized more frequently because of its increased occurrence and its widened geographic scope.

E. coli produces shiga-like toxins known as verotoxins (verotoxigenic E. coli or VTEC) because the toxin kills Vero cells in tissue culture. All verotoxin-producing E. coli produce one or more toxins. In structure and activity, they resemble shiga toxins produced by Shigella dysenteriae; hence the name shiga-like toxins. They are known, too, as the shiga toxin-producing E. coli (STEC).

Shiga-like toxin-producing E. coli induces hemorrhagic colitis (entero-hemorrhagic E. coli), the disorder responsible for the grossly bloody diarrhea noted in the 1982 investigation. STEC was dubbed "the hamburger bug" because STEC was identified in early outbreaks with undercooked hamburgers.

Some E. coli strains are especially well adapted to resisting acid more than other strains. This feature gives them a selective advantage to resist stomach acids. If they survive in the stomach, they pass into the intestine, through the small bowel, and enter into the large bowel. There, they divide, attach to intestinal cells, and produce shiga-like toxins. The toxins are able to cross the intestinal epithelial cell barrier, enter into the bloodstream, and then move to distant sites, including the kidney and brain. The toxins inflict great tissue damage in such organs.

SOURCES OF *E. COLI* O157:H7 AND ITS TRANSMISSION

E. coli O157:H7, as it has emerged, is now present in a large number of farm and wild animals. The feces of infected animals can contaminate soil, crops, food animals, and water supplies. The infection can be transmitted from person to person by the fecal-oral route.

At one end of the high-risk scale are very young children, especially those in day-care centers, and at institutions for severely mentally retarded persons. At the other end of the high-risk scale are the elderly, especially those in hospitals, nursing homes, and assisted-living facilities.

Persons also at high risk are those who recently have been given antibiotic medication, those with previous gastrectomy, and individuals with occupational exposures to cattle, handling ground beef, or testing stool specimens. However, in the general public, everyone is at some risk.

Most foodborne outbreaks from E. coli O157:H7 are associated with foods of bovine origin, especially ground beef. Thomas Kaper and his colleagues at the University of Maryland School of Medicine, in Baltimore, researched *E. coli* O157:H7. Kaper concluded, "With thousands of cattle on hundreds of farms going to tens of slaughterhouses, to one hamburger plant where everything is mixed together to allow cross contamination . . . it's no surprise that [*E. coli*] O157:H7 emerged."

Contaminated beef has been the main food source of *E. coli* O157:H7, but the pathogen is associated, to a lesser extent, with lamb, pork, veal kidney, venison, chicken, and turkey. At times, dairy foods have been contaminated with products such as unpasteurized milk, semi-soft cheeses, cheese curds, and yogurt.

As the problem of *E. coli* O157:H7 grew, it was not confined to foods of animal origin. The pathogen began to turn up in minimally processed, bagged, leafy vegetables such as lettuces, mesclun (a mixture of young salad greens), and spinach; in unpasteurized apple juice and in fresh orange juice; and in salad sprouts from alfalfa or radish seeds. Because animals are reservoirs for the pathogen, their feces contaminated nearby wells used for drinking water, and nearby water bodies used for swimming.

Contamination from Farm to Fork

Because contaminated meat is the main source of *E. coli* O157:H7, it receives the most attention. Meat can be contaminated from farm to fork, through a long and intricate chain. The meat animal starts at a feedlot, and from there goes to a slaughterhouse, processing plant, through a series of movements in packaging, shipping, distributing, and storing at wholesale and retail levels, to its final destination. Preparation may be done at a day-care center, school, recreational camp, military establishment, picnic, barbecue, church supper, family reunion, community center, restaurant, hospital, nursing home or other institutions, as well as in numerous individual homes. Each step in this chain provides opportunities for contamination of the meat with *E. coli* O157:H7 (and other foodborne pathogens).

The most common features of *E. coli* O157:H7-related meat outbreaks have been:

- The cooking heat was too low or the cooking time was too short. An infective dose of the pathogen may be present even when meat is only *slightly* undercooked.

- There might have been cool spots on restaurant grills during times of peak use.

- A newly introduced slow-cook procedure, adapted for frozen cryovac vacuum-packed roasts might have used insufficient cooking time with commercial frozen precooked meat patties.

- Roast beef was served and eaten rare or medium rare.

- Meat was held at room temperature, sometimes even for short periods of time.

These findings suggest that fewer *E. coli* O157:H7 bacteria are needed to cause illness than for *Salmonella*, which often is associated with more gross food-handling errors. Even minor errors of temperature or time calculations can be risky with *E. coli* O157:H7.

Changed Agricultural Practices and *E. coli* O157:H7

Changes in agricultural practices are factors to consider in the prevalence of *E. coli* O157:H7, a problem largely associated with cattle and foods derived from them. Formerly, on family farms, cattle were grazed on grass, their normal diet. Now, cattle are reared intensively in huge livestock lots. *E. coli* O157:H7 is more prevalent in cattle feces and on cattle hides in such an environment than previously recognized. In 2000, U.S. Department of Agriculture (USDA) researchers found that 28 percent of

E. COLI O157:H7 NECESSITATES REWRITING OF FOOD SAFETY RULES

After *E. coli* O157:H7 emerged as a virulent pathogen, food technologists Robert L. Buchanan and Michael P. Doyle agreed that "the unusually virulent enterohemorrhagic strains of *E. coli*, including the O157:H7 serotype, have prompted food microbiologists to rewrite the rule book on food safety. These pathogens are more significant than other well-recognized foodborne pathogens for reasons including the severe consequences of infection that affect all age groups, their low infectious dose, their unusual acid tolerance, and their apparent special but inexplicable association with ruminants that are used for food."

—*Scientific Status Summary of the Institute of Food Technology,*
  Oct 1997

live cattle entering slaughterhouses were shedding *E. coli* O157:H7 in their feces. At the initial state of processing, before evisceration, 43 percent of the cattle carcasses were contaminated with *E. coli* O157:H7.

Feed is another factor associated with *E. coli* O157:H7. In lieu of grass, the cattle are fed an abnormal and indigestible high-energy diet such as corn or soybeans, which makes the cattle more susceptible to *E. coli* O157:H7. The antibiotics added to the feed destroy the beneficial microorganisms normally present in the animals' rumens, and allow *E. coli* O157:H7 to flourish.

Reducing *E. coli* O157:H7 in Animals

A simple switch in cattle feed—from corn to hay—for the last five days before slaughter, can reduce the risk of *E. coli* O157:H7 in meat eaten by humans. This was the finding, reported in 1998, of a study conducted jointly by the USDA's Agricultural Research Service and Cornell University's Plant, Soil, and Nutrition Research at Ithaca, New York. The researchers found that cattle fed corn tended to develop heartier, acid-resistant strains of *E. coli* in their digestive tracts. Acid resistance facilitates the passage of bacteria through the gastric stomach and allows the bacteria to colonize in the human colon. Switching to hay just before slaughter reduced the occurrence of these strains. The research revealed a previously unknown mechanism that enables the bacteria to develop acid resistance. Some undigested grain ferments in the animal's colon, producing volatile fatty acids. *E. coli* bacteria, including the O157:H7 strain, develop genetic defenses that help the bacteria to thrive in this low-pH environment. But cattle digest hay (and grass) readily. As a result, acid levels in the colon remain low, and discourage the development of acid-resistant bacteria.

Of course, the implications of these findings were startling. Changed feeding practices in food animals were causing human infections. To prevent the problem, animal-feeding practices would need to be altered drastically, with a return to former feeding practices.

This preliminary finding reported in 1998 was confirmed later, and reported in 2003, in the *Journal of Dairy Science*. The researchers noted that up to 80 percent of dairy cattle in the United States carry *E. coli* O157:H7. However, contaminated fecal matter could be prevented from entering the food supply, achievable by a change in feeding practices. Instead of using inappropriate feed containing corn or soybeans, by switching to hay as briefly as five days, *E. coli* O157:H7 in cows was found to decline a thousandfold.

Despite these dramatic findings, confirmed once again, the use of high-energy feed with corn or soybeans has continued. The practice puts more weight on the animals quickly, even though their health suffers and their meat becomes riskier for humans who consume it. However, the findings reinforce the soundness of the practices of grass-grazing animals in summer, and hay-feeding animals in winter. Some farmers and consumers are interested in reverting to such normal feed. At present, the movement is modest. But as people recognize the association between feeding practices and human health, the movement will grow.

Feeding practices when the animals are transported from feedlots to

CONTROLLING *E. COLI* IN PIGS WITHOUT ANTIBIOTICS?

Because *E. coli* is increasingly antibiotic resistant, Roger B. Harvey, a veterinary officer at the USDA's Food and Feed Safety Research Laboratory in College Station, Texas, led a team effort to find alternatives. The group attempted to develop recombined porcine continuous-flow (RPCF). This is a mixed culture of beneficial and commensal bacteria (that is, in a symbiotic relationship in which one species of bacteria benefits, while another species is unaffected).

The team's approach was to colonize the intestinal tracts of newly born and young weaned pigs with a mixture of commensal bacteria obtained from other pigs, in order to establish a healthy gut flora much more quickly than otherwise would occur. These beneficial bacteria attach to intestinal walls and block sites so that disease-causing bacteria such as *E. coli* cannot attach and compete for needed nutrients. Some of the colonizing bacteria also produce bactericidal compounds that work against the pathogens, and reduce the pathogens' ability to adhere and colonize in the pigs' intestinal tracts.

The RPCF mixture of beneficial bacteria was found to reduce mortality, morbidity, and medication costs due to *E. coli* in the treated pigs, compared to the untreated pigs. The treatment showed promise as a replacement for antibiotics. —*Agricultural Research,* March 2004

slaughterhouses are another factor associated with *E. coli* O157:H7. They may be given no food for as long as two days during the travel, then given half rations on the third day, followed by another two days without food, according to Mark Rassmussen, at the USDA's Agricultural Research Service's (ARS) Animal Disease Center in Ames, Iowa. The dietary stress caused by periods of fasting affects the levels of pH and volatile fatty acids in the animals' rumens, and creates an ideal environment for *E. coli* O157:H7 to thrive.

After the animals are slaughtered and the meat is processed, the type of meat product is another factor associated with *E. coli* O157:H7. The public has been advised—rightly or wrongly—to decrease consumption of fats contained in foods from animal sources. This advice has led to a profitable line of numerous low-fat versions of traditional offerings, such as low-fat ground meats, and low-fat milk and other dairy products. The consequence has been higher levels of *E. coli* O157:H7, which is more likely to develop in fat-reduced products than in their traditional counterparts. Typically, decreasing the fat content involves increasing the water content. Vegetative bacteria are more heat resistant in foods with higher water activity, and *E. coli* O157:H7 has a higher survival rate.

The addition of ingredients (such as carrageenan, starch, and soy protein) to replace fat in ground beef increases the survival of pathogens such as *E. coli* O157:H7 during extended periods of storage and subsequent cooking. Yet another risk factor with fat-reduced ground beef is that it may require higher internal temperature in cooking than traditional ground beef.

E. COLI O157:H7: A "DISEASE OF PROGRESS"

The changes in agricultural practice and their impact on pathogens caused Dennis G. Maki, professor of medicine at the University of Wisconsin School of Medicine, to remark that infection from *E. coli* O157:H7 is "what we call a disease of progress." Maki explained that this pathogen has caused an increasing amount of food- and waterborne diseases in recent years because of the tremendous changes in how we produce food in the developed world.

The human health consequences from *E. coli* O157:H7 can be devastating, as learned by anyone who has experienced it, or watched a family member or friend suffer through it. The infectious connections are more varied, more extensive, and more serious than those inflicted by other

MINIMALLY PROCESSED FOODS AND *E. COLI*

The need for adequate cooking of food to kill *E. coli* O157:H7 was demonstrated with beef gravy, by Vivay K. Juneja and a team at the USDA's Food Safety Research Unit in Wyndmoor, Pennsylvania. They cooked intentionally contaminated *E. coli* O157:H7 gravy at low heat (114°F) from ten to fifteen minutes. The bacteria were heat shocked at this temperature, which was insufficient to kill them. Then, the researchers cooked the gravy to a final internal temperature of 140°F. The bacteria *survived longer* in the gravy cooked this way than in gravy cooked adequately from the beginning of the cooking procedure.

This finding suggested that minimally processed foods might increase the risk for *E. coli* O157:H7 viability and growth. Frequently, only mild heat is used with minimally processed cook-in-a-bag refrigerated foods, including filled pasta products (ravioli, tortellini, cannelloni, etc.), moussaka, lasagna, and chili con carne. The slow-heating rate and low-heating temperatures used to prepare such foods expose pathogens that may be present to conditions similar to heat shock, which would make them *more* resistant. Also, the induced heat resistance is a concern with meat products kept in warming trays before final heating or reheating, or where equipment failure interrupts the cooking cycle during processing.

common foodborne infections. The general public is only vaguely aware of the health consequences of this virulent pathogen.

E. coli O157:H7 and Hemorrhagic Colitis

In the early 1970s, hemorrhagic colitis was recognized and described by various terms such as "evanescent colitis," "transient ischemic colitis," and "transient hemorrhagic colitis." After *E. coli* O157:H7 was identified as one cause of this disorder, it was renamed hemorrhagic colitis.

E. coli O157:H7 can cause a distinctive hemorrhagic colitis that was uncommon until this strain emerged. The frequent identification of *E. coli* O157:H7 in the stools of people with hemorrhagic colitis—usually absent in stools of healthy individuals—helped investigators to recognize the presence of this pathogen in contaminated foods, and the animal sources of the foods.

Typically, *E. coli* O157:H7-induced hemorrhagic colitis begins with non-bloody diarrhea and severe abdominal cramps. About half of the patients vomit. About one-third experience some fever, but it is not especially high. High fever is more common in persons who are severely affected.

Usually by the second day of the illness, the stools become bloody. The amount of blood in the stools can range from mere streaks to being essentially all blood. The bloody stools continue from two to four days. People may be so seriously ill that they require hospitalization.

In persons who experience nonbloody diarrhea, the illness may end six days after it began. Also, there have been reports of asymptomatic infections.

Occasionally, *E. coli* O157:H7 goes from the intestinal tract to other sites in the body. For example, the pathogen was isolated from the glans (soft tip of penis) of a ten-month-old boy twenty-eight days after he developed bloody diarrhea from *E. coli* O157:H7 infection. In other rare cases, the pathogen has been identified in blood or in urine. In one reported case, after insertion of a urinary catheter, the urine became infected with *E. coli* O157:H7, which led to hematuria (blood in the urine). If a wound provides the pathogen with access to the abdominal cavity rather than the intestines, the consequence can be peritonitis, a severe infection of the membrane lining the walls of the abdominal and pelvic cavities.

PREVENTING *E. COLI* INFECTION

A study at Rutgers State University in New Brunswick, New Jersey, suggested that specific tannin compounds present in cranberries may prevent *E. coli* from adhering to the lining of the urinary tract. This action would allow the urine to flush out the bacteria from the bladder and void it from the body. —*New England Journal of Medicine*, Oct 1998

E. coli O157:H7 and Hemolytic Uremic Syndrome

Hemolytic uremic syndrome (HUS) is one of the consequences of *E. coli* O157:H7 infections. It is a multisystem disease, especially affecting the kidneys. Any organ in the body can be affected. HUS can induce numerous disorders, including:

- High fever and kidney failure

- Gross anal dilation (a stretching of the organ far beyond its normal dimension)

- Complications, such as intussusception (a prolapsed portion of the intestine)

- Microangiopathic hemolytic anemia (a disorder of the small blood vessels)

- Neurologic disorders, including symptoms such as seizures, jerking, confusion and lack of comprehension or articulation, and impairment of the senses

- Thrombotic thrombocytopenic purpura (a serious and sometimes fatal disorder marked by clotting of the blood platelets, and seen in bruise marks and skin discoloration)

Ten months after one outbreak of *E. coli* O157:H7-associated food-borne illness, nineteen out of thirty-seven of the persons affected had significantly extra-renal abnormalities, including pancreatitis, colonic necrosis (death of cells), glucose intolerance, adult respiratory disease syndrome, and liquid in the lungs. Of these patients, 57 percent required dialysis and 76 percent required transfusions. Three of the children died.

HUS may or may not be preceded by diarrhea. The diarrhea-associated HUS, which is the more common form, may be connected with *Shigella dysenteriae* type 1 infection, as well as with shiga-like toxin-producing *E. coli* infection. The less common nondiarrheal form of HUS may be associated with *Streptococcus pneumoniae* infection.

HUS may be misdiagnosed. At times, it has been mistaken for other health problems, ranging from appendicitis to blocked blood vessels in the colon.

The shiga-like toxin produced by *E. coli* O157:H7 sets up a main barrier to fighting the pathogen effectively with antibiotics. Actually, antibiotic treatment may harm, rather than help, by exacerbating *E. coli* O157:H7-caused HUS. Antibiotics cause *E. coli* O157:H7 bacteria to increase their release of shiga-like toxins. Antibiotics stress the bacteria and coax the DNA from the toxin-encoding virus out of the bacterial DNA. Then, the virus replicates in large numbers inside the bacteria, and causes the release of toxins. Eventually, the bacteria burst, and the toxins make their way to the kidneys and other organs.

E. coli: Gene Mutations and Their Potential Transference

The movement of *E. coli* O157:H7 among other *E. coli* strains is a major public health concern in the United States and elsewhere. There is an enormous potential for the spread of shiga-like toxin genes to non-O157:H7 strains of *E. coli.*

E. coli has an exceptionally high number of mutations. These genetically flawed microbes take up DNA from other bacteria because they are unable to repair the errors in their own DNA. The result is that their evolution is speeded up significantly. This development may explain, in part, the ability of new *E. coli* strains to thrive in salted foods such as sausages and in acidic foods such as cider.

MASSIVE OUTBREAKS OF *E. COLI* FROM MEAT SOURCES

The largest recorded outbreak to date from *E. coli* O157:H7-contaminated hamburgers occurred in 1993 in the Pacific Northwest. Although all food-borne outbreaks result in suffering and anguish, these outbreaks were especially tragic because so many young children were affected by illness, long-term health problems, and deaths. More than 500 persons were made ill; a third required hospitalization; and most of the victims were children under ten years of age. Four very young children died, and more developed the complications with the hemolytic uremic syndrome (HUS) described earlier.

The hamburgers, shipped to Jack in the Box restaurants, were distributed by Vons Meat Service, located in El Monte, California. The meat, from more than a dozen slaughterhouses, had been federally inspected and met federal standards.

A spate of earlier outbreaks from *E. coli* O157:H7-infected meat in Walla Walla had resulted in Washington being the first state to require that all *E. coli* O157:H7 infections be reported to state health officials.

The Jack in the Box outbreaks led to several actions. Foodmakers, Inc., the parent company of Jack in the Box, instituted changed practices in food handling in the restaurants that strengthened food safety. Nationally, some consumers, outraged by the outbreaks that had been publicized widely, formed STOP (Safe Tables Our Priority), an organization with a goal to improve the nation's food safety. The USDA, reacting to public criticism, attempted to strengthen meat safety regulations. In response, the meat industry brought a lawsuit against the agency. The industry protested the USDA's proposed microbial testing program for *E. coli*

O157:H7 in meat, and declared that the program was unscientific and its cost not justified. Many parents of the children affected by the *E. coli* O157:H7 outbreaks brought a class action suit against Jack in the Box. The suit ended two years after the outbreaks, with a settlement of $18 million. The long-term fallout was continued parental grief from the loss of young children, or coping with the chronic health problems inflicted from the outbreaks on the surviving children.

The Jack in the Box outbreaks were followed by other *E. coli* O157:H7-associated outbreaks. One group of outbreaks resulted from the consumption of unpasteurized apple cider made from unwashed windfall apples that probably had been contaminated with animal feces. Another group of outbreaks resulted from the consumption of sprouted seeds from radishes and from alfalfa. (These outbreaks will be discussed later.)

Another Massive Multistate Outbreak with *E. coli* 0157:H7-Contaminated Beef

In 1997, four years after the large Jack in the Box outbreaks, other large *E. coli* O157:H7 outbreaks occurred. Contaminated ground beef was suspected. Many people in Colorado were made ill. This time, the Hudson Company was involved. Its processing plants in Columbus, Nebraska, were suspected. Meat had been shipped to at least forty-eight contiguous states. Burger King had been Hudson's largest customer.

The Hudson Company had used a common practice called "reworking" of meat. Meat from one day that was not processed was held over to the next day to be reworked for processing. The company kept poor records. Workers at the plant had lied to USDA inspectors about the extent of the potentially contaminated meat that had been shipped from the plant. Initially, the company recalled 20,000 pounds of ground beef. The volume of the recalls kept expanding. The numbers went from 1.2 million pounds of beef to an ultimate 24 million pounds of beef. At the same time, the total recall was the largest in the history of U.S. meat recalls. (It was topped in 2008 by a meat recall of 143 million pounds suspected of contamination.)

The USDA closed the Hudson's plants in Columbus. In September 1997, the Hudson Company was sold to its long-time rival, Tyson Foods.

Cooking Hamburgers Safely: Not an Easy Call

Color alone is not a reliable guide for the "doneness" in cooked ground

MEAT RECALLS IN 2007: *E. COLI* O157:H7

To grasp the extent of the problem of *E. coli* O157:H7 contamination of the meat supply in the United States, this is a listing of recalls conducted by the USDA's Food Safety Inspection Service for possible contamination by this pathogen during a single year, 2007.

- **January 29, 2007:** The Natural State Meat Company, Batesville, Arkansas, 4,240 pounds of ground beef products recalled

- **March 2, 2007:** Tyson Fresh Meats, Pasco, Washington, 16,743 pounds of ground beef recalled

- **April 20, 2007:** Richwood Meat Company, Inc., Merced, California, 107,943 pounds of ground meat products recalled

- **May 10, 2007:** PM Beef Holdings, LLC, Windom, Minnesota, 117,500 pounds of beef trim recalled

- **May 11, 2007:** Davis Creek Meats and Seafood, Kalamazoo, Michigan, 129,000 pounds of beef products recalled

- **June 8, 2007:** Tyson Fresh Meats, Inc., Sherman, Texas, 40,440 pounds of ground beef products recalled

- **June 9, 2007:** United Food Group, LLC, Vernon, California, expanded final recall of 5.7 pounds of fresh and frozen ground beef

- **July 21, 2007:** Abbott's Meat, Inc., Flint, Michigan, 26,669 pounds of ground beef products recalled

- **July 25, 2007:** Custom Pack, Inc., Hastings, Nebraska, 5,920 pounds of ground beef and buffalo products recalled

- **September 5, 2007:** Fairbank Reconstruction Corporation, Ashville, New York, 884 pounds of ground meat products recalled

- **September 29, 2007:** Impero Foods & Meats, Inc., Baltimore, Maryland, 65 pounds of ground beef products recalled

- **October 6, 2007:** Topps Meat Company, LLC, Elizabeth, New Jersey, expanded final recall of 21.9 million pounds of ground beef

- **October 6, 2007:** Cargill Meat Solutions Corporation, Butler, Wisconsin, 845,000 pounds of ground beef products recalled

- **October 13, 2007:** Arko Veal Company, Forest Park, Georgia, 1,900 pounds of ground veal products recalled

- **October 13, 2007:** J & B Meats Corporation, Inc., Coal Valley, Illinois, 173, 554 pounds of frozen ground beef products recalled
- **October 24, 2007:** Blue Ribbon Meats, Hialeah, Florida, 8,200 pounds of frozen ground beef products recalled
- **October 27, 2007:** Del-Mar Provision Company, Inc., Buffalo, New York, 50 pounds of ground beef products recalled
- **November 1, 2007:** General Mills Operations, Wellston, Ohio, 3.3 million pounds of frozen meat pizza recalled
- **November 3, 2007:** Cargill Meat Solutions Corporation, Wyalusing, Pennsylvania, 1,084,383 pounds of ground products recalled
- **November 24, 2007:** American Food Group, LLC, Green Bay, Wisconsin, 95,927 pounds of various coarse and fine ground beef products recalled
- **December 17, 2007:** Snapps Ferry Packing, Afton, Tennessee, 102 pounds of patty and bulk ground beef products recalled
- **December 27, 2007:** Texas American Food Service Corporation, Fort Worth, Texas, 14,800 pounds of ground beef products recalled

beef. Naturally occurring factors may affect the color of cooked beef: the age of the animal; the part of the animal from which the meat was taken; how much air to which the meat has been exposed; whether the meat had been frozen previously; or if seasonings had been added before the meat was cooked.

Although conventional wisdom held that "pink" hamburgers were undercooked and "brown" hamburgers were safe to eat, USDA research subsequent to the rash of outbreaks from *E. coli* O157:H7-tainted hamburgers in the mid-1990s, found that color was unreliable. The USDA studies showed that the color test could give consumers very misleading impressions about the safety of ground beef when it is cooked. The centers of many of the hamburgers tested turned brown before reaching a safe internal temperature of 160°F, which is sufficient to destroy *E. coli* and other pathogens that may be present in the meat. Premature browning is caused by beef that has undergone oxidation, which causes the meat pigment, myoglobin, to turn brown at considerably lower heating temperatures than the researchers expected. A small number of the hamburgers tested turned brown at temperatures as low as 135°F, yet the meat would not be cooked safely at this temperature.

Both freezing and thawing had some influence on the meat's tendency to brown prematurely. Two-thirds of the hamburgers made from previously frozen meat turned brown at lower final cooking temperatures. The amount of total fat, the pH of the meat with added seasonings, and the amount of the meat after shrinkage from cooking, were contributing factors in browning hamburger prematurely.

There was more confusion. Pinkness in the cooked ground beef did not indicate necessarily that the meat was cooked insufficiently. Nearly half of the hamburgers tested, after cooking, retained some pinkness when they were cooked at 160°F, and almost 20 percent of the hamburgers cooked at 175°F showed some pinkness in some areas. A large number of the hamburgers tested received a borderline score that straddled the line between pink or brown. This finding added more ambiguity.

There were more uncertainties. Half of the samples the USDA tested were fresh meat; the other, frozen for a week and then thawed by various techniques. The samples were fried to a range of end-point temperatures and then evaluated for meat color, the pinkness of the juice, and the cooked texture. The researchers admitted that the study had limitations, because there is no uniformity in the judgment of color by food preparers. Also, the study turned up an hitherto unnoted observation. Meat from fresh beef became browner in appearance after it was removed from the grill and allowed to sit for several minutes. In contrast, the hamburgers made from the previously frozen beef, appeared increasingly pink after they were removed from the grill!

The findings suggested that temperature, not color, is the appropriate indicator of doneness in cooked hamburgers. Also, the juice should be clear.

After the USDA learned about the prevalency of premature browning, the agency removed the advice from its informational materials. Instead, it recommended the use of a thermometer. This advice was not greeted enthusiastically by focus groups. Consumers found meat thermometers to be a hassle. Many people in the focus group agreed that if they were made ill after eating hamburgers, they would more likely stop eating them than to start using a thermometer. Also, taking the internal temperature of hamburgers is far from simple. Hamburgers are not homogenous throughout. Their protein, fat, and moisture temperatures may vary.

Hamburger-juice color appears to be a more reliable indicator of cooked hamburger safety. According to Donald Kropf, professor of animal science at Kansas State University, the juice should be *clear*.

With all the various aspects investigated, the experts were silent on one important factor: the shape of the patty. Common sense dictates that the thicker the patty, the greater the chance that the interior may not be cooked adequately. The thinner, flatter patty will cook more thoroughly throughout.

FOOD OUTBREAKS OF *E. COLI* O157:H7 FROM NON-ANIMAL SOURCES

Meat and other foods from animal sources are the main foods in *E. coli* O157:H7 outbreaks. However, with the increased spread of the pathogen, produce is being contaminated more frequently with *E. coli* O157:H7. These are some of the occurrences in recent years. Every outbreak has its own distinctive features.

Outbreaks of *E. coli* O157:H7 from Leafy Vegetables

Some of the outbreaks have occurred with lettuce, mesclun, coleslaw, and spinach. In the outbreaks with lettuce, raw manure-contaminated soil and irrigation water were found in fields adjacent to where the crops were grown.

A small lettuce farm, Fancy Cutt in Hollister, California, grew mesclun greens, such as radicchio, frisée, and arugula. In 1998, its mesclun sickened more than sixty people in Illinois, Connecticut, and New York. Investigators found that several features on the farm could have contributed to the mesclun contamination by *E. coli* O157:H7. Wall openings could have allowed chickens or other animals to track infected feces into the area where the mesclun was processed. Cattle were kept near the processing shed. A nearby well supplied water that could have been contaminated. A broken filter system could have acted as a breeding ground for the bacteria, and the recirculated wash water for the greens might have been contaminated. Handwashing facilities were inadequate for the mesclun handlers. Any one or more of these factors might have been involved.

Cabbages were cut in Kentucky Fried Chicken restaurants to make coleslaw, until eleven people were made ill by *E. coli* O157:H7. The contamination was traced to a field where the cabbages were grown. In addition, the restaurants used improper washing procedures with the cabbages.

Since 1996, nearly two-dozen outbreaks of *E. coli* O157:H7-contaminated fresh leafy vegetables have occurred. Much of this produce is grown on farms in central California. The most recent multistate outbreak with *E. coli* O157:H7 occurred in 2006 with ready-to-eat bagged spinach. Nearly 200 cases of illness were reported to the Centers for Disease Control and Prevention (CDC), and resulted in more than 100 persons being hospitalized, and accounted for at least three deaths.

Investigation of the outbreaks identified environmental risk factors, and the areas that most likely were involved. But the investigators were unable to determine definitely the cause(s) of the contamination. Investigators learned that feral pigs, wandering across a free-range cattle ranch, may have picked up *E. coli* O157:H7 from cattle excrement, and carried it into neighboring spinach fields. Also, irrigation wells used for the crops and surface waterways were exposed to feces from cattle and wildlife.

DNA analysis of the *E. coli* O157:H7 that contaminated the spinach was found to match the DNA of the pathogen that contaminated the spinach processed by Natural Selection Foods of San Juan Bautista, California. As a result, nearly 100 victims of the outbreaks sued Natural Selection Foods.

Fallouts from the Outbreaks

By 2006, the CDC estimated that *E. coli* O157:H7 was causing some 73,000 infections and more than sixty deaths yearly in the United States. These outbreaks, in addition to many others from numerous foodborne pathogens, led to renewed calls for a single independent food safety agency. At present, there is great disparity between the federal food safety resources at the USDA and the Food and Drug Adminstration (FDA). The USDA has about 7,000 people who inspect some 6,000 processing plants daily. The FDA has only some 800 inspectors who can visit a specific processing plant, on average, only *once every five years*. Because of the enormous difference in resources, some members of Congress, the Government Accountability Office (GAO), and numerous public interest groups, repeatedly call for the creation of a single agency to supervise food safety. However, both the USDA and the FDA continue to resist such change.

The bagged spinach outbreaks occurred during the same period of time as numerous recalls were occurring with lettuce, bottled carrot juice, egg salad, ground beef products, and turkey, from a variety of foodborne pathogens. U.S. Representative Rosa L. DeLauro (D-CT) one of the ardent sponsors of legislation to create a single agency for food safety remarked that "the system is broken, and Congress needs to act to protect public health."

A "1960s Health Food" Becomes a Contaminated Food of the Late 1990s

In 1998, a series of *E. coli* O157:H7 outbreaks, as well as *Salmonella* outbreaks, occurred with a food dubbed as the "1960s health food": alfalfa sprouts. The CDC, in tracking outbreaks with contaminated alfalfa from 1995 to 1998, found that the sprouts had resulted in some 1,300 confirmed cases of food poisoning in California, Kansas, Michigan, Missouri, New Mexico, and Virginia. One death was reported. Some who became ill had bloody diarrhea. Some required hospitalization for HUS. One person developed thrombotic thrombocytopenia purpura (described earlier in this chapter). The CDC suggested that there were thousands more unreported cases. These outbreaks followed earlier ones in Japan in 1996, from contaminated radish sprouts. About 6,000 people had been affected by the largest *E. coli* O157:H7 outbreak that Japan had ever experienced.

Contamination with sprouted seeds may occur from contaminated seeds, or during the growing, harvesting, processing, storing, shipping, or sprouting phases. Also, germinating seeds for sprouting are conducted in a moist, humid environment—a favorable breeding ground for bacteria. Also, the sprouts may be rinsed in contaminated water.

In the aftermath of the outbreaks, the FDA issued an advisory that young children, the elderly, and persons with compromised immune systems should avoid eating raw sprouts. The commercial sprouting industry instituted several strategies to improve the safety of the product. To kill *E. coli* O157:H7 and other pathogens that might be present, the sprouts were sanitized. However, the FDA still regarded the product as a potential health risk.

Unpasteurized Fruit Juices and *E. coli* O157:H7

In recent years, there have been recalls of fruit juices due to *E. coli* O157:H7 contamination. Some cases involved orange juice; others, unpasteurized apple juice (cider). Well-publicized outbreaks occurred in 1996, with unpasteurized cider from Odwalla in Dinuba, California, a major nationwide supplier of fresh fruit juices. Nearly seventy people were made ill from *E. coli* O157:H7-contaminated cider. One young girl died. Four children developed kidney failure. The outbreak triggered nine lawsuits, some brought by individual plaintiffs and one as a class action suit against Odwalla. Among the plaintiffs were the parents of a four-year-old girl made severely ill with HUS, and whose kidneys were damaged permanently. Another set of parents brought suit because their two-year-old daughter suffered from colitis, anemia, and renal failure. She was on kidney dialysis during most of her hospitalization. In addition to the lawsuits, Odwalla also faced a federal grand jury probe.

The likely source of the outbreak was attributed to contact of the apples with animal feces prior to cider processing. Typically, this might occur in apple orchards where farm animals or wild animals might graze. Commonly apple "drops" gathered from the ground are used to make cider. Traditionally, cider was not pasteurized, and the Odwalla cider was not pasteurized.

FERMENTATION DESTROYS *E. COLI* O157:H7 IN UNPASTEURIZED CIDER

The acidity of fermented apple cider does not differ significantly from unfermented fresh apple cider. However, the fermentation reduced the number of *E. coli* O157:H7 cells to an undetectable level after three days at 68°F (120°C), according to the findings of Jeffrey Semanchek and David Golden, from the Department of Food Science and Technology at the University of Tennessee in Knoxville. The researchers found that the combined effects of pH, sulfur dioxide, carbon dioxide, and ethanol in the fermented cider was an effective means of destroying the *E. coli* O157:H7 without pasteurizing the cider.

—*Journal of Food Protection*, Dec. 1996

The outcome of this episode was that Odwalla began to pasteurize its cider. For other processors who continued to sell unpasteurized cider, the FDA required a statement on the cider's label to read: "WARNING: This product has not been pasteurized and, therefore, may contain harmful bacteria that can cause serious illness in children, the elderly, and persons with weakened immune systems."

Odwalla settled the lawsuits, and paid $1.25 million as a criminal fine. This sum was shared by STOP (Safe Tables Our Priority), the University of Pennsylvania, and the Joint Institute for Food Safety and Applied Nutrition.

E. COLI O157:H7 AS A WATERBORNE INFECTION

E. coli O157:H7 is a waterborne as well as a foodborne infection. The CDC reported that of all waterborne outbreaks from infectious organisms, *E. coli* O157:H7 causes the most severe illnesses.

E. coli O157:H7 is hardy and can survive for many weeks in municipal water reservoirs, lakes, ponds, and other bodies of water, especially in cold temperatures. Also, the cells of *E. coli* O157:H7 can enter into a viable but nonculturable state and survive long periods of time at room temperature.

In 1991, sewage contamination of a public water supply, containing *E. coli* O157:H7, resulted in a large outbreak in a rural town in Ireland. Some 11,000 people were made ill. Untreated human sewage had leaked from a nearby sewage pipe into one or two town wells.

E. coli O157:H7 has been found to survive for up to a month in tap water. An outbreak of HUS occurred in Saitama, Japan, among young

E. COLI O157:H7 AS A MAJOR PUBLIC HEALTH PROBLEM

"Seldom has a single bacterial strain had such a wide-ranging impact on the regulatory community," wrote Stanley T. Omaye in *Food Technology* (May 2001). Omaye continued, "There is just cause, however, as the disease caused by [*E. coli*] O157:H7 and its relatives can be so devastating. Numerous and rigorous new rules have been imposed on several industries as a direct result of *E. coli* O157:H7. It has changed the way consumers and food service workers view ground meats, sprouts, certain fresh vegetables, and other commodities. The emergence of new STECs [shiga toxin-producing *E. coli*] may compound an already vexing problem for regulators and consumers. Steps taken now to prepare for the emergence of new STECs may save lives later."

children in a kindergarten. They drank unchlorinated water from the school well. Seven children developed neurological symptoms, including generalized seizures, impaired consciousness, urinary incontinence, gaze nystagmus (involuntary eye movements), phrenic nerve palsy, action tremors, and vertigo. Two of the children died.

Swimming in contaminated water has been implicated in several waterborne *E. coli* O157:H7 outbreaks in the United States. Infections usually occur when swimmers swallow some of the water.

CHAPTER 5

Campylobacter: An Infection of Public Health Significance

Harold, the first time on his own, prepared his meal. After cutting pieces of raw chicken, he washed the cutting board and knife but did not scour them. He rinsed his hands under running tap water. Then he cut tomatoes, peppers, and cucumbers for a salad with the same knife and cutting board. He cooked the chicken hastily, wanting to view the football game on television. As he watched and ate, he thought that the chicken was slightly undercooked, but he did not want to interrupt viewing the game by returning to the kitchen to cook the chicken to doneness, so he continued to eat it. After two days, Harold developed gastrointestinal upset for a few days. Then, it subsided. However, later he began to experience numbness, pain, progressive weakness, and ultimately, paralysis.

*C*ampylobacter (in Greek, "campyo" means curved, and "bacter" means rod) are slender, spiral, curved rods, with a characteristic corkscrew-like appearance viewed microscopically. The bacterium has darting mobility by means of a single flagellate at one, or at both ends.

Campylobacter has been recognized as an infective bacterium for more than a century. Originally, *Campylobacter* was classified with the genus *Vibrio* as *Vibrio fetus* (see Chapter 11). In 1886, in Germany, pediatrician and bacteriologist Theodor Escherich—for whom *Escherichia* was named—observed microscopically the organisms in the stool samples of infants with diarrhea. However, the human infection was regarded as a rare, and perhaps opportunistic pathogen. In 1913, two investigators, John McFadyean and Stewart Stockman, identified *Campylobacter,* which at the time was known as "related *Vibrio,*" in the fetal tissues of aborted sheep. In 1957, the pathogen was classified as a subspecies of *Vibrio fetus.*

In that year, E. O. King isolated related vibrios from blood samples of diarrheal children. The finding was still regarded as rare, and perhaps opportunistic.

In 1972, clinical microbiologists in Belgium were the first to isolate *Campylobacter* from stool samples of diarrheal patients. By then, a laboratory technique had been developed for American veterinarians to make diagnoses of *Campylobacter* from stool specimens of animals. The technique was applied to human stool specimens. It was discovered that *Campylobacter* was neither rare nor opportunistic, but rather was widespread and a major cause of human diarrheal illness.

CAMPYLOBACTER STRAINS

Formerly, it was thought that only a few *Campylobacter* strains were important to investigate, monitor, and control. Later, scientists and health officials worldwide began to recognize that other less-known strains also warranted attention. Although these strains have attracted attention only recently, they may not have emerged recently. Rather, they may have been in existence for a long time.

The *Campylobacter* strains most studied are those identified as causes of human diseases: *C. jejuni, C. coli, C. fetus* subspecies (ssp.) *fetus,* and *C. fetus* ssp. *coli.* Two of these strains will be discussed later in the chapter, in terms of the health consequences from their infections. *C. pylori,* originally regarded as a *Campylobacter* strain, later was reclassified in the genus *Helicobacter,* as *Helicobacter pylori* (see Chapter 20).

SOURCES OF *CAMPYLOBACTER* INFECTIONS

The intestinal tracts of many creatures serve as vast reservoirs for *Campylobacter* bacteria, and indirectly serve as sources of infections in humans. The prime source is poultry, both farm-raised chickens, turkeys, and ducks, as well as all varieties of wild fowl. Also, the pathogen is present in the intestinal tracts of farm animals such as cattle, sheep, swine, and goats, as well as in companion animals such as dogs, cats, rodents, and monkeys. The foods most frequently contaminated are poultry, raw milk, and untreated water.

Animals that carry *Campylobacter* in their intestines may be healthy. The problem of human infection results from food contaminated by the feces shed by *Campylobacter*-containing animals.

TRANSMISSION FROM PERSON TO PERSON

Campylobacter can be transmitted person to person. Anyone who has direct contact with infected animals, especially poultry, can become infected, and in turn, infect others. Food handlers, poultry raisers, food preparers, slaughterhouse workers, and veterinarians are all at risk. Person-to-person contact can be from an infected infant to siblings and caregivers. At day-care centers, infection can be passed from one child to another. Also, *Campylobacter* can be transmitted by homosexual contacts.

Animals may carry *Campylobacter* in their fur or pelt after shedding the pathogen in their stools. Young children who fail to wash their hands after petting dogs or cats, or animals at petting zoos, can become infected with *Campylobacter,* and also can infect others.

PERSONS AT HIGH RISK FOR CAMPYLOBACTERIOSIS

Anyone can become infected with *Campylobacter* bacteria. Those at high risk are persons with underdeveloped immune systems such as newborn infants, and those with weakened immune systems such as elderly people. Other groups at high risk include cancer patients on immunosuppressive therapy, or persons with underlying illness. For example, people with AIDS are nearly forty times more at risk for *Campylobacter* infection than are members of the general population.

SYMPTOMS OF CAMPYLOBACTERIOSIS

To many people, the symptoms of campylobacteriosis seem like "the flu." The infection begins with some common symptoms of foodborne illness, including headache, malaise, stomach cramps, muscle aches, and fever, up to twenty-four hours before the beginning of intestinal symptoms. Then, the infection shows symptoms of classical gastroenteritis: nausea, vomiting, abdominal pain, and copious watery diarrhea. Frequently, blood is in the stools. Fever can go as high as 104°F.

The illness usually lasts less than a week, but the stools keep shedding the pathogen for several weeks. Not all cases of *Campylobacter* require treatment, which usually is an antibiotic. As will be discussed shortly, the number of pathogens resistant to standard "first-line" antibiotics used for diarrheal disease has become a major problem. The medical community advises that antibiotics be restricted for use only with the most severe cases of campylobacteriosis.

SOME HEALTH CONSEQUENCES OF CAMPYLOBACTERIOSIS

Persons who recover from campylobacteriosis without complications are fortunate. For some, the consequences can be severe and with various outcomes. Specific strains of *Campylobacter* can lead to certain disorders. These will be discussed shortly. But for campylobacteriosis, in general, some people may experience these consequences:

* Convulsions (in children)

* Pneumonia

* Severe colitis with tenesmus (painful and ineffectual straining for stool movements or urination)

* Toxic megacolon (enlargement of the colon due to chronic constipation)

* Urinary tract infections

* Various organ inflammations, including arthritis, endocarditis (heart), cholecystitis (gall bladder), meningitis (brain), pancreatitis (pancreas), and inflammation of the lymph nodes

Occasionally, *Campylobacter* bacteria get into the bloodstream, and infect other parts of the body several weeks after the original infection subsides. This consequence is more common in persons with a specific gene known as HLA-B27 than those without it.

Less frequently, infections occur outside the intestinal tract. These conditions include bacteremia (bacteria in the blood), septic arthritis, and septic abortion.

SOURCES OF *CAMPYLOBACTER* CONTAMINATION

Campylobacter Contamination in Poultry

With poultry, *Campylobacter* is passed down from one generation to the next. If the mother hen has *Campylobacter* bacteria in its intestines, the pathogen gets into the membrane. The baby chicks are exposed to *Campylobacter* when they push through the membrane just inside the eggshell.

Baby chicks share feed and water with each other. Also, baby chicks eat droppings from each other. If some chicks are contaminated with *Campylobacter,* the pathogen is spread to other chicks.

Throughout the 1990s, very high rates of *C. jejuni*-contaminated raw poultry—sometimes up to 100 percent of chickens or turkeys—were found at the retail level. Due to some newly instituted practices, more recent levels of contaminated poultry has dropped somewhat, but still, much poultry is contaminated.

Some people buy organic chickens in the belief that such birds are likely to be less contaminated than their counterparts. Organic chickens may have better quality, but testings in the United States found no difference in safety. In 2001, a team in Denmark actually found *higher* levels of *Campylobacter* bacteria on organic broiler chickens than on intensively reared ones. It was thought that free-range poultry are apt to contaminate feed and/or water with their feces.

HARMLESS BACTERIA COMBAT *CAMPYLOBACTER*

Dosing newly hatched chicks with harmless bacteria may lead to poultry that is uncontaminated by two major food-poisoning organisms, *Campylobacter* and *Salmonella*.

Laboratory studies conducted by the USDA's Agricultural Research Service found that the number of these two pathogens present in the chicks' intestines was reduced up to a hundredfold or more. First, an aerosol spray of the harmless bacteria was applied as the chicks were hatching. Then, a second treatment was added to their first drinking water.

The harmless bacteria were extracted from the intestines of adult chickens, and prepared in an oxygen-free environment. Growth of the culture in the absence of oxygen encouraged proliferation of these protective bacteria, which colonized in the chicks' intestines and crowded out the disease-causing foodborne pathogens.

—USDA's *Quarterly Report of Selected Research Projects*, Jan–Mar 1994

The best safeguard for poultry consumers is to *assume* that raw chickens and turkeys are contaminated with *Campylobacter,* but to recognize that the pathogen is killed readily by cooking the poultry thoroughly. Also, food preparers need to avoid cross-contamination of raw poultry with other foods and practice thorough handwashing after handling raw animal food.

Even cooked poultry is not always safe, if it is cooked inadequately. There have been cases of *Campylobacter*-contaminated poultry in barbecued chicken. Although the exterior of the birds was blackened, the interior of the birds was undercooked. Also, in 1992, an outbreak in the metropolitan Los Angeles area of *Campylobacter* infection was traced to ready-to-eat processed turkey.

Antibiotics and Poultry Infections

In 1991, the Farm Animal Concerns Trust (FACT) called for "standards for pathogen-free farming . . . to be created and enforced" to control *Campylobacter* in raw poultry. FACT, which described itself as a group "opposed to intensive livestock and poultry husbandry methods that reduce food safety and economic opportunities for family farms," reported that food safety "will never be optimal while crowding and unsanitary farming remain unregulated."

The use of antibiotics with livestock was instituted in an attempt to achieve pathogen-free farming by means of medication, and at the same time, permit the continuation of intensive animal rearing.

SPICES INHIBIT *CAMPYLOBACTER*

Spices have been shown to have an inhibitory effect on *Campylobacter* and other foodborne pathogens. Oregano, sage, and ground clove were chosen to be tested for their effect on growth of *Campylobacter fetus* ssp. *jejuni*. These spices commonly are used in preparing meats and meat dishes which have been involved in outbreaks of this illness. Kurt E. Deibel and George J. Banwart in the Department of Microbiology at Ohio State University tested the spices at concentrations between 0.1 and 1.0 percent, over a sixteen-hour incubation period. The tests showed that at a concentration of 0.5 percent of oregano or sage, cell death occurred in the pathogen. At a concentration of 0.5 or 1.0 percent of ground clove, there was neither decrease nor increase of *C. fetus* ssp. *jejuni* cells. The study suggested that appropriate concentrations of specific spices may reduce or kill *C. fetus* ssp. *jejuni*.
　　　　—Deibel and Banwart, Institute of Food Technologists, June 23, 1982

In 1995, the Food and Drug Administration (FDA) approved the use of fluoroquinolones, a group of antibiotics, with food animals. By 1999, the

Minnesota Department of Health found an increase in the number of *Campylobacter* infections in humans resistant to antibiotics. Its study concluded that antibiotic use in poultry was contributing to antibiotic resistance in people. The Centers for Disease Control and Prevention (CDC) found an increased resistance to fluoroquinolones correlated with the increased use of these antibiotics in poultry. The CDC also found that people with fluoroquinolone-resistant *Campylobacter* infections were more likely to suffer *severe infections* accompanied by bloody diarrhea and require hospitalizations, than people with nonresistant *Campylobacter* infections.

In 2000, the FDA announced that it proposed to withdraw its previous approval for two antibiotics from the fluoroquinolone group for use with livestock. These antibiotics, also used for human health, had become ineffective. This proposal was unprecedented. It was the first time that the agency proposed withdrawing approval of an antibiotic used by the livestock industry. Also, it was the first time that the FDA had proposed banning any antibiotic due to bacterial resistance.

According to an FDA statement, the agency's decision was based on several factors. Of prime importance was that using fluoroquinolones in poultry causes the development of fluoroquinolone-resistant pathogens in poultry. *Campylobacter* bacteria in poultry were harming consumers who might eat undercooked poultry. Another factor was the information contained in a study that had been released in 2000, Risk Assessment on the Human Health Impact of Fluoroquinolone-Resistant *Campylobacter* Associated with the Consumption of Chicken. The document was a joint effort by the CDC, the U.S. Department of Agriculture (USDA), the National Chicken Council, the U.S. Census Bureau, and the University of Pennsylvania Medical Center. The group concluded that annually some 11,500 people infected with *Campylobacter* would have a fluoroquinolone-resistant illness resulting from the antibiotic's use in poultry. Likely, some of these patients, especially young children and the elderly, would have prolonged illnesses and complications that would be life threatening.

Because treating individual infected chicken or turkeys with antibiotics was too expensive, fluoroquinolones were added to the drinking water of the entire flock. According to the FDA's risk assessment about 24 percent of the poultry being processed were contaminated with fluoroquinolone-resistant bacteria.

The fluoroquinolones, approved for use with poultry and cattle in

1995, as mentioned earlier, by 2000 had been in use for five years. By then, the incidence of fluoroquinolone-resistant bacterial infections in humans had risen dramatically. Polymerase chain reaction techniques had allowed epidemiologists at the CDC to trace specific subtypes of *Campylobacter* from chickens to an infected hospital patient. From the evidence that the CDC gathered, the agency had been urging the FDA for several years to ban fluoroquinolone use in poultry.

After the FDA's proposal to withdraw its previous approval for use of fluoroquinolones with livestock, there were protests from the affected interests. For several years, there were heated debates, countless investigations, studies, risk assessments, conferences, reports, and so on. In 2005, the FDA banned an antibiotic in the fluoroquinolone group for use with poultry. The banned antibiotic (Baytril) is chemically similar to another antibiotic (Cipro), which is prescribed commonly to treat foodborne illness in people. The FDA reported that use of Baytril in poultry reduced the effectiveness of Cipro in treating *Campylobacter* infection in humans.

Prior to the ban, Baytril had been given to poultry for therapeutic purposes. When a respiratory infection was found in a few birds, the antibiotic had been administered to the entire flock.

The FDA's ban was hailed by some groups. For example, Margaret Mellon, director of the Food and Environment Program of the Union of Concerned Scientists, regarded the decision as "precedent setting" and the first step "to cancel some of the nontherapeutic uses of human-use antibiotics in agriculture."

David Wallinga, director of the Antibiotic Resistance Project at the Institute for Agriculture and Trade Policy, reported that "Cipro is an essential antibiotic and we cannot allow its effectiveness to be compromised by squandering it on poultry."

The FDA's ban was greeted as bad news by affected industries. A statement issued by the Animal Health Institute, representing the manufacturers of animal health products, reported that "the loss of these products leaves poultry producers without an important tool to treat sick poultry, and it will reduce animal health and welfare while increasing animal death and suffering."

Campylobacter Contamination in Dairy Products

Raw milk is another major vehicle of *Campylobacter* contamination. Numerous outbreaks have been reported. Some cases have involved

ARE RAW MILK CHEESES SAFE?

Government regulations in the United States, United Kingdom, and elsewhere now require that all milk used to produce cheeses be pasteurized, due to numerous outbreaks associated with cheeses made from unpasteurized milk. Verner Wheelock, a spokesperson for the Specialty Cheesemakers Association, questioned the justification for these draconian measures. Wheelock contended that the outbreaks resulted from *post-production* contamination, and that pasteurization, in itself, was no guarantee of safety. Wheelock argued that lactic acid, present in raw milk, is effective in combating pathogenic bacteria. Many pathogens are unable to survive the production process with semi- and full-ripened cheeses. Wheelock cited a Swiss study demonstrating that *C. jejuni* as well as *Staphylococcus aureus*, *Escherichia coli*, *Listeria monocytogenes*, and *Salmonella* Typhimurium, injected into raw milk at the beginning of semi- and full-ripened cheese production, had all but disappeared two days after cheese manufacture. Another piece of persuasive evidence, according to Wheelock, was that many raw milk cheeses are produced and eaten in France, yet the number of food poisoning cases from such products is exceedingly low.

school tours to visit dairies, where the children have been given samples of raw milk to drink. A 1984 outbreak in California involved a dairy that was producing *certified* raw milk, which holds to a high standard. Other cases of *Campylobacter*-contaminated milk involved improper pasteurization due to faulty equipment.

One unusual source of *Campylobacter*-contaminated milk was reported in 1990. In South Wales, United Kingdom, bottled milk was delivered to the doorsteps of homes. There was evidence of tampering with the foil bottle caps, and people were being made ill from the milk. Cameras were set up, and photographs revealed that magpies and jackdaws (carrion crows) were pecking through the bottle caps to sip the milk. The birds were contaminating the milk with *Campylobacter.*

Campylobacter Contamination in Water

Water is another important source of *Campylobacter* infections. The first recorded waterborne outbreak from *Campylobacter* in the United States was in 1978, in Bennington, Vermont, and involved drinking water. Some 2,000 to 3,000 residents out of its total population of some 10,000 were sickened by *C. fetus*. The municipal water system was found to be contaminated by water from unfiltered sources.

Another large *Campylobacter*-associated waterborne outbreak occurred in 1995 in the United Kingdom. A food processor inadvertently discharged wastewater, which was pumped into a public water supply. The incident resulted in the largest outbreak of waterborne gastroenteritis ever reported in the United Kingdom.

Other waterborne *Campylobacter* outbreaks have occurred in the United States at various sites and under different conditions. In one case, at a county fair, vendors used unchlorinated water from a shallow well to make beverages and ice. In another instance, water from a duck pond, visited by wild birds, leaked into nearby oyster beds, and contaminated raw oysters with *C. jejuni*. In another outbreak, shellfish beds were contaminated with *Campylobacter* by runoff from sewage diverted from a failed septic system. The result was shellfish-related infections in humans who ate the shellfish.

In Northern Ireland, nearly half of all raw mussels, cockles, and scallops tested were found to be contaminated with strains of *Campylobacter.*

Unlike tap water, bottled mineral water may not be treated. Numbers of different organisms found in mineral water can survive for considerable lengths of time, especially in uncarbonated water, supplied in plastic bottles, or bottled by hand. Cases of campylobacteriosis, as well as cholera, typhoid fever, and traveler's diarrhea, have been traced to such products.

A waterborne outbreak of campylobacteriosis occurred from colonic irrigation at a chiropractic clinic, and resulted in the illness of thirty-six people and six deaths. Investigators found that the colonic irrigation machine was contaminated with *Campylobacter,* as well as with *Shigella* and *Salmonella,* and resulted in bacterial infection. The contaminated colonic irrigation machine was seized by the police. Even after standard cleaning, water samples taken from such devices have shown contamination from high levels of pathogens.

Campylobacter Contamination in Other Foods

As noted, poultry, milk, and water are the main *Campylobacter*-contaminated items. Others occur less frequently. There have been a few outbreaks with beef, raw calf's liver (consumed in "nutritional therapy"), and eggs. On rare occasions, vegetables have been implicated. The cases were likely from cross-contamination, as with a restaurant episode when lettuce was contaminated by its contact with raw chicken. Occasionally, fruits are implicated. Supermarkets offer sliced or cubed watermelon, papaya, or other fruits. Some of these ready-to-eat convenience products have been found to be contaminated with *Campylobacter*. The addition of lemon juice to cut fruit can reduce, but does not eliminate, all live *Campylobacter* bacteria that may be present.

An unusual *Campylobacter* outbreak occurred in 1995 in a Louisiana restaurant. *Campylobacter* survived for days in refrigerated garlic butter, intended for use on French bread. The heat used to melt the garlic butter was insufficient to kill the *C. jejuni* present. The pathogen made thirty patrons ill, four of which required hospitalization.

SOME CONSEQUENCES OF *C. JEJUNI* INFECTIONS

C. jejuni has certain characteristics. A small number of its cells can lead to infection. In experiments, as few as 500 cells caused infection in healthy volunteers; probably a smaller number of cells can cause infection in immunocompromised individuals.

C. jejuni infection is more common in summertime than during other seasons. The incidence of infection increases in times of floods, droughts, climate change, and rising sea levels. According to the CDC, *C. jejuni* infections are increasing worldwide. It is an infection of major public health concern, and one that has become increasingly resistant to antibiotic treatment.

C. jejuni is neither aerobic nor anerobic. It requires from 2 to 15 percent oxygen, and from 3 to 5 percent carbon dioxide to survive.

Compared to other foodborne pathogens, *C. jejuni* is fragile. It is killed readily by heat in thorough cooking of food, and by treatment of municipal drinking water. Unlike other foodborne causes of gastroenteritis, such as *Salmonella*, *Escherichia*, or *Staphylococcus*, *C. jejuni* does not multiply in food.

The acute infection inflicted by *C. jejuni* is gastroenteritis. It is difficult to distinguish *C. jejuni*'s role in this condition from that of other foodborne pathogens which also inflict gastroenteritis.

C. jejuni is the leading cause of bacterial gastroenteritis reported in humans in the United States. *C. coli*, less common and less severe, causes illness in humans, but unlike *C. jejuni*, *C. coli* also can infect swine. Both *C. jejuni* and *C. coli* are difficult to differentiate. They are similar genetically, and exchange DNA with each other. Clinical manifestations between the two strains are quite similar.

Because *C. jejuni* induces gasteroenteritis, there can be other gastrointestinal consequences. Some are infrequent, such as *C. jejuni* found in the bile of patients who undergo surgical therapy for cystitis. Occasionally, *C. jejuni* causes urinary tract infections. The bacteria survive only briefly. Now and then, *C. jejuni* enteritis leads to acute pancreatitis. In cases of cholecystitis (inflammation of the gall bladder), *C. jejuni* bacteria are found in the bile ducts of some patients. *C. jejuni* can cause spontaneous bacterial peritonitis (inflammation of the peritoneum, the membrane that lines the abdominal and pelvic cavities) in patients with cirrhosis (inflammation of the liver) due to alcoholism. Also, *C. jejuni* infection can cause peritonitis in patients who are ambulatory (not bedridden) and undergo peritoneal dialysis.

C. jejuni infections can have numerous consequences for some people. Many of the body's organs, tissues, or systems may be involved.

C. jejuni infections can have dermatologic effects. Erysipelas is a contagious disease of the skin and subcutaneous tissues that results from infection. In some patients with *C. jejuni*, an erysipelas-like cellulitis has been reported in patients with hypogammaglobulinemia (an abnormally low level of serum globulin due to infection), and in patients with recurrent *C. jejuni* bacteremia (presence of bacteria in the blood). Occasionally, patients with *C. jejuni* enteritis develop erythema nodosum (an acute inflammatory skin disease, marked by red nodules on the shins, due to oozing of blood and serum).

C. jejuni infections can lead to rheumatic effects. There may be a ten-day interval between *C. jejuni* enteritis and the development of arthritic conditions. About 3 percent of *C. jejuni* infections result in reactive arthritis, usually affecting the knees, ankles, and wrists. In rare instances, *C. jejuni* infections lead to septic arthritis, osteomyelitis, and infections in prosthetic joints in persons who already are ill.

C. jejuni infections can lead to septic abortions and miscarriages in women. *C. jejuni* bacteria have been identified in fetuses and in maternal blood. In cases of septic abortions, *C. jejuni* infections can lead to other inflammatory illnesses, including myocarditis and pneumonia. Fatalities are rare.

C. jejuni infections can lead to neurological disorders. The bacteria can induce acute motor axonal polyneuropathy. (Axons are long, thin extensions of nerve cells. They carry the nerve impulses. Polyneuropathy is a disorder resulting from numerous functional and/or pathological changes occurring in the peripheral nervous system.) Acute motor axonal polyneuropathy is a paralytic disorder. However, the neurological disorder most often associated with *C. jejuni* infection is Guillain-Barré syndrome (GBS).

In 1982, *C. jejuni* was recognized as a triggering agent in many GBS cases. By then, the mounting evidence was overwhelming. It was found that the risk of developing GBS after being infected by *C. jejuni* was a hundred times higher than in the non-infected population.

C. JEJUNI AND GUILLAIN-BARRÉ SYNDROME

Guillain-Barré (pronounced GHEE-yan-BAH-ray) syndrome (GBS) is a disorder in which the body's immune system attacks parts of the peripheral nervous system. At first, there are varying degrees of weakness or tingling sensations in the legs, frequently spreading to the arms and upper part of the body. These symptoms may increase in intensity until the muscles fail to function and paralysis sets in. Sometimes, the condition is called acute flaccid paralysis because the muscles become floppy. In such cases, the disorder is a life-threatening medical emergency with impaired breathing, and an abnormal blood pressure, and heart rate. The individual may be placed in a respirator, and monitored closely for blood pressure and heart beat, blood clots, and infections. Fortunately, most patients recover from such medical emergencies, but they may continue to experience weakness to some degree. However, some cases result in fatality.

GBS can affect anyone, at any age, and both sexes are equally prone to this disorder. The syndrome can develop over the course of hours or days, or up to three or four weeks. Most people reach the stage of greatest weakness within the first two weeks after the symptoms appear. By the third week of the illness, most patients are at their weakest. Then the body's immune system begins to attack the body itself. Usually the cells of the immune system attack only foreign materials and invading organisms. However, in GBS, the immune system begins to destroy the myelin sheath

What is the mechanism that causes *C. jejuni* to cause initial nerve damage and an inability to function in individuals with GBS? The myelin sheath, described in the inset below, is composed of various molecules. One of the major components is polysacchararides, comprising a string of different types of sugar molecules. The *C. jejuni* bacterium has a similar string of sugar molecules on its outer coat. Thus, when an individual is infected with *C. jejuni*, the body regards the bacterium as foreign and begins to generate an immune response to the invader. Unfortunately, these same antibodies that are made to bind to the sugars on the outer coat of the bacterium also bind to the sugars on the myelin. This process is known as molecular mimicry. (To find out more about molecular mimicry, see the inset on page 11.)

that surrounds the axons of many peripheral nerves, or even attacks the axons themselves. The function of the myelin sheath is to help protect the axons so that they can transmit nerve signals, even over long distance.

In GBS and in other diseases in which the myelin sheath is injured, the nerves are unable to transmit signals efficiently. This accounts for the muscles losing their ability to receive and respond to the brain's messages that need to be carried through the nerve network. Also, with inefficient signaling, the brain receives fewer sensory signals from the rest of the body, and results in the body's inability to sense heat, pain, and other sensations. Alternatively, the brain may receive inappropriate signals that result in a feeling of tingling, "crawling skin," or painful sensations. Because the signals to and from the arms and legs must travel the longest distance, they are most vulnerable to malfunctions.

It was observed that the disorder can strike people shortly after they have had symptoms of a respiratory or gastrointestinal infection. Occasionally, surgery or vaccination triggers the syndrome. All these signs point to viral or bacterial infections.

If GBS is preceded by a viral infection, it is thought that the virus has changed the nature of cells in the nervous system so that the immune system treats them as foreign cells. Also, it is possible that the virus makes the immune system itself less discriminating about which cells it recognizes as its own, and allows some of the immune cells, such as certain types of lymphocytes, to attack the myelin.

After antibodies have bound to the myelin coating, a cascade of events begins. New immune cells arrive and they begin to attack the myelin. This interferes with proper nerve functioning. As a result, this interference triggers the beginning of clinical signs of GBS.

In some cases, the infected individual may have some antibodies present from a previous exposure to *C. jejuni*, but at a level too low to have caused an infection at the time. However, following the second infection, the exposure to *C. jejuni* acts as a booster to the immune response, and leads to a rapid development of the syndrome as the antibody levels rise rapidly to a point at which they can bind to the myelin and begin to interfere with nerve function. This finding is important, in view of attempts to make vaccines against *C. jejuni*. It should be apparent that any vaccine that would lead to antibody production would *increase* the likelihood of triggering GBS following *C. jejuni* infection.

In 1995, the USDA's Economic Research Service estimated the annual cost in the United States from *Campylobacter*-caused GBS. At the time, the cost ran as high as $1.8 billion, not including the cost of lost productivity. With steeply increased medical costs since 1995, no doubt current figures are far higher. It is obvious that the foodborne and waterborne sources of *Campylobacter* contamination need to be addressed. Changes in agricultural practices, food handling, and water purification are needed for *Campylobacter* control.

SOME CONSEQUENCES OF *C. FETUS* INFECTIONS

In 1913, *C. fetus* was recognized as an animal infection that could cause abortions. In 1919, *C. fetus* was identified with abortions in cows; in 1947, abortions in cattle; and in 1967, abortions in sheep. Relatively late, in 1984, *C. fetus* finally became recognized as an infection that could cause human abortions, premature labor, and septicemia (blood poisoning) in the newborn human. Also, *C. fetus* was identified in the vaginas of infected pregnant women, and in their stools two days after they gave birth.

C. fetus rarely causes diarrheal illness, but it can produce systemic illnesses such as bacteremia and sepsis in immunocompromised persons. Most commonly, *C. fetus* is identified in the bloodstream of infected humans. *C. fetus* induces fever. The infection can lead to grave health disorders, such as thrombophlebitis (inflammation of veins and associated with blood clots); endocarditis (inflammation of the lining of the heart and the connective tissue bed on which the heart rests); aneurysm (a sac formed by local dilation of an artery or vein); septic arthritis; osteo-myelitis (inflammation of bone); meningitis (inflammation of the brain); and abscesses. Bacteremia, although an infrequent consequence, is more likely to be a consequence of *C. fetus* than *C. jejuni*.

C. fetus ssp. *fetus* can infect vascular aneurysms, especially the vascular endothelial surfaces. This strain lacks the ability to produce endotoxins or cytotoxins. It does not display the invasiveness shown by other enteric pathogens (examples, *Vibrio cholerae* or *Shigella sonnei*).

Persons who are especially vulnerable to *C. fetus* ssp. *fetus* are the elderly, those who already are ill from other causes, immune-suppressed patients, and individuals recuperating from open-heart surgery.

ESTIMATING *CAMPYLOBACTER* INFECTIONS

Estimates about *Campylobacter* rates of infection vary from year to year, and from different groups making the estimates. The lack of preciseness is reflected by one estimate, made in 1997, by the USDA's Agricultural Research Service of 2 to 8 million cases of campylobacteriosis—quite a wide range. The CDC's estimates are based on *reported* cases. The agency admits that for every reported case, many more are unreported. Thus, the CDC estimates may be significantly below actual numbers.

Collecting estimates from various sources (CDC, FDA, USDA, and the Institute of Food Technology), there appears to be from 2 to 2.5 million cases of *Campylobacter* infections each year in the United States. These numbers have held steady through the 1990s and 2000s, up to the present.

The estimates for the numbers of deaths inflicted by *Campylobacter* range widely, from 100 to 500 deaths yearly. Estimates for hospitalizations are made less frequently. They are about 10,000 yearly.

Regardless of the lack of precision in these figures, they do give an overall impression. *Campylobacter* is an infection of public health significance.

CHAPTER 6

Shigella: Person-to-Person Bacterial Transmission

Lydia, aged eighty-two, needed some assistance. She moved into the home of her son, Phil, and his wife, Ellie. Lydia was happy to spend more time with her three-year-old grandchild, Phoebe. The arrangement worked well, and permitted Ellie to return to the workplace. She was secure in the knowledge that her daughter was well cared for by Lydia.

After a few weeks, Lydia had an unfortunate fall. She required temporary hospitalization to receive physical therapy and other treatment that would be difficult in a home setting.

Ellie and Phil had to make a difficult decision. Either Ellie could quit her job and care for Phoebe at home, or continue to work and place Phoebe in a day-care center. Money was short, especially because Lydia's health insurance and Medicare failed to cover much of the costly medical bills.

Reluctantly, Ellie and Phil decided to enter Phoebe in a day-care center. They chose one that was affordable and close enough to Ellie's workplace so that she could deliver and pick up her daughter before and after work.

Phoebe enjoyed playing with other children at the center, and eating snacks and lunch with them. In Phoebe's third week at the center she complained to Ellie that her stomach hurt. At home, Phoebe began to throw up. She had some fever. Then, she had diarrhea.

Ellie decided to stay home and nurse Phoebe. She notified her workplace and the day-care center. The director of the center thanked Ellie for keeping Phoebe home. She related that one working mother had deposited her child and left hastily. It was obvious that the toddler was ill. The director strongly urged Ellie not to have Phoebe return until she was well. Ellie gave her assurance.

Phoebe recovered in a week. During that time, Ellie resisted visiting Lydia, not wishing to infect Lydia with whatever Phoebe had picked up. However, Phil continued to visit his mother regularly.

After Phoebe was fully recovered, Phil developed stomach cramps, headache, and fever, followed by vomiting and diarrhea. He stayed home for a week, and kept a distance from Phoebe. He did not visit his mother.

Ellie, who had planned to return to work, stayed home to care for Phil. She decided to keep Phoebe home as long as possible, to save the cost of the day-care center. Ellie's days were full, attempting to care for Phil, and keeping Phoebe occupied and away from Phil. Soon, Ellie was not feeling well. She had symptoms similar to those experienced by Phoebe and Phil. By now, Phil felt well enough to return to work, and he arranged to have Phoebe return to the day-care center. Although it was out of his way, he could drive Phoebe to and from the center. Meanwhile, Ellie was home alone, coping with her illness. After a week, Ellie felt well enough to return to work. By then, Ellie and Phil's finances were stressed.

Meanwhile, Lydia developed stomach cramps, vomiting, and diarrhea. The hospital staff immediately isolated her. However, Lillian, an eighty-nine-year old patient who had shared the room with Lydia, also became ill, with symptoms similar to Lydia's. Lillian had some chronic health problems before she entered the hospital. Now, she became gravely ill. Antibiotic treatment was ineffective. She weakened, and within several days, Lillian died.

The infection had been passed person to person. It began with a diapered toddler at the child day-care center, passed along to other children and healthy adults, and on to a frail, elderly woman.

*S*higellae are aerobic, rod-shaped bacteria that infect humans, and produce shigellosis. Some strains produce shiga toxins and induce dysentery. The shiga toxins were mentioned previously in connection with *E. coli* O157:H7 in Chapter 4. The shiga toxins are named after a Japanese bacteriologist, Kiyoshi Shiga (1870–1957).

Traditionally, shigellosis has been associated with areas of poor sanitation and poor nutrition. Often, it affects infants and young children in such settings. However, shigellosis has become a public health problem in affluent areas, too, and results from food and water contamination by infected persons. Shigellosis is highly infective, and is transmitted from person to person by the fecal-oral route. In turn, infected individuals transmit the infection via food and water. The infection can spread to community outbreaks of shigellosis. In regions where shigellosis is endemic, such as in Central American countries, the infection can be spread even from one village to another.

SHIGELLA STRAINS

Four strains of *Shigella* account for most food- and waterborne outbreaks of shigellosis. *S. sonnei* and *S. flexneri* are the most common. *S. sonnei* accounts for about 75 percent of the outbreaks, especially in cases at child day-care centers. Outbreaks with *S. flexneri* have declined somewhat. Neither *S. sonnei* nor *S. flexneri* normally infect species other than humans. Less common strains are *S. boydii* and *S. dysenteriae*. Other strains exist, but they are rare. *Shigella* strains have become resistant to first-line antibiotic treatment.

HOW *SHIGELLAE* INFECT HUMANS

The *Shigella* bacteria break through the barrier of the gut and colonize within the intestinal walls, or slip through those walls and reach other tissues. Once inside a host cell, the *Shigellae* enter between cell transport systems. They harness actin (a key mobility molecule) to propel themselves. The *Shigellae* move smoothly within the intestinal cells, pushed by their acquired action tails. Each *Shigella* hurls itself against the cell's membrane, strongly enough to distort the membrane and indent an adjacent cell. At the area of distortion, the *Shigellae* make contact with membrane junctures that form part of a cell-to-cell transport network. The bacteria use cadherin, a molecule that bridges these junctures, and the *Shigellae* move from cell to cell. As described by one researcher, the action is like people having a party that spreads from one train car to the next through the connecting doors of the train.

Shigellae can spread without leaving the interior of the cells. This feature allows *Shigellae* to evade the immune system, and increases the pathogen's virulence. The gastrointestinal illness is induced when *Shigellae* invade the cells that line the intestinal tract.

SHIGELLOSIS IN THE UNITED STATES

In 1965, the Centers for Disease Control and Prevention (CDC) began a national surveillance program for *Shigella*. By the mid-1980s, some 300,000 to 450,000 cases were being reported annually. By the late 1980s, the number of reported outbreaks increased in all regions of the country, especially in places of large populations with low incomes; in minority groups; and among young children and young women of childbearing age. There was an increase in community-wide outbreaks. The number of cases doubled from 1986 to 1988, with an infection rate of 5.4 persons per 100,000 being infected in 1986, to 10.1 persons per 100,000 in 1988. The number of people infected in 1988 was the largest number since the CDC began its national surveillance program. Also, the reported numbers were only those that were laboratory-confirmed cases, and did not include many more people who were infected but not brought to medical attention. Public health workers suggest that actual numbers may be two to three times higher.

FACTORS IN THE RISE OF SHIGELLOSIS

The rise in the number of shigellosis cases was attributable to several factors. People were in settings where more people were in person-to-person contacts. Former homemaking women were entering the workplace and more young children were placed in child day-care centers. More of the elderly, formerly cared for at home, were in nursing homes. There was more institutionalization of others with special needs, such as mentally disabled persons of all ages. There was growing recognition that male homosexuals were infecting each other through anal-oral contacts.

Another factor in the rise of shigellosis was the transformation in food preparation and in lifestyle. Large central kitchens prepared food that was widely distributed. If only one food preparer was infected, many people, in numerous states, could become infected. *Shigella* is one of the most infectious pathogens. As few as 10 to 100 organisms may be all that are necessary for infectivity.

Americans were choosing to eat out more frequently, or to carry home convenience foods prepared by others. These lifestyle changes increased the risk for shigellosis and other foodborne illnesses.

The changed pattern from preparing modest-sized batches of foods locally, to centralized food processing of massive amounts for widespread distribution is another high-risk factor for shigellosis (and many other foodborne illnesses). Many outbreaks have occurred due to this changed pattern. For example, a shigellosis outbreak at the U.S. Naval Hospital in Bethesda, Maryland, in a cafeteria used by active-duty staff, resulted from salads prepared in a large centralized plant. Another shigellosis outbreak affected troops deployed to Saudi Arabia during the Gulf War in 1993, resulting from foods prepared in a large centralized plant elsewhere, and widely distributed. Other outbreaks have involved airline food prepared at centralized plants or chain-restaurant food prepared at centralized locations.

By 1996, shigellosis was among the most common notifiable disease infections. It was especially prevalent among children younger than five years of age. Shigellosis infected 46.3 persons per 100,000 population—a steep rise from 5.4 persons a decade earlier.

In March 2007, the CDC released the most recent estimates for shigellosis (reported in 2005). The reported cases were down to 16,000 annually. Although this figure is lower than the 1980s and 1990s, it is an increase over the all-time-low of approximately 14,000 cases reported in 2004.

In 2003, an outbreak of a *S. sonnei* strain emerged that caused a prolonged and widespread community outbreak of shigellosis associated with child day-care centers in three states. The strain had become antibiotic resistant, which does not bode well for the future status of shigellosis outbreaks.

SIGNS, SYMPTOMS, AND HEALTH CONSEQUENCES

Shigellosis usually begins within three days after exposure to the infective agent, but the period can be as short as one day, or as long as seven days. The infection begins with abdominal cramps, and diarrhea, marked by voluminous amounts of watery stools. These symptoms may be accompanied by fever. The diarrhea tends to worsen as the illness progresses. Bloody mucus may be present in the stools. The abdominal pain continues, with vomiting, headaches, and continued fever. Usually, the symptoms last for five or six days, but can last as long as three weeks.

Some children do not develop the usual gastric intestinal symptoms, but have headache, high fever, abdominal cramps, and even convulsions.

Usually, shigellosis clears up on its own without complications. However, in some cases, severe infections in the very young or the very old may require treatment. Unfortunately, *Shigella* has become resistant to mainline antibiotics.

Oral DNA Vaccine from *S. flexneri*?

Molecular biology enabled researchers to identify and isolate specific antigens (usually proteins or protein fragments) from viruses, bacteria, or other infectious agents. Now, a revolution in vaccinology may develop, with oral DNA vaccines (also known as naked DNA vaccines). They offer promise as alternatives to traditional forms of vaccines. Injection of genes that encode antigens can stimulate immune responses to the antigens. Cells readily process the foreign DNA, synthesize the encoded antigens, and stimulate immunologic responses against them. The immune response may be more protective than those obtained by direct injection of the antigens.

In the past, vaccinologists created DNA vaccines by copying the DNA of a bacteria such as *S. flexneri.* Now, they attempt to deliver the DNA of the bacteria into the body to produce enough copies of a gene to use as a vaccine. Researchers bend the required DNA into genetic plasmids, and add the plasmids to bacteria. As the bacteria multiply rapidly, the plasmids are copied along with the bacteria's own DNA. The researchers kill the bacteria, and purify the plasmids for later use in injectable vaccines.

Now, the attempt is being made to simplify this complex process by having *S. flexneri* both copy and deliver the plasmids. However, it is difficult to get *S. flexneri* to synthesize the immune-stimulating antigens of another organism. Instead, researchers are trying to get the pathogen to serve as a delivery vehicle by infecting a host's cells with plasmids. *S. flexneri* causes problems in humans if the organism replicates after invading cells.

To transform *S. flexneri* into a safe oral DNA vaccine for humans, genes crucial for replication are deleted from the organism. Without these genes the bacteria are too weak to replicate.

Another approach is to encapsulate plasmid DNA in microscopic spheres of a biopolymer called PLG. The spheres protect the DNA of an oral vaccine from intestinal acids and enzymes. Later, the biodegradable spheres disintegrate and release the encapsulated plasmids into the fluid interior of cells.

Oral DNA vaccines show promise. One concern is that the foreign plasmids might disrupt the function of a cell's normal genes.

For some individuals, shigellosis may lead to toxic megacolon, an enlargement of the colon. For others, consequences may be reactive arthritis, neuromuscular disorders, or a compromised immune system.

The *Shigella* can survive in the human intestine for months after the symptoms of the infection have subsided. Such individuals are asymptomatic carriers, who continue to be infective agents, either by direct contact with other people, or indirectly, by contact with food or water.

At times, medical determinations of shigellosis cases have been misdiagnosed, and mistaken for conditions such as acute ulcerative colitis, bacteremia, pseudoappendicitis, pseudomeningitis, or mesenteric lymphadenitis.

HIGH-RISK SETTINGS FOR *SHIGELLA* INFECTION

Child Day-Care Centers

Child day-care centers account for many shigellosis outbreaks. Studies have shown that children under three years of age who attend such centers are twice as likely to become infected by shigellosis, as children who are cared for in their own homes. Other studies have shown high rates for another age group. Children under six years of age attending such centers have a shigellosis rate of 7.4 per 1,000 children, compared with 0.6 per 1,000 children kept at home.

Several factors contribute to the high shigellosis rate at child day-care centers. Toddlers who attend might not yet be toilet trained. Their diapers are reservoirs for fecal contamination. Staff members who change diapers may also prepare foods. Unless high standards of hygiene are maintained, *Shigella* can be transmitted. Toys, furniture, eating trays, and other fomites, readily become contaminated, unless they are sanitized frequently. Many young children put objects or their fingers into their mouths. Children are in close contact with each other during activities. Working parents may deposit their infected child at the center rather than lose pay in attending an ill child at home.

Large Group Gatherings

Whenever people gather together in large numbers, there are potentials for outbreaks of shigellosis (as well as other foodborne outbreaks). For example, more than 3,000 cases of shigellosis occurred in New York City during a Passover holiday observance of Jews. Other outbreaks took place in upstate New York, New Jersey, and Ohio, at private Hebrew day schools. Educational programs were launched that emphasized the importance of handwashing after defecation and before food contacts.

PREVENTING SHIGELLOSIS IN CHILD DAY-CARE CENTERS

According to the CDC, "handwashing with soap and running water may be the single most important preventive measure to interrupt transmission of shigellosis. Soap and running water should be readily accessible to all persons during community outbreaks of shigellosis. Because young children are most likely to be infected with *Shigella* and are most likely to infect others, a strict policy of supervised handwashing for young children after they have defecated and before they eat is crucial. Institutions where hygiene may be suboptimal (for example, schools, child-care centers, and homeless shelters) can amplify transmission of shigellosis into the community and should be targeted for intensive control efforts. Excluding persons with diarrhea from handling food and limiting use of home-prepared foods in large gatherings will reduce the risk of large outbreaks caused by foodborne transmission.

"Antimicrobials [i.e., triclosan, discussed in Chapter 21] have a limited role in the control of epidemic shigellosis and are not a substitute for hygienic measures in reducing the secondary spread of shigellosis . . . Prophylactic use of antimicrobials cannot be recommended to prevent illness in persons who are exposed but not ill. In addition, using antimicrobials to treat patients with mild shigellosis to reduce the spread of secondary infections is not known to be any more effective in preventing *Shigella* infections than handwashing with soap and water; moreover, the practice can lead to the development of resistant strains that complicate therapy . . ."
—*Morbidity & Mortality Weekly Report,* CDC, Aug 1990

Another setting for an outbreak was at the Nantahala National Forest in North Carolina, at a reunion of Rainbow Farm. More than seventy-five people who attended were made ill, and in turn they made fourteen more persons ill by contact. Investigation showed that the illnesses were from *S. sonnei.* The investigators found that the outbreak was from poor hygiene in the setting. There was an insufficient amount of safe potable water. The trench latrines were inadequate to meet the needs of the participants. Weather conditions may have been a contributing factor. There was frequent rainfall during the event.

Infected Food Handlers and Preparers

Contaminated foods are those that often result from contact by infected food handlers and preparers. Outbreaks have occurred with raw produce such as iceberg lettuce, green onions, parsley, and uncooked baby corn.

If an infected food preparer chops, dices, or mixes raw foods and blends them with other ingredients to form dishes that require no further cooking, such dishes are at high risk for *Shigella* transmission (and other food pathogens). For example, there have been cases of contaminated salads, containing a protein food (such as shrimp, tuna fish, or chicken) or a carbohydrate food (such as potato, made into potato salad). Such salads are served cold, without reheating the cooked foods. At the beginning, the ingredients may be safe, but can acquire *Shigella* through being handled by an infected person.

Contaminated Water

Drinking water, or water used for recreational purposes, such as for swimming in lakes or pools, or wading pools for young children, can become contaminated by fecal matter from people. Often, the fecal contamination in drinking water comes from untreated water sources. The recreational water may be contaminated by toddlers who are not yet toilet trained.

Natural disasters, severe flooding, and windstorms may be factors in waterborne shigellosis. One outbreak at a resort was caused by contaminated water and ice supplied by a well. High spring rainfall had raised the water table, and *Shigella* were spread through the groundwater. The tap water and ice from a machine at the resort sickened patrons with *S. sonnei*.

LARGE OUTBREAKS OF SHIGELLOSIS

Cruise Ships

Large outbreaks of shigellosis have occurred on cruise ships. Confinement of large numbers of people with lots of person-to-person contact make an ideal setting for spreading infection.

On an Italian cruise ship, of 1,322 passengers, 330 were made ill with shigellosis. The outbreak was the fourth one for the vessel.

Another shigellosis outbreak occurred on the Viking Serenade, a cruise ship of the well-known Royal Caribbean Cruise Lines. During a round trip voyage from San Pedro, California, to Ensenada, Mexico, 586 of 1,589 passengers, and 24 of 594 crew members suffered from diarrhea and vomiting. One seventy-eight-year-old passenger was so ill that he was taken off the cruise ship and hospitalized in Mexico. He died in the hospital. The record showed that he had a history of health problems, including a heart disorder and diabetes. As a result of the outbreak, the cruise ship company cancelled two subsequent cruises in order to sanitize the ship.

Two shigellosis outbreaks are worth studying in greater detail. Both have unique features, and serve as instructive tales.

The Mysterious Case of Infected Muffins

Contamination of food with *Shigella* bacteria occurred in a large Texas medical center, and the contamination appears to have been an intentional act. An unsigned email on computer screens invited laboratory workers at the center to enjoy muffins. All the workers who accepted the offer and who ate boxed, commercially prepared muffins, experienced severe gastroenteritis. Another worker took the muffin home and shared it with a family member. Both became ill. Some of the persons who had eaten the muffins required hospitalization.

Investigation suggested that the ill people were suffering from *S. dysenteriae* type 2 culture, a strain of *Shigella* that had been in the laboratory storage freezer. During examination, the investigators found that the freezer showed signs of tampering. Six beads of *Shigella* were missing from one of the vials that originally had contained twenty-five beads. Stool specimens of nine patients identified their *S. dysenteriae* type 2 to be an identical match with the same strain found in an uneaten muffin, and in the stored vials.

The investigators suspected, but could not prove, that some worker with the skill to culture the organism from the bead, and who had access to the laboratory freezer, intentionally had contaminated the muffins.

Sleuthing the Case of the Five-Layered Bean Dip

As food preparation and distribution involve more and more components, outbreak investigations have become more complex. For example, a shigellosis outbreak in 2000 was multistate. At first, it affected people in the Northwest, then in California. As the outbreaks continued, there were cases in ten states. Antibiotic-resistant *S. sonnei* was identified in the stools of more than 400 people.

The incriminated food was a five-layered bean dip, manufactured by Señor Felix's Mexican Foods, in Baldwin Park, California, and distributed widely under various brand names. The dip, itself, had several components, processed in other plants, and then assembled into the final product. It consisted of beans, salsa, guacamole, nacho cheese, and sour cream. Each layer was prepared and refrigerated before being manually assembled into the finished dip. The preservative, sodium benzoate, was added to individual layers, but was not used for the products shipped to the Northwest states, where many people wanted to buy "preservative-free" food products.

The beans were the only cooked ingredient in the final dip. Because the various ingredients came from different sources, the investigators needed to check each one. At the cheese plant, the cheese paste layer was prepared in large batches once or twice a week. Blocks of cheese were hand-cut into chunks, and then fed into a device that converted them into cheese paste. The investigators found that the device was difficult to clean properly, and that there was cheese buildup. In addition, the cheese plant had numerous violations of good manufacturing practices. The plant lacked standard operating procedures, and reflected inadequate cleaning and sanitizing of processing equipment, and inadequate refrigeration of products.

Inspectors questioned employees at the cheese plant, and learned that one employee was responsible for hand-breaking the cheese and feeding it into the paste-maker device. He reported having had a stomach upset during the period of time when the contaminated dip was being manufactured. He was an hourly employee, with no paid sick leave.

This outbreak is instructive. In reporting the investigation of this large multistate shigellosis outbreak from a commercially prepared food product, Akiko C. Kimura, from the California Department of Health Services, wrote:

> *The evolving epidemiology of foodborne outbreaks reflects changes in the way that food is processed and distributed. The consumer can be educated to cook or wash minimally processed products such as raw meats,*

eggs, and fresh produce thoroughly before eating. However, in the case of a ready-to-eat product such as this dip, the responsibility to ensure safety of the product before opening rests with the growers, manufacturers, distributors, and retailers. Increasing emphasis is being placed on improving food safety through identifying and controlling potential hazards. These establishments also need to provide frequent, linguistically appropriate food-safety training for all employees and remove financial disincentives [i.e., not providing salary for sick leave] for employees with gastrointestinal illnesses.

In this outbreak, a virulent drug-resistant organism was rapidly disseminated through a commercially processed product . . . This outbreak . . . illustrates the vulnerability of the food supply, which is increasingly characterized by centralized production and broad distribution.

PART THREE

Significant Foodborne Pathogens

CHAPTER 7

T. gondii:
An Underrated Parasite

Louise was in her third trimester of her first pregnancy. She felt well and energetic. She went into her small vegetable garden to do some weeding. She found it awkward to wear gloves and besides, she enjoyed the feel of the soil as she shook it loose from the weeds. As she entered the garden area, a stray cat sped away. She had seen it before, and felt that the creature helped keep rodents and raccoons from damaging the vegetables.

When Louise returned to the house, she washed her hands hurriedly, and began to do some housecleaning. With her husband at work, she decided to empty the litterbox of their house cat. Besides being an amiable companion, the cat was a good mouser. Whenever the woman heard mice in the walls of their remodeled old farmhouse, she opened the door to the attic or cellar, hoping that the cat would catch the mice.

After doing chores, Louise rested, and then began supper preparations. She would cook a pork roast in the microwave oven. She was glad that pork roasts were now certified trichinae-free. That assurance allowed her to cook the roast to a juicy pinkness, rather than the former cooking of such roasts to dry grayness for "doneness."

Louise gave birth to an apparently healthy infant. However, it soon became apparent that the infant suffered loss of vision and hearing. Later, it became obvious that the child also was mentally retarded.

The Centers for Disease Control and Prevention (CDC) estimates that more than 60 million people in the United States are infected with parasitic *Toxoplasma gondii*, but are unaware of their infection because they are asymptomatic. Many people have never even heard of the infection. Yet, the U.S. Department of Agriculture (USDA) considers toxoplasmosis to be the third most important pathogen in the United States.

T. gondii costs Americans billions of dollars annually. Yet the estimates do not include the emotional price of families with *T. gondii*-infected infants, who may have sight or vision impairments, as well as mental retardation. Nor do these estimates include losses associated with AIDS patients who may also be infected with *T. gondii,* or other persons affected due to organ transplants or blood transfusions. Their already weakened immune systems are weakened further by *T. gondii* infections.

Regarding parasitic diseases such as *T. gondii* "during the last several years" wrote Jerry D. Smilack at the Mayo Clinic in Scottsdale, Arizona, in 1989, "we have been witnessing the profound interplay between the human immune system and the pathogens hitherto rarely appreciated." He cited toxoplasmosis, among others, as "infections few clinicians might have anticipated diagnosing, now are seen routinely in many medical centers. It is trite but true that all practicing physicians must become familiar with these pathogens."

T. gondii infects half of the world's population. Each infected person carries thousands of these parasites. Many *T. gondii* reach the brain, where they can do serious damage. Toxoplasmosis may occur as a silent infection, or as a chronically significant condition.

THE COMPLEX LIFE CYCLE OF *T. GONDII*

T. gondii can survive asexually in the first phase of its life cycle in any warm-blooded animal. The pathogen does not discriminate. It can live in animals as diverse as farm animals such as pigs, sheep, and cattle; in bats, rodents, deer, buffalo, kangaroos, crows, and sea otters; or in humans. *T. gondii* will lay its oocysts (egg-like cysts) that will hatch and grow in any mammal. Depending on the ambient temperature, the oocysts form within two to twenty-one days.

In the second phase of its life cycle, however, which is sexual, *T. gondii* is very discriminating. By some means, the parasite must find its way into the intestinal tract of a member of the feline family. It matters not whether it is a domestic cat or a feral cat, a jungle cat, puma, bobcat, or cougar. Any will do nicely. When the feline is infected, the oocysts, enclosed within a protective wall, infect the cat's intestinal epithelium. After the intestinal infection is established, more oocysts are produced and the cat can infect soil and water, which then can infect humans and other mammals. Cats, not yet infected, can become infected by ingesting oocysts embedded in the muscles and other organs of their prey. In the cat, as in all other creatures infected, the oocysts first infect the gut and then spread to other sites where they become established. Infected cats can develop toxoplasma pneumonia, encephalitis, hepatitis, pancreatitis, or myocarditis, but they do not transmit these disorders to humans. The real hazard to humans is the cat that is shedding oocysts in its stool.

T. gondii's Ultimate Goal

Once T. gondii have been able to get into a cat's intestines, it can produce oocysts. A single cat can shed 100 million oocysts in its droppings. The oocysts can infect humans, other mammals, and birds.

After the oocysts are in the human body, they spread quickly. Within hours, they can be detected in the heart and other organs. They are able to penetrate the blood-brain barrier and enter the brain. All this is made possible because T. gondii dissemble the immune system. The parasites hijack dendritic cells, common in the gut and part of the immune system. Commonly, if dendritic cells come into contact with pathogens, they respond by going to the lymph nodes or the spleen, where they communicate with other immune cells. However, when the dendritic cells are at the mercy of T. gondii, they go through the body but ignore signals from other immune cells to commit suicide. Instead, the dendritic cells carry the parasites into the brain and other organs, like Trojan horses. Unlike other pathogens, T. gondii are able to enter almost every type of cell in the bodies of thousands of host species. The parasites slip into the cells by latching onto the cells' surface and pulling the membrane over themselves. Once inside the cells, the host does not recognize the pathogen as a foreign body that it should destroy. Killing its host is not in T. gondii's interest for its own survival.

After acute infection, T. gondii continue to live in tissue cysts in humans, especially in muscles and brain. Individuals with immune deficiencies, such as patients with malignancies, may experience a rupture of the T. gondii cysts, leading to reactivation of diseases, including encephalitis or disseminating toxoplasmosis. Immunoglobulin IgG antibodies appear early after the infection. They reach a peak within six months after the infection begins, and remain detectable for life.

Transmission of T. gondii from Cats

When infected cats defecate, they release the highly contagious oocysts. Farm or feral cats can contaminate crops and pasture land on farms or in home gardens. The oocysts can survive in soil for more than a year, and are viable even after freezing and thawing. They can contaminate food crops and drinking water.

On farms, cats can contaminate animal feed stored in uncovered bins. The farm animals or wild animals and birds that eat infected rodents, or other creatures that wander into the area also can become infected.

People who eat raw or undercooked meat and poultry, or unwashed produce may become infected. The USDA estimates that half of all *T. gondii* infections in the United States are caused by raw or undercooked infected meat.

Pork, especially, is problematic. Only one *T. gondii* cyst is necessary to infect a pig. Some of the most common ways of preparing meat are unable to destroy any *T. gondii* oocysts that may be present, because the necessary temperatures are either not reached at all, or not maintained long enough. A temperature of 140°F (60°C) for ten minutes is the minimal temperature required to kill the oocysts. It has been shown that pork cooked in microwave ovens may still contain viable *T. gondii* as well as other foodborne infectious organisms, including *Salmonella*, *Listeria*, and *Trichinella*.

How *T. gondii* Find Their Cats

It is not always easy to find a cat. Through evolutionary adaptation, the *T. gondii* parasite has developed some sophisticated ruses to achieve its goal. It has learned to manipulate the non-cat host's behavior in order to reach a cat's intestines. How does it do it?

T. gondii has learned cleverly how to go from one host to another by creating a way to get infected rodents to be eaten by cats. The parasite manipulates the rodents by diminishing their wariness of cats, and actually to find cats alluring. This rodent brain rewiring produces a fatal attraction.

Zoologist Manuel Berdoy led a team at Oxford University to monitor rats exposed to cat odors. Normally, rats avoid such smells. Yet infected rats seemed to lose their fear, and at times, even preferred cat fragrances to other odors. The rats' personality change marks the ability of a parasite to manipulate its victimized mammal. If infected rats lose their fear of cats, it is easier for cats to catch them. The end result is that *T. gondii* achieve their goal of reaching cats' intestines.

Several years later, there was a follow-up to the Oxford University research, conducted by a team at Stanford University in California. Led by Ajai Vyas, the team demonstrated in laboratory studies that rats carrying the parasite *T. gondii* lose their fear of the smell of felines. Intentionally infected rats displayed normal types of fear responses except that they had lost their fear when exposed to the smell of bobcat urine. That reaction demonstrated that *T. gondii* have a remarkable specific behavioral effect on their hosts. *T. gondii* chose to form oocytes on the rats' amygdala, the fear center in the brain.

Both the Oxford and Stanford studies raised the question: does infection with *T. gondii* alter the human brain, too? Parasitologist Jaroslav Flegr at Charles University in Prague, the Czech Republic, gave psychological questionnaires to people infected with *T. gondii*, and to controls. He found a small but statistically significant tendency of infected individuals to be more self-reproaching and insecure than the controls. Personality differences intensified with long periods of infection.

Flegr found that men who showed immunologic signs of a prior *T. gondii* infection scored comparatively higher than uninfected men in traits such as suspicion of authority, and a propensity to break rules. Women who showed immunologic signs of a prior *T. gondii* infection scored comparatively higher than uninfected women in traits such as warmth, self-assurance, and chattiness. Flegr speculated that there might be a biological basis for the stereotypic "cat lady" (the loopy friendly neighbor who keeps scores of cats, loves them as children, and is inured to their odors).

CAN *T. GONDII* INFLUENCE GENDER SELECTION IN HUMAN POPULATIONS?

Parasitologist Jaroslav Flegr and his colleagues studied the medical records of more than 1,800 infants born in maternity clinics in Prague, where the infants are tested routinely for antibodies to toxoplasmosis. The usual sex ratio is 104 boys to every 100 girls. The 454 pregnant women who tested positive for *T. gondii* infections gave birth to 290 boys and only 187 girls. The women with the highest antibody levels had more than twice as many boys as girls. Flegr suggested that the parasitic infection may suppress the maternal immune system, which sometimes reacts against male embryos and causes more boys to be miscarried.

Other scientists suggest that *T. gondii* may influence the human brain in other ways. At present, this idea is not accepted widely, but several studies have suggested a correlation between *T. gondii* and schizophrenia. Robert Yolken, director of Stanley Laboratory of Developmental Neurovirology at Johns Hopkins University in Baltimore, Maryland, and his team reviewed medical records of military personnel. Soldiers who developed schizophrenia were twice as likely as other soldiers to show signs of *T. gondii* infections, confirmed by their blood samples.

SOURCES OF *T. GONDII* AND ITS TRANSMISSION

The USDA's certification program with pork as trichinae-free permits food preparers to cook pork to pinkness rather than as previously recommended, to be well done. (See Chapter 16 on Trichinosis.) This development concerns Jitender P. Dubey, at the USDA's Animal Parasitology Institute in Beltsville, Maryland, and an expert on *T. gondii*. In the early 1970s, he identified the essential role of cats in *T. gondii's* life cycle. Dubey suggests that with the trichinosis scare on the wane, consumers may be tempted to serve rarer pork. This practice will not assure that *T. gondii*, which may be present as well as the trichinae in the pork, will be killed. Also, as mentioned in the discussion of trichinae, ground beef may be contaminated with pork, intentionally or unintentionally. Undercooking may result in live *T. gondii* as well as live trichinae in the meat.

Dubey noted, too, that 43 percent of sows and 24 percent of market hogs are exposed to *T. gondii* infection. These percentages make undercooking of pork a risky business.

In 2007, the USDA analyzed more than 6,000 samples of retail meat samples of cuts of pork, beef, and chicken. Each sample weighed a minimum of 2.2 pounds. Ground meats and sausages were not included in this testing program. The researchers found the prevalence of live *T. gondii* in pork sold in retail meat cases nationwide in about four out of a thousand samples. None of the beef or chicken sampled contained live *T. gondii*. It is thought that improved hygiene practices and attempts to keep farm cats out of the barns are features responsible for a lower incidence than formerly of *T. gondii* in pork.

Also, in 2007, the CDC announced that *T. gondii* infects about 23 percent of the U.S. population, aged twelve or older—about 50 million people. Of these about 15 percent show symptoms of *T. gondii*.

Awareness of *T. gondii* infections may have reached farms, but awareness needs to be extended to homes, too. Just as it is necessary to cover feed boxes on farms, it is necessary to cover children's sandboxes when not in use, and to keep stray cats and other creatures out of the vegetable garden. It is not a good idea to handle stray cats or to adopt them. Keep housecats indoors and discourage them from catching rodents.

The litter box needs to be handled very carefully. The Food and Drug Administration (FDA) offers some suggestions:

- Empty the litter box daily. The oocysts require several days to become infective.

- Wear rubber gloves.

- Use disposable plastic liners. Seal the litter bag tightly with a twist tie and dispose of the liner in a plastic garbage bag. If you do not use a plastic liner, after emptying the box, disinfect it with scalding water and allow it to remain in the box for five minutes.

- After you remove the rubber gloves, scrub your hands with hot, soapy water.

- If you are pregnant, it is wise to let someone else clean the litterbox (this topic will be discussed shortly).

There are additional precautions. If you have companion animals, make certain that beds are not shared by animals and people. Keep the animals' food dishes separated from household dishes, and wash them separately. Do not permit animals to lick the remnants of food from plates and bowls used by humans. Teach children to wash their hands thoroughly after touching companion animals, or in visits to petting zoos or farms.

During food preparation, wash your hands thoroughly after handling any raw meats. Avoid hand contact with eyes and mucous membranes. *T. gondii* can penetrate mucous membranes in as little as fifteen seconds. Human bodily fluids such as saliva and breast milk may be infected. To date, sexual transmissions from semen or vaginal fluid have not been demonstrated. Bodily fluids from animals, including saliva, milk, blood, urine, and nasal and conjunctival secretions, can be infectious.

Young kittens are more likely to transmit *T. gondii* than older cats. Cats generally become infected from eating rodents, birds, or raw meat. Feed house cats canned or dry commercial food, or table food that is not raw or undercooked.

Infected cats shed oocysts for only about a week, but when they shed, they release millions of them. Cats can be reinfected, even though they have very high levels of antibodies against *T. gondii* from a previous infection even years earlier.

T. gondii transmission may occur inadvertently in hospital settings, with blood transfusions or organ transplantations. The unfortunate incident with the celebrated tennis player, Arthur Ashe, is an example. He had brain surgery in 1982, and had been given a blood transfusion. In 1992, suddenly one of his arms was paralyzed. A biopsy revealed the presence of toxoplasmosis, and a blood test confirmed that he was infected with HIV, the virus that causes AIDS. It is thought that both infections were due to the earlier blood transfusion.

Water, too, may be a transmission vehicle for toxoplasmosis. Municipally treated drinking water has been identified in outbreaks of *T. gondii* infections. Some outbreaks have resulted from unfiltered municipal drinking water supplies, especially in developing countries. However, the world's largest recorded toxoplasmosis outbreak to date occurred in a developed country, Canada. The outbreak occurred in British Columbia in March 1995. The public water supply was suspected as the most likely source of the infection. It was thought that infected domestic or feral cats (or possibly cougars) had defecated into the watershed and heavy rains had washed oocysts into the reservoir. By the end of the outbreak, at least 112 people including twelve infants were infected with *T. gondii*. A number of patients reported flu-like symptoms, exhibited retinal spots, and tested positive for the disease.

T. GONDII RISKS AND CONSEQUENCES

Individuals with compromised immune systems are at highest risk. Estimates are that about 80 percent of people over sixty years of age with impaired immune functioning are infected with *T. gondii*. Many are asymptomatic.

T. gondii infection is linked to numerous health problems, including ocular lesions, jaundice, enlarged liver, convulsions, central nervous system problems, encephalitis, Hodgkin's disease, mental retardation, myocarditis, hearing loss, and pneumonia.

T. GONDII INFECTION AND THE HEART

Latent toxoplasmosis can lead to cardiac failure. H. Werner at the Robert Koch Institute in Berlin, Germany, demonstrated how toxoplasma cysts in human heart muscle led to cardiac problems. In resting metabolism, the cysts secrete antigenic substances into surrounding tissues. This can lead to lesions, especially of the gangliocytes, and result in impaired cardiac function. The cysts probably survive for decades in the tissues. Werner reported that tachycardia with hypotension and cardiomegaly (enlargement of the heart), arrhythmia, systolic murmurs, and other symptoms of cardiomyopathy, possibly could be explained by *T. gondii* infection.

T. gondii Infection and Pregnancy

T. gondii infection in pregnant women can result in spontaneous abortions (miscarriages) or stillbirths. If the birth is carried to term, it can result in offspring with numerous grave health problems. These linkages are well established by the medical evidence.

Several thousand infants in the United States are born each year with congenital toxoplasmosis. The pregnant woman is most vulnerable in acquiring *T. gondii* infection during the first trimester; her fetus, in the third trimester. The parasite may take weeks to move from mother to fetus. Toxoplasma-specific antibodies also are transported across the placenta. They can be measured in blood samples of newborn infants.

Many cases of congenital toxoplasmosis are avoidable if pregnant women would avoid two practices: shun raw or undercooked meats, and refrain from cleaning litter boxes of cats. If it really becomes necessary for a pregnant woman to clean a litter box, then the CDC recommends that she wear rubber gloves, a face mask, and wash her hands thoroughly after removing the gloves. Similarly, if she gardens, she should wear rubber gloves before handling soil or sand, and wash her hands thoroughly after removing the gloves.

About two-thirds of the infants infected at birth with toxoplasmosis may not show any obvious signs of the infection. However, after a few months or even a few years, there may be subtle and nonspecific signs, such as odd behavior, changes in personality, and dips in IQ. There may be varying degrees of neurologic defects, ranging from learning disability to mental retardation, seizures, deafness, and blindness. About 10 percent of infants with congenital toxoplasmosis suffer nerve damage and encephalitis, with or without cerebral calcification and hydrocephalus sufficiently severe to require hospitalization. Another 10 percent of these infants die as a result of generalized infection or severe encephalitis.

An infected woman may pass the infection along to one child, but not to subsequent offspring, if she has built up immunity. If she has not built up immunity, then subsequent offspring also may be infected. There is still another scenario. The infected mother may build up enough immunity to *T. gondii* to protect the fetus from miscarriage, but not enough immunity to protect it altogether from the ravages of the infection.

T. gondii Infection and the Eyes

Peter Lou, an opthalmologist, and his colleagues at the University of Toronto, Canada, reported that toxoplasmosis inflicts greater eye damage than previously appreciated. The team described three siblings, all with toxoplasmosis-type eye damage: scarring on retina, poor vision, or blurred vision.

George A. Stern at the Francis I. Proctor Foundation for Research in Ophthalmology in San Francisco, California, and Paul E. Romano at McGaw Medical Center at Northwestern University in Chicago, Illinois, reported on two siblings who suffered toxoplasmosis-type scars on their retinas at birth. Both had poor vision. The older child also had mild retardation. The younger child also had moderate psychomotor retardation. Both children, as well as their mother, showed signs of immune reactions against *T. gondii*. In the period between the births of these two children, the mother had suffered five miscarriages.

In some countries, notably France and Italy, pregnant women are required to be tested for toxoplasmosis. This procedure is not routine in the United States.

T. gondii Infection and Schizophrenia

T. gondii infection increases a person's risk of developing schizophrenia, according to the findings of epidemiologist Dave W. Niebuhr and his colleagues at Walter Reed Army Institute of Research in Silver Spring, Maryland. The team studied 180 U.S. military personnel discharged with diagnoses of schizophrenia. The researchers analyzed the blood samples of the individuals collected before and after physicians diagnosed the mental disorder, and looked for elevated levels of antibodies that fight *T. gondii*. The researchers also analyzed blood samples of 532 military recruits with no psychiatric disorders. Of those who developed schizophrenia, 7 percent had been infected with *T. gondii* before their diagnoses. Five percent of the healthy group showed *T. gondii* infections. Although the percentage difference between the two groups is small, those exposed to *T. gondii* had a 24 percent greater chance of developing schizophrenia than did those who did not have the infection.

Previous research had identified *T. gondii* infections in some people with schizophrenia, but had not shown that the infection *preceded* the mental disorder.

Niebuhr's team emphasized that the parasite may foster schizophrenia only in those who are genetically predisposed to this mental illness. Most people infected with *T. gondii* never develop schizophrenia.

TESTING FOR TOXOPLASMOSIS

The symptoms of toxoplasmosis are so similar to other infections that it may not be on the checklist of suspects. Signs of the infection may include fever, headache, swollen lymph glands, cough, sore throat, nasal congestion, loss of appetite, and skin rash.

If toxoplasmosis is suspected, it can be confirmed with tests of blood and amniotic fluid of the pregnant woman, and ultrasound of the brain for both the mother and fetus.

Tests not necessarily for pregnant women, but for toxoplasmosis infection, include histologic examination, and skin testing several months after the original infection, for delayed hypersensitivity to toxoplasmosis antigens. Serology tests detect specific antibodies. Once formed, such antibodies may persist for many years. Lymph nodes can be examined for any changes.

The CDC notes the limitation of serology tests for toxoplasmosis. No assay exists that can determine exactly when the initial infection occurred. A substantial proportion of positive IgM test results probably will be false-positive.

To test farm animals for toxoplasmosis, enzyme immunoassay tests are performed with swine, either on site or in laboratories.

Is Toxoplasmosis Underdiagnosed?

The USDA reported that some 86 percent of all foodborne illnesses in the United States are undiagnosed. There is reason to believe that many toxoplasmosis cases either are not recognized or they are misdiagnosed. There are several close parasitic relatives that infect animals, including *Neospora, Hammondia, Besnoitia,* and *Sarcocystis*. Like *T. gondii* all these parasites form cysts and can cause miscarriages in cattle, sheep, goats, and nonhu-

ENCEPHALITIS OR TOXOPLASMOSIS?

Acute encephalitis caused by *T. gondii* was diagnosed in 1983 outbreaks of central nervous system toxoplasmosis in Belgium, the United States, Canada, and Haiti. The cases from the different countries showed similarities in many aspects of opportunistic infections occurring in homosexuals and in drug addicts. The cases, studied by Benjamin J. Luft and colleagues, found that only two out of the ten patients were homosexual and only one was a heroin addict. Nine of the patients died.

Diagnosis of central nervous system toxoplasmosis was difficult. The infection had not been suspected. Clinical manifestations of the disease varied. There was no specific antibody response. Luft and his team emphasized the importance of considering toxoplasmosis in attempting to diagnose any case of encephalitis of unknown origin.

man primates. It is not known if these parsites can infect humans, too. We know far less about their actions or their potential public health risks than we do about *T. gondii.*

Is Toxoplasmosis Misdiagnosed?

Some parasitic infections are misdiagnosed as other health disorders. For example, what is thought to be a brain abscess may be, in reality, a *T. gondii* infection. AIDS patients may be diagnosed as having central nervous system lymphoma. In reality, they may have toxoplasmosis. A proper diagnosis is important because the treatments differ for these two conditions. A correct diagnosis can be determined only by histologic evaluation of tissue by performing a brain biopsy.

Ulcerative colitis may be amoebic colitis. A peptic ulcer or a hiatal hernia may be a *Giardia lamblia* infection. Epilepsy may be an advanced case of cysticercosis. Cyst-like lesions in the oral cavity can be the encapsulated larval stage of pork tapeworm, beef tapeworm, *Trichinella spiralis* or *Ascaris lumbricoides.*

Another long-unrecognized protozoan, capable of parasitizing many of the same hosts as *T. gondii*, for decades has masqueraded as a particularly virulent form of *T. gondii*. In the late 1990s, parasitologist Jitender P. Dubey, mentioned earlier, identified and named *Neospora caninum*, isolated from tissues of dogs that had died from a virulent toxoplasmosis-like disease. He was able to grow the pathogen in a laboratory at USDA's Agricultural Research Service (ARS) in Beltsville. He demonstrated that the pathogen would induce severe toxoplasmosis-like disease in dogs. Dubey also showed that the same pathogen could induce paralysis or death in cats, rats, mice, and gerbils. He was able to identify the same pathogen in livestock such as calves and sheep. Although similar to *T. gondii*, *Neospora* can infect many tissues. *Neospora* is found most commonly in the brain and spinal column; *T. gondii*, in the brain, muscles, and eyes. Microscopically, the two pathogens look similar, except that *Neospora* cysts are much thicker than *T. gondii*'s. Unlike *T. gondii*, the outer wall of cats' intestines may not be the primary host for *Neospora*, according to Dubey's findings. Given the similarity of both pathogens, however, Dubey suspects that *Neospora*, too, may be an important infectious organism that targets humans.

CHAPTER 8

Listeria: Devastating for Some Individuals

Ready-to-eat sliceable turkey became a popular convenience food, available at deli counters in food stores. In 2002, an outbreak of Listeria mono-cytogenes *infection affected forty-six individuals in eight states after consuming such turkey. The illness began for these people with flu-like symptoms. A week later, they experienced diarrhea. Two to eight weeks later their symptoms varied, and included abdominal pain, nausea, vomiting, high fever, chills, severe headache, backache, and stiff neck.*

Ultimately, the outbreak caused seven deaths, and stillbirths or miscarriages in three pregnant women among the affected people. The pregnant women who survived faced possible additional health problems such as septicemia (blood poisoning) or Listeria *meningitis. Their fetuses, if also infected, faced similar possible additional health problems after birth.*

Listeriosis is an infection caused by the bacterium *Listeria monocytogenes*. In common parlance, often *L. monocytogenes* is shortened to *Listeria*.

Listeria is a foodborne disease that has a low rate of infection. However, for some individuals, it is far more severe than other foodborne illnesses. In 2006, the Centers for Disease Control and Prevention (CDC) estimated that each year 2,500 Americans suffer grave illnesses from listeriosis, and 500 of them die. *Listeria's* mortality rate is far higher than for other foodborne illnesses.

The CDC surveillance network FoodNet tracks emerging foodborne illnesses. FoodNet reported that *Listeria* infections had the highest hospitalization rate of all foodborne diseases. Despite the relatively few number of cases, listeriosis accounts for nearly half of all reported deaths from foodborne illnesses.

Until 1986, there had been no systematic monitoring program for liste-

THE ORIGIN OF THE NAME

Listeria is named after the celebrated English surgeon, Joseph Lister, the first Baron Lister of Lyme Regis (1827–1912). He used carbolic acid to prevent septic infections, and founded antiseptic surgery. *Monocytogenes* is derived from a symptom of infection: an increase in the disease-combatting white blood cells known as monocytes.

riosis. Now, it is a reportable disease. Doctors are expected to report cases to state health authorities.

A HIGHLY ADAPTABLE BACTERIUM

Listeria bacteria have several unusual characteristics. They are described as facultative. This means that they are highly adaptable, and adjust to new environments. For example, they can cope with cold and hot temperatures that would kill many other bacteria.

Listeria bacteria are psychrotropes. This means that, unlike most other bacteria, they can thrive and grow in extremely cold temperatures—as low as minus 40°F. They can thrive on cold surfaces and overtake other bacteria that are less resilient. The temperature in refrigerators is one at which *Listeria* not only grow and thrive in stored foods, but also on the surfaces within the appliance.

Listeria bacteria survive some degree of heat processing of foods that might kill many other pathogens. *Listeria* bacteria are anaerobes. In the absence of air, they can thrive and grow in vacuum-packaged foods. However, *Listeria* also can grow aerobically. Foods contaminated with *Listeria* appear, smell, and taste similar to noncontaminated foods. *Listeria* bacteria are more resistant to salt, nitrite, and acids to a far greater degree than other microorganisms.

Listeria is pervasive in the environment throughout the world, except in Antarctica. It can be found in soils, dust, water, mud, streams, sewage plants, wild and domestic animals, silage, animal feed, and humans. *Listeria* has been isolated from many mammals, birds, ticks, and crustaceans. Doctors have found *Listeria* in the feces of about 1 percent of the general population, in 5 percent of slaughterhouse workers, and in 26 percent of those who had contact with listeriosis patients.

Because *Listeria* bacteria are distributed so widely, there are many opportunities for food contamination. In 1988, the World Health Organization (WHO) convened the Informal Working Group on Foodborne Listeriosis and noted, *"L. monocytogenes* should be considered as an environmental contaminant whose primary means of transportation to humans is through a contamination of foodstuffs at any point in the food chain—from source to kitchen."

Listeria has been recognized since 1911 as an infective organism in animals. Formerly, it was thought that transmission of the pathogen to humans occurred from contact with farm animals. But scientists were puzzled by the finding that the infection also appeared in urban communities, far from farm animals. By 1928, the first case of human infection was identified. However, it was only as recently as 1983, that *Listeria* was identified as a foodborne pathogen. In that year, *Listeria* was found to contaminate coleslaw in Nova Scotia, Canada, and result in an outbreak of illness. It was thought that the cabbage from which the coleslaw had been made, had been stored in a cold environment after it had been grown and harvested from fields fertilized with raw sheep manure. However, the conjecture was never confirmed.

THE LONGEVITY OF *LISTERIA*

Despite the efforts of food retailers and food-processing plant managers to maintain a clean, safe environment for food, strains of *L. monocytogenes* have been found to persist for a year or longer. "This is disturbing because this points the finger at retail stores and some processors as a continuing source of food contamination," reported Brian D. Sauders, a member of a team studying *Listeria*, led by Martin Wiedmann at Cornell University in Ithaca, New York.

Sauders and Wiedmann examined specific strains of *L. monocytogenes* that had been identified in 125 foods in fifty retail food stores and in seven food processing plants in New York State, examined by inspectors from the State's Department of Agriculture and Markets. The inspectors had found the bacteria during routine surveys of sanitary inspections, and also as a result of consumer complaints between 1997 and 2002.

—*Journal of Food Protection,* July 2004

The Nova Scotia outbreak was a harbinger of events that followed. The characteristics of *Listeria*, combined with the growing popularity of ready-to-eat and minimally processed convenience foods, often encased in newly introduced vacuum packaging, inevitably led to *Listeria*'s emergence as an important foodborne infection. It was the beginning of sporadic as well as large-scale outbreaks. Listeriosis continues to be an ever-present hazard and a public health concern.

Many microbiologists believe that pathogenic organisms, long with us, have exchanged their genetic codes with previously non-pathogenic ones and this exchange has given rise to new ones. *Listeria* fits into this pattern. As a facultative pathogen, it has emerged only in the last few decades as a virulent foodborne pathogen.

A BRIEF HISTORY OF *LISTERIA*

Listeria was isolated in 1926 by three scientists at Cambridge University, England. They discovered the pathogen in an epidemic among rabbits and guinea pigs. The scientists named it *Bacterium monocytogenes*. The same pathogen was called Tiger River disease by researchers who reported an outbreak among gerbils at the South African Institute for Medical Research in Johannesburg. Doubtless, the same organism had been isolated from human patients, too, but called by different names.

The name of the bacterium was changed to *Listeria monocytogenes* in 1940, subsequent to a meeting of scientists in New York.

A staggering number of *L. monocytogenes* strains exist. In an early outbreak of listeriosis in France, some 12,000 different *L. monocytogenes* strains were identified in various delicatessen foods. More than 200 types of foods, mostly ham, pâté, jellied meat, and certain cheeses were found in this outbreak, which had been caused by jellied pork tongue. The virulent strain of *L. monocytogenes* was found to be type 4b in this outbreak. Subsequently, this strain has been identified in other outbreaks.

According to Martin Wiedmann, mentioned earlier, of many strains of *L. monocytogenes*, to date, five strains are virulent, and specific subsets may be more virulent in certain individuals.

INDIVIDUALS AT HIGH RISK FOR *LISTERIA* INFECTION

Listeriosis may affect healthy people yet result in few or no symptoms. The infection may be experienced merely with flu-like symptoms and not even be identified as listeriosis. However, for some groups of people, the infection is a high risk, even if they are infected with only a few *Listeria* bacteria.

Once *L. monocytogenes* bacteria infect the body, they become intracellular within the circulating lymphocytes. They exert an effect on tissues that normally are resistant to infection, such as the central nervous system, gravid uterus (uterus in pregnancy), and placenta.

Healthy Pregnant Women

Healthy pregnant women and their developing fetuses are at great risk for listeriosis. During pregnancy, the immune system is dampened in order to protect the developing fetus from being rejected by the maternal organism. If the pregnant woman becomes infected with *Listeria*, the pathogen can be carried, intrauterine, through her placenta, and affect her fetus as well. Half of all reported listeriosis cases are with pregnant

LISTERIA'S GENES ARE SEQUENCED AND ITS DNA ARE FINGERPRINTED

In 2001, the USDA announced that scientists had new information about *Listeria's* genetic makeup, which could help find ways to reduce the risk of food contamination and subsequent illness due to this pathogen. The researchers began to investigate the total genetic structure of *L. monocytogenes* serotype 4b strain, and completed the initial phase of examining fragments of the genome. The next phase would be to construct a complete genome map from the fragments.

PulseNet is a detection system that gives scientists an ability to fingerprint the DNA of *Listeria* and other foodborne bacteria, and then compare the fingerprint to see if the *Listeria* is from a common source. Pulsinet was established by the CDC in 1997 to track the virulent pathogen, *E. coli* O157:H7 (see Chapter 4). The detection system is useful as well for *Listeria*.

MODIFYING *LISTERIA* BACTERIA
TO UNDERSTAND THEM BETTER

By making a small modification in *L. monocytogenes*, German scientists created a strain that can infect mice. Andreas Lengeling and Wolf-Dieter Schubert at the Helmholtz Center for Infectious Research in Braunschweig, Germany, reported that their redesigned strain of *L. monocytogenes* would permit them to study the foodborne disease in easy-to-handle laboratory mice.

Guided by the structure of the curved *L. monocytogenes* invasion protein InlA, which binds to its human intestinal receptor, the researchers mutated two key amino acids in the protein InlA. The mutant form binds more tightly to the human receptor than a wild-type protein, and also binds to the previously incompatible mouse version of the receptor. Upon ingestion, mutant *L. monocytogenes* infect mice and provide a model of the disease. The scientists are using this model to study why pregnant women are so highly susceptible to listeriosis. —*Cell*, 2007

women and their fetuses. Pregnant women are twenty times more at risk from listeriosis than are healthy nonpregnant women.

In the pregnant woman, listeriosis may spread to her central nervous system, with symptoms such as headache, stiff neck, confusion, and loss of balance. Convulsions can occur. The infection can progress to *Listeria* meningitis, an inflammation of the membrane covering the brain's spinal cord, and to encephalitis, an inflammation of the brain. In fulminant form, *Listeria* meningitis is indistinguishable from bacterial meningitis. It can be identified only through laboratory testing, especially by analyzing the cerebrospinal fluid. Nearly half of all listeriosis cases reported to the CDC from 1980 to 1982, took the form of meningitis, which if untreated has a fatality rate as high as 90 percent. However, if the woman is given an effective antibiotic the treatment not only helps her, but also may prevent or cure infection in the infant as well. Untreated, the woman may suffer a miscarriage, have a premature delivery, or later, a stillbirth.

Listeriosis may be acquired *in utero* or during passage of the fetus through the birth canal. The newborn infant that survives, but is infected, generally has septicemia, meningitis, or encephalitis. The mortality rate is high.

Studies from June 1985 through December 1992, conducted by the Los Angeles County Department of Health Services, found that women with twin gestational pregnancy had nearly four times the risk of developing such complications compared to women with a single fetus. Triplet pregnancies carried an even higher risk. An increased incidence of listeriosis also was found in pregnant women up to thirty-five years of age, compared to older nonpregnant women.

Aging Adults and Others at High Risk

In older children and adults, especially those over sixty years of age, complications of listeriosis usually involve the central nervous system and the bloodstream. Bacteremia, which may result, is the presence of bacteria in the bloodstream. Other effects may include febrile gastroenteritis, pneumonia and endocarditis (inflammation of the lining of the heart and its valves). Skin contacts with *L. monocytogenes* can cause localized abscess or skin lesions.

The number of people at risk may increase with a larger aging population. People living longer with cancer and other serious health conditions that impair functioning of the immune system are at increased risk for listeriosis. The immune system is compromised by chemotherapy and by treatment with corticosteroids. HIV/AIDS patients are 200 to 300 times more susceptible to listeriosis than the general public. Individuals given drugs to prevent organ transplant rejection are at high risk of listeriosis. So, too, are individuals with heart disease, diabetes, cirrhosis of the liver, rheumatoid arthritis, ulcerative colitis, patients undergoing renal dialysis, and individuals with drug or alcohol addiction.

SOURCES OF *LISTERIA*

Production advances over the last few decades have increased the risks of *Listeria* contamination in meat processing, according to Larry Borchert, science advisor to the American Meat Institute Foundation. The advances actually have made processed meat products more susceptible to *Listeria* contamination than formerly. In the past, sodium chloride levels in such foods were higher, averaging 3.5 percent, compared to the current level of only about 1 percent. Nitrite, added in the past to processed meat, averaged 80 parts per million (ppm), compared to the average current level of 10 ppm. Formerly, *Listeria*, if present in such foods, required some twenty hours for a new generation of bacteria to grow; under current conditions,

only eleven hours. To make processed meat products safer, Borchert recommended surface application on frankfurters of liquid smoke and its
components such as phenols, carbonyls, and acids. Although such substances may help to combat *Listeria*, as toxic additives, they pose another
type of health problem. Other suggestions to combat *Listeria* contamination of processed meat products include: surface applications of herbal
compounds of eugenol (the principal component of clove oil) or clove
extracts, and rosemary; lactates; or trisodium phosphate rinses.

Ready-to-Eat Foods

Processed meat products such as frankfurters, luncheon meats, fermented
sausages, and prosciutto are regarded as ready-to-eat foods. Yet, if they
are not reheated thoroughly, such products can cause listeriosis. Other
ready-to-eat foods that carry some *Listeria* risks are those available at
delicatessen counters, including refrigerated pâtés, meat spreads, and
smoked seafood.

Other ready-to-eat foods that may be contaminated with *Listeria*
include poultry products; cold-smoked meat, poultry, or fish; and raw or
undercooked fresh meat, poultry, or fish (such as mackerel and pollock).
Listeria contamination has been found with imported and domestic seafoods, including cooked frozen crabmeat, raw and cooked shrimp, and
cooked surimi (a restructured imitation shellfish product made from
"trash" fish and other ingredients).

Newer Food Packaging

The introduction of modified atmosphere packaging (MAP) added a new
risk factor for *Listeria* contamination. This type of packaging retards but
does not stop bacterial growth entirely, nor does it kill any *Listeria* that
may be present in packaged meat, poultry, or fish. Additional steps must
be taken to control the organism, according to the results of a study led by
Douglas L. Marshall at the Louisiana State University Agricultural Center
in Baton Rouge. The team concluded that "such steps include vigorous
plant sanitation, proper cooking temperatures, proper packaging methods, and strict temperature control during refrigeration and storage." The
team found that the effectiveness of MAP to inhibit *Listeria* decreased
with increasing temperature (*Journal of Food Protection*, Nov 1991).

Injured *Listeria* bacteria may be more resistant to eradication efforts
with foods in the real world than from the laboratory-cultured *Listeria*

cells used in scientific studies. One of the researchers of this study, Yuquian Lou, in the Department of Food Science and Technology at Ohio State University, reported this finding at the 1994 annual meeting of the Institute of Food Technologists. Lou noted that the injured cells of *Listeria* synthesize enzymes called "heat-shock proteins" which help them to repair themselves. After the cells recover, they retain these proteins. This makes the cells even more resistant to further stresses. As a result, the cells that have undergone stress have *dramatically increased resistance to heat*. The implication of this finding is that food-safety standards, set without considering this factor, might involve overly optimistic assumptions about the conditions under which these pathogens can be eradicated.

Listeria-Contaminated Dairy Products

Listeria-contaminated dairy products can result from conditions on dairy farms. Infected cows, with no obvious signs of listeriosis infection, can shed large numbers of *L. monocytogenes* in their milk for months. A cow's teats, a farm worker's hands, and farm equipment may be contaminated by contact with infected animals, and subsequently contaminate milk and dairy products made from it.

Listeria bacteria exposed to some degree of heat, such as in milk pasteurization, may be injured but still survive and repair themselves. This finding, according to researchers Diane H. Meyer and Catherine W. Donnelly in the Department of Nutrition and Food Science at the University of Vermont in Burlington, "is highly significant from the point of view of the dairy industry and the customer." They cited the likelihood of temperature deviation above 41°F (5°C) during milk processing, packaging, distribution, and marketing, as well as temperature abuse by retailers and consumers. Meyer and Donnelly reported that "all of the above manipulations increase the milk to temperatures which expedite markedly the rate of repair of injured *L. monocytogenes*. Even though the milk is subsequently cooled to 41°F (5°C), our results suggest that the overall rate of repair . . . would be accelerated. Individuals consuming this milk at a later time could be exposed to viable *Listeria* capable of causing disease." The two researchers found that heat-injured *Listeria* is capable of repair both in whole and low-fat (2 percent) milk (*Journal of Food Protection*, June 8, 1992).

In the mid-1980s, when listeriosis was rampant, a 1986 survey revealed that 7 percent of some 1,000 dairy farms checked were producing

Listeria-tainted milk. After strengthening controls, by the late 1980s, the incidence of *Listeria* contamination at dairy farms dropped to 2 percent.

Listeria has been especially prominent as a problem with soft-ripened cheeses. Mexican-type soft cheese such as queso blanco, queso fresco, and queso panela have accounted for deaths in pregnant women. (This will be discussed shortly.)

Other *Listeria*-contaminated soft-ripened cheese, implicated to a lesser extent, include brie, camembert, feta, mozzarella, and blue-veined Roquefort and liederkranz. *Listeria* contamination has not been identified with hard cheeses such as cheddar, romano, parmesan, or swiss, or with processed cheese slices, or acid-containing dairy products such as cottage cheese.

Incidents with dairy foods, other than cheeses contaminated by *Listeria*, have included both pasteurized and unpasteurized milk, products made with raw milk, cream, butter, ice cream, ice milk, and novelty ice cream products such as ice cream bars.

In late December 2007, two elderly men died from listeriosis after drinking pasteurized milk processed by a Massachusetts dairy. Other persons were made ill by the contaminated milk. State health authorities urged consumers not to drink milk produced by the processor, which was sold under several brand names. Investigators thought that the *Listeria* contaminated the milk after it was pasteurized, possibly during bottling or when flavoring was added.

Listeria-Contaminated Produce

Produce, too, is vulnerable to *Listeria* contamination. On occasions, raw celery, tomatoes, lettuce, cucumbers, radishes, cabbages, and potatoes have been found to be *Listeria* tainted. However, the main concern is with ready-to-serve packaged raw produce and other minimally processed foods. Once produce is cut, if *Listeria* is present, the produce readily supports *Listeria* growth. Take an apple for example. If it is eaten whole, the skin serves as a barrier to many pathogens, including *Listeria*. But demand for fresh-cut produce, including apple slices, makes produce vulnerable to potentially harmful microorganisms. Cutting produce causes wounds that permit pathogens to penetrate raw produce. Kenneth C. Gross, leader of the U.S. Department of Agriculture's (USDA) Horticultural Crops Quality Laboratory of the Agrcultural Research Service (ARS) in Beltsville, Maryland, demonstrated that *L. monocytogenes* can grow on fresh-cut apple slices, precut and packaged for consumer convenience.

Other *Listeria*-Contaminated Convenience Foods

Other convenience foods have had a record of *Listeria* contamination. Included are such diverse products as rice salad, refrigerated cookie dough, chocolate milk, frozen ready-made sandwiches, and ready-to-eat sandwiches distributed in vending machines and convenience stores. Products with extended shelf life, such as commercially formulated salads and spreads may be convenient but they are especially vulnerable to contamination.

Other Sources of *Listeria* Contamination

Other sources of *Listeria* contamination are not as well recognized. For example, use of a microwave oven is risky. The appliance may heat the microorganisms present in a food to a temperature that actually *spurs* their growth rather than kills them. Stephen F. Dealler and Richard W. Lacey at Leeds University in England measured the core temperature of frozen dinners microwaved according to the package directions. They found that microwave radiation induces the flow of an ionic current on the surface of foods with high-salt concentrations. The ions may absorb the microwave energy and act as a shield, reducing the waves' penetration. This finding explains why microwaved food often boils on its surface, but remains cool on the inside. Dealler and Lacey recommended that people using microwave appliances should microwave foods longer, and at a lower power than the packages instruct, and then allow them to remain for a few minutes in the microwave oven to help ensure that harmful pathogens have been killed.

Foods may become contaminated with *L. monocytogenes* from the fingertips of food handlers. A research group led by Anna M. Snelling at the Department of Microbiology at Leeds University in England intentionally applied the pathogen to the fingertips of volunteers in order to measure the survival time and factors affecting the organism. *Listeria* proved to be remarkably resistant and persistent (even more than *E. coli*), after food handlers washed their hands with soap or with a water-based chlorhexidine hand cleanser. Neither substance decontaminated *Listeria* from the volunteers' fingertips. A previous study, cited by the team, had examined the hands and gloves of workers who processed chilled turkey meat in an abattoir. *L. monocytogenes* had been found on 10 percent of the hands and gloves of people who handled carcasses after chilling and portioning the turkey, and on 16.7 percent of persons who packaged the turkey cuts.

Listeria lurks in the home kitchen, too. Kitchen dishcloths may be a source of *Listeria* contamination. In a study in Great Britain, 11 percent of all kitchen dishcloths in use were contaminated with *Listeria*.

If kitchen sponges are used, they should be replaced frequently. One-time use of paper toweling, when possible to substitute for kitchen dishcloths and sponges, probably is a better choice.

REPEATED LISTERIOSIS OUTBREAKS

Ever since *L. monocytogenes'* emergence as a recognized foodborne pathogen, there have been repeated outbreaks, affecting many people. As might be expected, many of the outbreaks have been associated with two categories: soft-cured cheeses and ready-to-eat meat, poultry, and pork products. Also, as might be expected, pregnant women, fetuses, and other high-risk groups have suffered the most.

The outbreaks are not limited to the past, but continue into the present. Nor is foodborne *Listeria* confined to the United States. Outbreaks have been reported in European countries of France, Switzerland, Finland, Spain, and England, and also have been reported in Australia and Israel.

Major Outbreaks in Europe

Actually, the early outbreak in France, in 1992, with jellied pork tongues (mentioned earlier in this chapter) was a forerunner of subsequent outbreaks, here and abroad, with ready-to-eat meat products. The French outbreak, caused by *L. monocytogenes* serotype 4b, made 279 people ill. One-third of the cases were pregnant women and newborn infants. The outbreak resulted in twenty-two miscarriages and sixty-three deaths. The source of the outbreak—jellied pork tongues—was identified only eight months after the outbreak. Identification of listeriosis is difficult because the symptoms in infected people may not become apparent until weeks after the contaminated food has been eaten.

Still reeling from the 1992 outbreak, the following year France experienced another *Listeria* outbreak, also due to ready-to-eat meat. The new outbreak was traced to pork rillettes (potted minced pork). This outbreak affected twenty-five people, and resulted in four miscarriages and one death.

Between 1998 and 1999 France experienced a rash of *Listeria* cases. This time, the contaminated foods were raw cheeses: Mont d'Or and

Epoisses. There were extensive recalls. In one outbreak, two people died and one remained in critical condition. The outbreak led to a scandal. Three cheese executives were jailed. The government charged them with involuntary manslaughter and causing injury linked to a "deliberate failure to abide by safety regulations or cautions imposed by the law."

Another outbreak in France from cheeses tainted with *Listeria* serotype 4b resulted in 108 persons reported ill, five miscarriages, and twenty-one deaths. All the deaths involved high-risk groups: fetuses, the newborn, and the elderly. Soft Brie was the suspected cheese.

Switzerland, a country like France renowned for its cheeses, also had numerous outbreaks with soft cheeses such as Vacherin and Mont d'Or. European countries that had cheeses imported from Switzerland reported a total of 111 persons made ill, and thirty-one deaths.

Major Outbreaks in the United States

Major outbreaks in the United States mirrored the European experiences. In the late 1980s and early 1990s, there were numerous outbreaks resulting from *Listeria*-contaminated foods.

One of the nation's deadliest outbreaks of foodborne illness occurred in California in 1985, from *Listeria* serotype 4b-contaminated soft cheese. The CDC counted 142 cases of listeriosis due to this outbreak, as well as birth defects in surviving infants. More than 100 lawsuits were filed by family members in behalf of the deaths of forty-seven adults, thirty infants, and seventeen stillborn fetuses.

Between 1988 and 1990, there were 165 confirmed cases of persons infected from *Listeria*-contaminated soft cheeses, in California, Georgia, Tennessee, and Oklahoma.

Ready-to-eat meats, poultry, and fish products also account for numerous, and some deadly, foodborne outbreaks from *Listeria*. The peak period of outbreaks occurred in the late 1990s and early 2000s—the time of the exploding availability of ready-to-eat products. However, the hazard continues to hang, like Damocles' sword, over Americans who continue to choose these convenience foods.

One of the worst outbreaks of *Listeria* serotype 4b occurred during the 1998 to 1999 period. Almost 100 illnesses were reported in eleven states, and resulted in six deaths. Two pregnant women miscarried. The foods responsible for the outbreak were frankfurters and ready-to-eat meat and poultry products, processed by Bill Mar Foods in Zeeland, Michigan, a plant owned by Sara Lee Corporation, and distributed under many different brand names. By the time the problem was resolved, Bill Mar Foods had recalled 15 million pounds of frankfurters and other ready-to-eat meats.

Soon after this outbreak, another *Listeria* outbreak occurred in late 1998, from frankfurters and luncheon meats, manufactured by another Sara Lee plant located in Wayne County, Michigan. The outbreak was widespread, in twenty-two different states. By 1999, the CDC reported more than 100 people had been made ill. There were miscarriages, stillbirths, and deaths. Once again, *Listeria* serotype 4b was identified.

This outbreak led to a class action lawsuit in behalf of the people who had been made ill and who had died. Sara Lee made a settlement of several millions of dollars, but did not claim any wrongdoing.

The attorney, Kenneth Moll, who had represented the victims, claimed that the CDC numbers of some 100 documented illnesses and twenty-one deaths were gross underestimations. Moll reported that he had information about some 400 additional cases of illnesses and some forty additional deaths attributed to the outbreak.

Parallel to the civil suit against Sara Lee, the U.S. Attorney General in Grand Rapids, Michigan, launched an investigation of criminal wrongdoing. The Michigan Justice Department initiated this action in behest of USDA officials.

The following year, another outbreak occurred in ten states, caused by *Listeria*-contaminated deli turkey meat. The outbreak resulted in twenty-nine persons made ill. There were three miscarriages and four deaths.

The rapid-fire succession of outbreaks caused by ready-to-eat foods caused the meat industry to release guidelines for safe handling of these products. Also, the USDA's Food Safety and Inspection Service (FSIS) called a public meeting to discuss *Listeria,* with emphasis on efforts by industry and government to combat the pathogen. The FSIS wanted to use public input to set short- and long-term strategies for research, regulations, education, and enforcement for *Listeria*. In addition, the FSIS hoped to discuss sampling and monitoring programs and recall procedures.

Despite these efforts, outbreaks continued. In 2002, an outbreak of *Listeria*-contaminated sliceable turkey deli meat affected forty-six persons and caused three stillbirths and miscarriages and seven deaths in eight states, mainly in the Northeast.

The repeated outbreaks prompted the FSIS to seek additional actions.

Although the FSIS tested thousands of ready-to-eat product samples yearly, no federal regulations existed to require meat plants to test specifically for *Listeria.* The FSIS proposed that meat plants do such testing. The suggestion was hailed by microbiologist Catherine Donnelly, mentioned earlier, who was serving on a national committee to advise the secretaries of Agriculture and Health and Human Services on food safety issues. Donnelly frankly admitted that "it has been frustrating to look at the need

CDC's Guidelines to Prevent Listeriosis

Guidelines to prevent listeriosis are similar to those for preventing other foodborne illnesses. The general recommendations are:

- Cook thoroughly raw food from animal sources such as beef, pork, and poultry.
- Wash raw vegetables thoroughly before eating.
- Keep uncooked meats, poultry, and fish separate from vegetables and from cooked foods and ready-to-eat foods.
- Avoid unpasteurized (raw) milk or foods made from raw milk.
- Wash hands, knives, and cutting boards after each handling of uncooked foods.
- Individuals at high risk for listeriosis may choose to avoid soft cheeses.
- Cook leftover foods or ready-to-eat foods (frankfurters, etc.) until steaming hot.
- Avoid foods from deli counters such as prepared salads, meats, and cheeses, and thoroughly reheat cold cuts before eating them.

Additional advice has been offered by others to pregnant women:

- Avoid soft cheeses.
- Do not eat refrigerated pâté, meat spreads, or refrigerated smoked seafood unless it is part of a cooked dish such as a casserole.
- Avoid refrigerated smoked seafood such as salmon, trout, whitefish, cod, tuna, and mackerel labeled "Nova-style," "lox," "kippered," "smoked," or "jerky" found in refrigerated sections or at deli counters in food stores and delicatessens.

for change versus the speed of change" regarding the need to strengthen controls that would reduce *Listeria* contamination.

RECALLS OF *LISTERIA*-CONTAMINATED FOODS

Despite a decrease in the number of foodborne outbreaks from *Listeria* from the late 1990s and early 2000s, the problem has not gone away. Numerous recalls of *Listeria*-contaminated foods continue to be made, which is an indication that the problem remains.

Recent recalls include:

- 2,768 pounds of ready-to-eat chicken products in Tennessee
- 45,500 pounds of onions in California
- Smoked salmon and cheese spread in Georgia
- Diced onions sold at Trader Joe's
- Raw milk in Pennsylvania
- Sprouts in Minnesota
- 7,000 pounds of ready-to-eat turkey products in California
- 10,000 cases of fresh sliced mushrooms from Pennsylvania
- 47,000 pounds of fully cooked ham and turkey products from Ohio

A Multitude of Voluntary Food Recalls

The number of *Listeria* outbreaks is large. The number of voluntary recalls by food processors due to known or suspected *Listeria*-contaminated food products, is even larger. Yet these voluntary recalls have not always been publicized. Understandably, companies do not wish to tarnish their images, and lose sales.

At times, the recalls are so great in volume and so widely distributed, that a quiet recall would be impossible. An example is a 2001 recall by Cargill of some 14.5 million pounds of ready-to-eat meat and poultry products.

To illustrate the extensiveness of voluntary recalls due to known or suspected *Listeria*-contaminated foods, let us examine three representative years: 1999 through 2001. These were some, but not all, of the voluntary recalls during that period.

- **In 1999:** Deli meats, frankfurters, beef wieners (numerous recalls), turkey frankfurters, sausage, smoked sausage, cooked sausage, ethnic sausages such as mortadella (an Italian cooked sausage made from pork, pork fat, beef, wine and spices), German-style bologna, bockwurst and knackwurst (seasoned sausages), liverwurst, salami, pastrami, corned beef, smoked corned beef, cooked corned beef, head cheese, sliced ham, cooked ham, fully cooked bacon products, oven-roasted turkey breasts, oven-roasted honey turkey breasts, smoked turkey breasts, skinless turkey breasts, chicken burritos, frozen chicken burritos, chicken salad, and reduced-fat milk

- **In 2000:** Frankfurters (numerous recalls), cooked sausages, dry sausages, ready-to-eat sausages, ready-to-eat smoked sausages, pork spread ham, sliced ham, sliced boneless ham, sliced salami, beef salami, beef bologna, pastrami, sliced roast beef, cooked roast beef, corned beef, corned beef rounds, cheeseburgers, chicken nuggets, chicken patties, roasted ground chicken meat, sliced turkey, and turkey breasts

- **In 2001:** Frankfurters (numerous recalls), chicken frankfurters, turkey frankfurters, chicken wings, partially boned roasted young duckling halves, imported Hungarian salami, sliced cooked beef, ready-to-eat beef sausages, ready-to-eat meat and poultry, ready-to-eat turkey products, and Mexican-style meat and poultry products

Recently, the U.S. Congress passed the Food and Drug Administration Amendment Act of 2007 (FDAAA). The legislation deals, in part, with food safety. The law introduces some new and significant provisions. Food processors are obligated to notify the FDA of reportable food incidents no longer than twenty-four hours after determining that a product is a reportable food and to investigate the causes of the contamination. In essence, this provision will make "voluntary" recalls passé. No doubt, the provision was intended to help the FDA focus its limited resources on inspection more effectively. The byproduct is that the provision offers greater transparency for the general public. No longer will voluntary recalls be muted.

The new legislation gives the FDA greater authority to ensure food safety. If a company fails to notify the agency of a reportable food, the lack of candor can result in criminal prosecution if the failure involves a significant risk of injury to consumers. Companies will not have the option to handle recalls quietly. They will need to share information with the FDA, possibly have the information posted on the FDA's website for public viewing, have follow-up discussions with the FDA, and likely be targeted for an inspection. This new legislation covers drugs and medical devices as well as foods. For serious problems such as *Listeria* contamination of foods, the new legislation, long overdue, will allow the public as well as the regulatory agencies to be aware of foods that may be risky and best avoided.

A Multitude of Class I Recalls

During the same period just noted, the FDA issued numerous Class I Recalls (for products that pose imminent and grave danger to human health) for *Listeria*-contaminated foods. Among them, ready-to-eat and minimally processed foods predominated.

The recall procedure has shortcomings as a safety measure. It is, as the old saw goes, closing the barn door after the horse has gone. The recall may protect people from subsequent shipments of harmful foods to the marketplace, but has failed to protect the people who already suffer from illnesses and deaths from the outbreaks.

A TOLERANCE FOR *LISTERIA*?

In 1989, with *Listeria*-contaminated food a widespread and serious public health problem, the USDA instituted a policy of zero tolerance for *Listeria* in ready-to-eat products such as frankfurters and luncheon meats. As a result, *Listeria*-related illnesses dropped by 44 percent during the period of 1989 to 1993. From then, it remained unchanged up to 1998. At the end of that year, however, the massive outbreak (described previously) from Sara Lee's ready-to-eat products of frankfurters and deli meats occurred.

Processors of such foods claimed that it was impossible to meet the policy of zero tolerance for *Listeria* in ready-to-eat foods. They claimed that *Listeria* contaminates moist areas, including floors, walls, drains, conveyors, cleaning materials, and equipment surfaces in plants. The organism grows well on minimal nutrients and at refrigerated temperatures, and can grow in biofilms that coat surfaces, and prevent *Listeria* from being removed by cleaning, or killed by disinfectants. *Listeria* can produce biofilm on a variety of surfaces commonly used in food-processing plants, including stainless steel, nylon, Teflon, and polyester floor sealant. Isabel Blackman and Joseph Frank, at the Center for Food Safety and Quality Enhancement at the University of Georgia, Athens, reported that, over time, *Listeria* bacteria accumulate on such surfaces to levels that could lead to the spread of the pathogen throughout a food-processing plant. The processors argued that it is difficult, if not impossible, to eliminate *Listeria* completely on a continuous basis from processing plants, even when Good Manufacturing Practices (GMP) and an acceptable program of Hazard Analysis and Critical Control Points (HACCP) are implemented.

Processors suggested that the zero-tolerance policy should be reevaluated, with a change both of direction and emphasis that the regulatory agencies should take to reduce the listeriosis incidence. The suggestions made by processors would shift the burden to consumers. To wit:

- The food industry has gone to great lengths to reduce the prevalence of *Listeria* in manufacturing facilities and finished products. However, there has not been a concomitant reduction in the incidence of listeriosis. The incidence is likely to increase, mainly because a large portion of the population will be in the high-risk group. The increase in listeriosis is not likely to be due, principally, to processed foods, but rather to food contamination during home preparation.

- Because of the widespread distribution of *Listeria* in households, consumers—especially the highly susceptible individuals—should be informed about the risks of storing sensitive foods in the refrigerator for long periods of time.

- Only a portion of the population is at high risk of serious health problems resulting from *Listeria* infections. That segment should be informed about which high-risk foods should be avoided, and educated about the proper handling and preparation of foods to eliminate *Listeria*.

The processors concluded that after considering the above facts, it would seem "prudent" for regulatory agencies to establish tolerance levels for low-risk populations of *L. monocytogenes* in low-risk foods that do not allow growth of the organism. As an example, processors felt that the zero-tolerance level of *L. monocytogenes* in foods such as uncooked fermented sausage or cheddar cheese was unrealistic. *Listeria* may survive at very low levels in such foods during processing and storage, but they do not grow.

As of 2009, the zero tolerance is still in effect by the two regulatory agencies, the FDA and the USDA. Any ready-to-eat food that contains any amount of *Listeria*, or any product that may have come in contact with a surface contaminated with the pathogen, is deemed adulterated.

Despite numerous attempts by government and industry to eliminate *Listeria*, recalls of food products are on the rise. This development is due, partly, to the increased scrutiny of food processing plants by the federal regulatory agencies. Also, it is due to enhanced disease surveillance by the CDC through its programs of PulseNet and FoodNet that increase the likelihood of tracing sources of infection back to food-product manufacturers.

In 2005 and 2006, FDA Class I Recalls for products testing positive for, or linked to *Listeria*, included potato and egg salads, frozen strawberries used as a primary ingredient for smoothies, raw milk, coleslaw, packaged fresh-cut fruit, prepackaged turkey sandwiches, smoked salmon and trout, radish, alfalfa, and bean sprouts, and various chicken, turkey, vegetable, and imitation seafood-flavored spreads and a dip. In addition, the USDA's FSIS' *Listeria* recalls since January 2007 included frankfurters, sausages, deli-style ready-to-eat pork, roast beef, chicken and turkey products, hog's head cheese, spicy Thai-style pasta salad with chicken breast, ham salad and dried beef, and ready-to-cook chicken breast strips.

Cases of *Listeria* could be greatly reduced if consumers would avoid purchasing ready-to-eat deli foods and other convenience items. As any nutritionist knows, such products are less nutritious than their counterparts as basic foods. Because the deli foods and other convenience items carry a risk of *Listeria* as well, they are best avoided by all health-minded people, and especially for high-risk individuals.

CHAPTER 9

Noroviruses: Their Increased Incidence and Virulence

Lester, Colin, and Richard were driving from Mississippi to Texas to attend a weekend business conference sponsored by their company. On route, they stopped for supper at an upscale seafood restaurant renowned for its oyster bar.

A card was attached to the tasseled menu in the restaurant that read, "Oysters 'R' in Season: Enjoy Fresh Louisiana Oysters." Among other items, Lester ordered half a dozen raw oysters; Colin, oyster stew; and Richard, fried oysters.

During the following evening at the hotel, Lester and Colin began to feel queasy. During the night they experienced diarrhea and vomiting. The following day, neither man felt well enough to attend the conference. Richard, who felt well, drove the men to a nearby medical doctor recommended by a staff member at the hotel. The two men hoped that the doctor could alleviate their acute digestive distress.

Later in the week, the men learned about large outbreaks of illness in a number of states, caused by contaminated Louisiana oysters. Lester and Colin were among those who had been affected. Although Richard had not felt ill at the time, he also developed similar symptoms several days after Lester and Colin felt better. Richard had driven Lester and Colin home. His close contacts during the long drive had exposed him to a highly contagious infection.

Food- and waterborne noroviruses are the major cause, worldwide, of nonbacterial gastroenteritis. In early times, these infectious viruses had various names in the medical literature, such as "acute infectious nonbacterial gastroenteritis," "epidemic diarrhea and vomiting," "epidemic collapse," and "epidemic nausea and vomiting." These names give clues to the signs and symptoms of these infections.

In 1929, the infection was known as "epidemic winter vomiting disease" as a syndrome experienced by humans, and now recognized globally as acute nonbacterial gastroenteritis.

The press created misnomers for the infection by calling it "intestinal flu" or "stomach flu." The infection may have flu-like symptoms. However, "flu" denotes influenza, a viral infection primarily involving the lungs; whereas, viral gastroenteritis such as norovirus (as well as hepatitis A and rotavirus) involves the intestinal tract.

At times, when pathogens are identified, they are named after the geographic location where they were investigated, such as Hawaii virus, Mount Snow virus, and Taunton agents. Thus, the prototype pathogen causing acute nonbacterial gastroenteritis was identified in 1972, after an investigation of an earlier outbreak in 1968, in an elementary school in Norwalk, Ohio. The pathogen was named the Norwalk virus. Subsequently, numerous outbreaks of nonbacterial gastroenteritis infection with similar symptoms were reported. At first, the agents were called "Norwalk-like viruses" (NLVs) or "small-round structured viruses" (SRSVs). Later, they were all grouped together as noroviruses (NOVs), a genus of viruses that acknowledge the originally recognized strain—the Norwalk virus.

Some strains are more virulent than others, and are more stable environmentally. They resist chlorination, freezing, and heating up to 140°F. As additional strains have become more virulent, the incidence of infection has increased.

THE NATURE OF VIRUSES

Unlike bacteria that attack the body, viruses invade the human cells where they divert the cells' genetic material from its normal functions to produce the viruses themselves. NOVs are host specific, and humans are the main reservoir. NOVs multiply in the cells of the human gut, pass through, and cannot grow again until they reach another human gut. NOVs withstand the low pH of the human stomach and the harsh conditions in the small intestine. Unlike bacteria in food, NOVs cannot multiply until they reach a human gut via person-to-person contact, contaminated food infected by a food preparer, raw shellfish infected by human sewage in coastal waters, or from seepage or runoff from land.

By 2006, two new strains within a genotype group of NOVs, G11.4 sequence emerged. It is thought that like the influenza virus, NOVs may evade their hosts' immune system through frequent genetic changes, and then go on to trigger new outbreaks. This idea is difficult to prove. To date, NOVs cannot be cultivated in the laboratory, and presently, no animal model is known to exist.

In 1972, NOVs had been found as the first viruses definitely associated with acute gastroenteritis (AGE). Infection from NOVs has been found to be the most common cause of AGE.

From the early 1970s to the early 1990s, researchers were unable to develop simple methods to detect these viruses and to find the sources in nonbacterial gastroenteritis outbreaks and hospitalizations. Of more than 2,500 foodborne outbreaks reported to the Centers for Disease Control and Prevention (CDC) from 1993 to 1997, less than 1 percent of the cases were attributed to NOVs, and 68 percent to "unknown origin." As a result, NOVs were largely ignored and relegated to a minor role of gastroenteritis at a time when high-profile outbreaks were occurring with some bacterial infections such as *Salmonella* Enteritidis and *Escherichia coli*. Efforts and funding to prevent foodborne illnesses were focused on bacterial, rather than viral agents. All that began to change as identification of NOVs became clearer and recognized as a growing public health problem.

THE GROWING INCIDENCE OF NOVS

By 2006, two new cocirculating G11.4 norovirus strains emerged nationwide. They probably contributed to an increased number of outbreaks. By late 2006, the CDC was receiving many requests from numerous public health departments for information about the perceived number of outbreaks of AGE, especially person-to-person transmission in long-term health-care facilities. No national surveillance system existed for AGE outbreaks, including those caused by NOVs unless foodborne transmissions were suspected. The CDC solicited information from all fifty states. Only forty states responded. The majority of their outbreaks had no laboratory confirmation. But epidemiologic and clinical evidence suggested that the infectious outbreaks were associated with NOVs. The CDC analyzed their data, and found, indeed, that NOV-associated AGE had increased nationally in the frequency of outbreaks, including fatalities in long-term care facilities.

Among the findings, the CDC noted:

- **In 2004 and 2005:** There were seventeen reports of NOV outbreaks in long-term care facilities, affecting 573 residents and 288 staff workers. Thirty-six persons required hospitalization. One person, age ninety, died from NOV-associated AGE. The outbreaks had been preceded by illnesses among food handlers in the long-term care facilities.

- **In 2005 and 2006:** Outbreaks in New York State increased 298 percent. The following year, in New York State, the number of outbreaks increased, from forty-two during the previous year, to 167 outbreaks (a fourfold increase).

- **In 2006 and 2007:** The city of Boston, Massachusetts, had eighteen NOV-associated outbreaks in child day-care centers, colleges, and health-care facilities, affecting 1,327 persons.

As a result of recognizing the growing incidence of NOV infections, the Council for State and Territorial Epidemiologists passed a resolution to require that all AGE outbreaks be reported nationally, regardless of the mode of transmission (foodborne or person to person). The program was scheduled for implementation in 2008 through a National Outbreak Reporting System. The Council noted that better surveillance was needed, with specific protocols to investigate the role of NOVs in diarrheal deaths, especially among the elderly. The Council also noted the need to develop and apply new and easy-to-use norovirus assays for routine clinical practice.

CaliciNet is a centralized database at the CDC. The system is used to collect and compare norovirus sequences in order to identify emerging strains; track more virulent strains in real time; determine the role of contaminated foods in emerging strains; and make the information widely accessible to state and local health departments.

ARE NOVS ZOONOTIC?

Recently, high-profile examples of zoonotic viruses—transmissible from animals to humans—include the emerged avian influenza virus (H5N1) and severe acute respiratory syndrome (SARS) coronavirus. If NOVs are zoonotic, too, it is important for public health officials to monitor emerging strains, track their virulence, and attempt to limit their infectiveness with humans.

By the 2000s, a vast genomic variety of NOVs was identified. By 2004, five genogroups and twenty-two genetic clusters were established. Mainly they were NOVs that affect humans. However, the norovirus genus also contains noroviruses that infect pigs, cattle, and mice. Therefore, it is possible that NOVs are zoonotic, and infections may be transmitted directly to humans through animal contacts, or indirectly through the food chain. If true, then infections in humans may be even more serious than previously recognized.

Strains of NOVs exist that are thought to be associated with animals. Their contribution to the incidence of human infection is unclear. The NOV G11.1 sequence has been identified in fecal samples of cows; G11.18 in swine; and G11.4 in humans. The human strain has been identified also in livestock, as well as in retail meat. This finding raises the possibility of indirect transmission of NOVs through the food chain. Also, human NOVs can replicate and induce immune response in gnotobiotic pigs (animals living in a controlled germ-free environment), indicating that swine could serve as a reservoir for human NOVs. In addition, the genetic similarity of NOV strains between humans and swine raises a possibility that swine-human recombinant strains could emerge if a person was infected simultaneously with swine and human noroviruses.

Cattle, too, can be infected with NOV, but the strain is less closely related to the human NOVs. Cow NOVs produce recombinants in a similar manner as human NOVs. Thus, it is possible that a cow infected with both bovine and human strains of NOV simultaneously could produce a more virulent recombinant virus.

In a Canadian study, led by Kirsten Mattison at Health Canada, Ottawa, researchers tested stool samples from pig and dairy farms as well as from retail meat samples for the NOV genome. The swine NOV strain (G11.18) sequence and the bovine NOV strain (G11.1) sequence were detected in the swine and bovine samples, respectively. The researchers also identified the human NOV strain G11.4 sequence in both types of animal samples. This was the first report of the human strain in animal stool samples. Also, the researchers identified the human strain in a retail sample of raw pork. These findings suggest a potential mechanism for zoonotic transmission of NOVs to humans through meat and dairy foods, and foods from infected pigs and cows. The finding also suggests the possibility that a more virulent recombinant swine/human or cow/human NOV could emerge.

The possibility that raw meat may be contaminated with NOVs highlights the importance of proper handling and thorough cooking of such foods. Also, it reinforces the need for pasteurization of dairy foods.

EXTENT OF NOV INFECTIONS

The CDC estimates that NOV infections account for some 23 million episodes of illnesses annually in the United States, with 50,000 persons requiring hospitalizations. These infections are responsible for 300 deaths yearly. As with many estimates of foodborne illnesses, these numbers may be far too low. Many people do not seek medical assistance. Not all cases are reported. Only outbreaks are publicized. Some cases are misdiagnosed. Autopses are not performed routinely. Deaths may be attributed to other causes.

Of all the people exposed to foodborne infections, generally from 20 to 40 percent of them will become ill. However, for people exposed to NOV infections, from 60 to 80 percent will become ill.

By the age of fifty years, about half of all Americans have NOV antibodies in their blood from previous infections by these viruses. Unfortunately, previous infections do not appear to offer much immunity. If immunity exists, it is short-lived for less than six months. People with NOV antibodies can be reinfected, repeatedly.

TRANSMISSION OF NOVS

NOVs are transmitted mainly by the fecal-oral route through person-to-person contact. The infection is highly contagious. Fewer than ten viral particles can infect a person. The particles can be food-, water-, or even airborne. About half of all foodborne outbreaks occur from infected food handlers. Waterborne outbreaks, especially with raw shellfish, occur from water contaminated by human or animal feces. Sources may be untreated sewage entering coastal waters, or from seepage and runoff from land. Airborne transmissions occur from droplets of vomit expelled by infected persons.

Fomites can be reservoirs for NOVs. Fomites are surfaces and inanimate objects that can be contaminated. They include food preparation surfaces, food trays, sinks, dishes, utensils, cutlery, kitchen sponges, dishcloths, towels, clothing, mats, floors, showers, cribs, high chairs, toys, and other objects. Insects that have been in contact with fecal matter and then alight on food can be transmitters of NOVs. This source of transmission highlights the need for screened windows and doors in areas where foods are prepared.

The incubation period of NOV infections averages twenty-four to forty-eight hours, with an acute onset of vomiting and nonbloody diarrhea that lasts from twelve to sixty hours. Even after the person recovers and all symptoms are gone, there is prolonged shedding of the virus for up to two weeks.

SETTINGS AND PEOPLE AT RISK FOR NOV OUTBREAKS

NOVs can cause very large outbreaks in confined quarters where people are in close contact with each other. For example, outbreaks have occurred at day-care centers, schools, military establishments, summer camps, hospitals, and nursing homes. Health-care facilities are especially vulnerable when they house immobile or incontinent residents in long-term care. Other outbreaks have occurred in contact sports such as football, on cruise ships, at family reunions, tourist resorts, and restaurants.

Groups at Risk

NOVs are not a common cause of fatal diarrhea in infants, but may add to the damage already inflicted on infants from other pathogens. Malnutrition accompanies childhood diarrheal diseases in developing countries, regardless of the origin of the disease. Infants and young children can have multiple attacks, which intensify malnutrition and the effects of all infections. NOVs infect mainly older children and adults, especially the elderly. Viral gastroenteritis can be a severe infection for persons who are immunocompromised; who have liver, gastrointestinal, or blood disorders, or diabetes, kidney disease, or cancer; and those who are alcoholics. The infection may be serious, or even fatal, for elderly debilitated persons, especially if they are severely dehydrated. Electrolyte imbalances may require aggressive treatment with intravenous fluids. Death from NOV infection is mainly among the elderly. The CDC made recommendations for health-care facilities:

- Maintain all contact precautions, including hand hygiene and use of disinfectants.

- Avoid having staff members, from units or facilities where patients are infected, attend units or facilities where patients are not infected.

- Group together all symptomatic patients and isolate them. Provide separate toilet facilities for well patients.

- Instruct visitors about appropriate hand hygiene.

• Close affected units or facilities and prevent new admissions or transfers.

Outbreaks on Cruise Ships

Martin Enserink described cruise ships as "floating mini-cities with ever changing populations of hundreds or thousands of people in a confined space," and they "are a viral mecca, just like many hospitals and nursing homes."

When NOVs or any other pathogenic outbreak occurs on a cruise ship, the infection is difficult to control. By the time health authorities learn about a possible problem on board, the ship may already have begun its voyage and reached a point of no return. A cruise ship provides an ideal setting for infections with a closed and crowded environment. Identifying and interrupting multiple routes of transmission are especially difficult. For example, crew members infected during the voyage can serve as reservoirs for infecting newly arrived passengers on the next voyage. Or debarking passengers, who are infected but as yet asymptomatic, can be transmitters to others. If the cruise ship stops at ports of call, passengers who debark briefly may become infected on land, or new passengers who embark may be infected. Also, replenished food supplies taken on board may be contaminated.

In 1973, the CDC established the Vessel Sanitation Program, which resulted in a steady decline in outbreaks of NOVs and other pathogens on cruise ships until 2001. Then, there was a reversal of the trend. Between 2001 and 2004, the number of outbreaks increased nearly tenfold.

Cruise ships were sanitized scrupulously between voyages. The procedures required a full week of thorough disinfection including fomites such as doorknobs, railings, and elevator press-buttons. Some cruise ships organized special "vomit squads" for rapid cleanups during episodes

PLANNING A CRUISE?

The Centers for Disease Control and Prevention (CDC) maintains a registry of the health and safety records of cruise ships. This information is available to the public. Before making a selection, you can compare the records of the various cruise ship companies, and their specific cruise ships. This registry probably is more reliable than information supplied by travel agencies that may promote certain cruise companies for their own profit.

aboard the ships. Even when there are no infectious outbreaks, some passengers vomit from seasickness during voyages.

Despite these efforts, NOV outbreaks on cruise ships continue to be a problem, and affect large numbers of passengers and crews. Investigations have shown that several newly introduced NOVs and more virulent strains have been responsible for recent outbreaks.

In 2006, there were forty-five outbreaks on American cruise ships in European waters. This was a sharp rise from previous years in the United States. In some cases, more than 40 percent of all passengers were ill. Some ships experienced outbreaks on three or more consecutive voyages, despite thorough sanitizing between trips.

Outbreaks in Military Settings

As noted, many people in confined areas provide a conducive environment for the spread of NOVs. Among these are military settings. The NOV outbreak in the U.S. Air Force Academy in 1988 is described later in this chapter as an example of sporadic waterborne-associated NOV infections.

In 1998, a NOV-associated foodborne outbreak occurred among U.S. Army trainees at El Paso, Texas. The illness was traced to an infected confection baker, who contaminated crumb cakes, pies, and cinnamon rolls. Other suspected sources were an ice cream dispenser and a carbonated beverage dispenser. The outbreak resulted in ninety-nine soldiers requiring hospitalization.

In 2002, twenty-nine British soldiers and staff at a field hospital in Afghanistan became ill. The hospital was closed to all but patients with NOV-associated gastroenteritis. Some patients suffered so severely that one was evacuated to a U.S. military hospital in Germany, and ten more flown to England. This resulted in a secondary spread of the infection through person-to-person transmission. Two medical staff members who accompanied and treated the patients on the flight to England subsequently developed NOV-associated gastroenteritis.

An Outbreak in a School Setting

In February 2007, the District of Columbia Department of Health was notified of an outbreak of acute gastroenteritis in an elementary school among students and staff members. The infection was identified as a NOV. Investigators were able to trace the infection to one classroom, where computers were shared among students and staff members. In all other classrooms, either the students used their own computers or shared library computers.

The outbreak was the first report of a NOV detected on a computer mouse and keyboard, which, according to the CDC, highlights the possible role of computer equipment in disease transmission and the difficulty in identifying and properly disinfecting all possible environmental sources of NOV during outbreaks. Because a 1:10 household bleach solution is caustic, only corrosive-resistant surfaces can be cleaned at this concentration. The CDC reported that laptop computer keyboards have been shown to withstand more than 300 applications of a bleach solution at 80 parts per million without visible deterioration of the equipment.

Outbreaks in Restaurants

In 2005, three outbreaks and clusters of community cases of NOV-associated foodborne infections were traced to a franchised restaurant in Michigan. An infected food handler had prepared submarine sandwiches. This one individual was responsible for multisite outbreaks:

- At a school staff luncheon, party-size submarine sandwiches were catered by the restaurant. Of the twenty-nine school staff members in attendance, twenty-three were made ill.

- At a company staff luncheon, at the same restaurant that had catered the school luncheon, fifty-five out of ninety-five persons were made ill. The suspected contaminated foods were lettuce, jalapeño peppers, and onions.

- At a lunch at the same restaurant, nine out of eighteen persons were made ill at a social service organization meeting.

- Of individual patrons at the same restaurant, twenty-five out of twenty-eight were ill. The investigators had contacted them during a traceback.

The investigators found that the infected food handler at the restaurant had vomited and had diarrhea. He may have acquired his infection by person-to-person transmission from his child, who had been with an ill cousin who had attended a child day-care center. In the traceback, all the people who had been made ill in these outbreaks shared the same strains of NOV.

An environmental health inspector learned that the restaurant in question had been cleaned thoroughly prior to a visit by corporate supervisors of the restaurant chain. The food preparation sink was being used for handwashing. The restaurant was cleaned once again, but new complaints of illness from patrons caused the health department to recommend that the restaurant be closed temporarily. The restaurant chain complied.

Investigations showed that the infected worker washed lettuce each morning in the same sink used by employees to wash their hands. The sink was not sanitized before and after handwashing.

A professional cleaning company was hired to sanitize the restaurant. Then, the restaurant was reopened, and no further cases of illness were reported.

Public health officials admit that public-eating establishments present challenges, and can place the public at risk. To prevent restaurant-associated NOVs, as well as other foodborne pathogens, small restaurants might have difficulty operating when an employee is absent, and might not be able to afford to pay leave for an ill employee. The employee may not be able to afford unpaid sick leave, or being fired for a temporary absence due to illness. There seems to be no solution to this dilemma.

This large multisite NOV outbreak in Michigan in 2005 was followed by another large restaurant outbreak in the same state the following year. In this instance, several ill food service workers in a national chain restaurant infected at least 364 patrons. One server had worked in the restaurant as a line cook. While preparing antipasto platters, pizzas, and salads, he vomited into a waste bin. The antipasto contained calamari, bruschetta, and mozzarella cheese sticks with marinara sauce. All these components were under suspicion, as well as mashed potatoes with garlic.

The restaurant was assessed and many deficiencies were noted. Because of the layout of the restaurant, there was no barrier to impede airborne spread of the NOV or other pathogens from the kitchen to the main dining area. The lack of barrier might also permit airborne spread of the vomit. The inspectors also found deficiencies with employee handwashing practices, cleaning and sanitizing food and non-food contact surfaces, temperature monitoring, maintenance of sinks, and poor cleanup procedure for vomiting incidents. The cleanup procedure was to use a quaternary ammonium-based sanitizer that was ineffective against NOVs. Instead, an effective bleach should have been used.

Despite the raised awareness, Michigan continued to have an increased number of NOV-associated foodborne outbreaks. The state had thirty-four cases in 2005, and 114 reports of suspected or confirmed NOV outbreaks in 2006. After all these cases, official guidelines were issued for environmental decontamination after any vomiting incident. The outbreaks in Michigan were replicated in other states as well.

SOME SPORADIC NOV OUTBREAKS

Each sporadic outbreak has some different characteristics that are instructive. Here is a sampling.

In 1982, there were two exceptionally large outbreaks of what, at the time, was termed the Norwalk virus (now norovirus) in Minneapolis, Minnesota. An infected food handler made an uncooked buttercream frosting in a large vat with his bare arms up to his elbows in the icing. The contaminated frosting was spread to pastries, and later to a catered banquet. The contaminated foods led to two large outbreaks. At least 3,000 people were made ill in the first outbreak; at least 2,000 in the second outbreak.

In 1995, NOV-contaminated coleslaw in a Mississippi restaurant sickened 75 percent of the patrons who had eaten it. Investigators found that an infected worker had added leftover coleslaw to a fresh batch, and mixed it in a large tub with—yes—his bare hands. Health officials recommended that food handlers use elbow-length gloves or long-handled utensils to keep food safe during preparation. Also, they suggested that the restaurant prepare coleslaw in small batches, expose the coleslaw as little as possible to warm temperature during its preparation, and store it in two-inch deep pans to ensure proper temperature when the coleslaw was refrigerated.

In an Alaskan NOV outbreak in 1999, at a restaurant-catered luncheon, the potato salad had been prepared two days before the event by a sick food handler. He had used—yes—his bare hands to mix ingredients in a twelve-gallon plastic container. A number of persons were made ill.

In 2006, West Virginia had already experienced twenty outbreaks of NOV-associated acute gastroenteritis—a sevenfold increase in the state for the same period a year earlier. Then, another outbreak occurred, at a family reunion. Attendees came from two other states as well as West Virginia. Some of them were infected with NOVs. Attendees contributed various foods to the meals. A number of attendees became ill after the reunion. The suspected foods were scalloped potatoes, chicken, and chocolate cheese balls. Also, there may have been person-to-person trans-missions, with handshakes, hugs, and kisses among the family members.

WATERBORNE NOV OUTBREAKS

Contaminated water, too, has been the source of some sporadic out-breaks. In what was described as a "nontypical" NOV outbreak in 1988, nearly half of 3,000 cadets and staff at the U.S. Air Force Academy in Col-orado Springs experienced gastroenteritis. Investigators traced the infec-tion to a likely source: celery cleaned in nonpotable water, and then added to chicken salad. The vegetable washing sinks at the Academy had been removed during kitchen renovations. Employees washed the veg-etables with water carried by a two-ply rubber hose. Frequently, the same hose had been used to unclog a floor drain that had caused sewage to back up into the kitchen. In addition to NOV identified in the drain water, three types of *E. coli* and sixteen types of *Citrobacter freundii* were identi-fied. These pathogens might have acted synergistically with the NOV and increased the virulence of the outbreak.

A waterborne NOV-associated outbreak of gastroenteritis occurred at an Italian tourist resort in 2000. The outbreak was traced to contaminated drinking water from a breakdown in the resort's water system. Tap water samples revealed contamination with fecal matter. Nearly 350 people were made ill, including sixty-nine staff members. Many of the staff members, who were involved in water sports, also were infected. There were multiple sites of exposure: at the beach, in showers, with tap water, and in drinks made with ice.

A summer camp in Wisconsin experienced a NOV-associated outbreak in 2001. Most of the toilet facilities were pit toilets. Handwashing facilities were limited to cool running water, with no soap or towels available at the pit toilets. Investigators suggested that person-to-person transmission caused the outbreak.

During the same year, another camp experienced a NOV-related waterborne outbreak. At a youth camp in Virginia, groups of campers shared water, outdoor showers, and flush toilets that drained into septic systems. At the beginning of the outbreak, six out of eighty campers in one group showed signs of gastroenteritis. Then, five more in another group of eighty campers showed similar signs. All the ill campers had an acute onset of malaise, nausea, vomiting, and diarrhea for twenty-four to forty-eight hours.

Intervention measures were effective at the youth camp to stop the spread of infection with and among groups. There was limited contact between the ill and the well campers. The former were excluded from camp activities such as archery, shooting, rappelling, and other sports involving shared equipment. Separate latrines and washing facilities were provided. Showers were used at specific times, and then thoroughly sanitized. Separate drinking water was supplied. Scrupulous hand washing was mandated for everyone. The infected campers remained in isolation for forty-eight hours after all their symptoms had subsided.

In 2004, a NOV-associated outbreak of acute gastroenteritis occurred in people who had used the pool of a Vermont swimming club. Investigation showed a combination of factors produced the outbreak. The pool water was contaminated with human feces. The chlorine, usually used to disinfect the pool, was not entering the pool due to a blocked feed tube. There were several lapses of pool maintenance procedures. Pool records showed that during the period of the outbreak, seven private groups had used the pool, including three mother-infant swimming classes; two groups from a local girls' organization; a birthday party of children five to ten years of age; and a class of preschoolers. In addition, members of the swimming club had used the pool during two defined open-swim sessions.

A traceback to many of the pool users showed that some had gastrointestinal illnesses before they used the pool. Of 189 persons interviewed, fifty-three showed signs of infection. Some had sought medical care, and one adult with severe vomiting was hospitalized.

Interviews with swimmers and staff indicated that there was poor pool maintenance. The water was visibly turbid and cloudy when the regular maintenance person was not on duty, during the time when the pool use was highest. A kink in the tube that supplied chlorine to the pool water was identified and repaired. Testing showed that the level of chlorine disinfection used was suboptimal, and subsequently, hyperchlorination was instituted. Investigators found a lack of staff training and response policies, and a lack of records of pool-chemistry monitoring.

NOVS AND SHELLFISH

Mollusks such as oysters, clams, and mussels filter food through the seawater in which they live. They siphon two to three gallons of water hourly. This procedure is known as depuration. The mollusks filter not only plankton and other foods, but also viruses, bacteria, human and animal feces, chemical contaminants, and any other substances that may be present in the water. They not only filter these substances, but also can store some, especially viruses.

NOVs are the primary pathogens related to shellfishborne gastroenteritis worldwide. NOVs are especially persistent in oysters, which may act as ionic traps that concentrate and retain numbers of viral particles. Depuration can reduce about 95 percent of bacteria in oysters but the process is able to reduce only about 7 percent of viruses.

The viruses are stored mainly in the pancreatic tissue (the digestive ducts) of oysters, and the viral particles bind specifically in the oyster's digestive tract.

Enteric viruses such as NOVs differ from enteric bacteria such as *E. coli*, in NOVs' strong resistance to sewage treatment. The viruses can survive under unfavorable conditions in seawater and can act as reservoirs for transmission into the environment.

Shellfish cultivated in coastal areas close to human activities can be contaminated. NOVs can survive in treated sewage, and be present in high concentrations during an epidemic season. The viruses can persist in shellfish for extended periods of time, and create shellfishborne outbreaks.

Because of the extremely low infective dose of NOVs, feces from a single infected harvester in a shellfish gathering area is able to contaminate a very large volume of surrounding water and result in outbreaks. Conditions for outbreaks are especially favorable when the tidal flow is low and the oyster beds are shallow.

There have been numerous outbreaks from shellfishborne NOVs, and outbreaks continue to be a concern for public health. The following discussion highlights some notable outbreaks. Each has certain significant features for public health officials and shellfish consumers.

Oysters Harvested from Florida

The area of Apalachicola Bay, Florida, is known for commercial oyster harvesting. In 1993, forty-five people experienced NOV-associated gastroenteritis in seven different outbreaks. The oyster aficionados who ate large quantities of the contaminated shellfish had a gastroenteritis attack rate of 91 percent. However, these outbreaks were but a prelude to a multistate outbreak two years later, from late December 1994 to early January 1995. The outbreaks extended to several states, and at least 2,000 people were sickened. It was the largest oyster-associated NOV outbreak of gastroenteritis ever reported. Once again, the Apalachicola Bay area was involved.

The outbreak had some notable features. Both the quality of the water in the Florida bed, and the edible portion of the implicated oysters, had met national standards. During the holiday season the Apalachicola Bay area was used heavily not only by the customary commercial harvesters but also by recreational fishermen. It was suspected that the contamination was caused by human sewage and other waste dumped overboard from some vessel. Florida had no regulation for onboard toilets for boats under twenty-six feet in length.

The area was closed for harvesting, and a massive voluntary recall of oysters was initiated. There was a delay in removing the contaminated oysters from all markets. Tags on the oysters permitted traceback to general harvest areas, but they were not detailed sufficiently to allow recalls from specific sites. Also, many tags were lost, having been discarded when the oysters were shucked. In some cases, the contaminated oysters were still being sold after the areas were closed and oysters being recalled. As one official commented, "The consumer is left with no assurance of safety."

The episode demonstrated the limitations of the existing controls and the need for improved indicators of viral contamination. It was difficult to determine when it was safe to reopen the oyster beds for harvesting. Also, some unethical workers continued to harvest and sell "bootlegged" oysters from the contaminated areas, and used counterfeit tags on the oysters to conceal the shellfish's true origin. This illegal practice probably led to additional cases of gastroenteritis.

The Apalachicola Bay outbreak of 1994 and 1995 had an additional notable feature. The people who ate only cooked oysters were as likely to become ill as those who consumed the oysters raw. Most of the oysters were steamed or roasted. The cooking did not always ensure the safety of the oysters.

Oysters Harvested from Louisiana

A number of NOV-related outbreaks of contaminated oysters have occurred in Louisiana. In 1977, an especially widespread series of outbreaks occurred in that state and affected people in other states where the oysters were shipped: Alabama, Arkansas, Florida, Georgia, Maryland, Missouri, Mississippi, North Carolina, Tennessee, Texas, and Virginia.

SAFETY MEASURES WITH SHELLFISH

Special care is needed for safe handling of shellfish. Buy shellfish from reputable sellers. Promptly refrigerate shellfish between 32°F and 40°F. If the shells open, tap them. Discard any that fail to reclose.

Store freshly shucked shellfish refrigerated in covered glass jars. Use shucked mussels and clams within one or two days; scallops within two to three days; and oysters, within five to seven days.

Keep commercially frozen shellfish in the freezer no longer than six months; home frozen, no longer than three to six months. Long freezing causes quality loss.

In cooking shellfish, place them in a covered pot and *continue to steam them for four to six minutes after the shells open. Safely cooked shucked shellfish normally require four to five minutes in a boiling mixture.* After cooking, shellfish should be opaque and plump. Scallops should be firm and milky white. Oysters should curl at the edges and be slightly shrunken.

Refrigerate leftover cooked shellfish promptly. Plan to use it within three days.

Cooking of clams requires special care. Briefly steaming clams—as commonly is done —is *inadequate* to inactivate viral agents that might be present in the shellfish. The shells of clams will open after being steamed for about one minute. However, *an additional four to six minutes of steaming are needed for the internal temperature to reach the level required to inactivate viruses.* Some public health officials suggest that restaurant food preparers should be required to steam clams for the longer period of time to ensure safety. A similar practice should be followed in the home kitchen.

Research indicates that higher cooking temperatures are needed to destroy NOVs than those needed to destroy bacterial pathogens also associated with shellfish-related illnesses. The boiling point (212°F) for four to six minutes destroys these viruses.

There were large numbers of harvesting boats, and many of the oyster beds were located in remote areas. Because of the isolation, authorities thought that the areas were far away from potential sources of sewage. Louisiana had no requirements for routine testing for fecal matter. Yet these remote areas were contaminated, not from sewage, but from the disposal of human feces, thrown overboard from fishing vessels. This practice was common among the harvesters.

The outbreaks were traced to a single ill worker, whose fecal and vomitus discharges went into a bucket that served as the toilet on the oyster harvesting boat. The investigation showed that *the waste from that one individual contaminated a large area, estimated to be a kilometer long, a hundred meters wide, and two meters deep.*

Some of the people who were made ill in these widespread outbreaks in 1997 had consumed the oysters raw; others, steamed. It was unclear as to how much heat had been used in cooking the oysters, such as in oyster stew, or the length of cooking time. It was recognized that cooking oysters at 140°F for thirty minutes had *little* or *no effect* on killing the NOV. The degree of heat and the length of cooking time probably were insufficient to kill the NOV in the contaminated oysters. Persons who ate fried oysters were not made ill.

As a result of repeated outbreaks, some states required the posting of notices at places where shellfish was sold at the retail level. Lousiana required the following: "WARNING: Raw oysters, raw clams, and raw mussels can cause serious illness in persons with liver, stomach, blood or immune disorders."

California and some other states required a similar notice on the tags of the sacks or containers of oysters from the Gulf of Mexico. The regulations specified that retail establishments had to display the notice on signs, menus, table tents, or other visible means at the point of sales.

Despite the popularity of raw shellfish offered at oyster bars, seafood restaurants, and other venues, eating raw or undercooked shellfish carries risk. Although the high risk for certain groups of persons is acknowledged, the risk for healthy people is not emphasized. It should be. Regardless of strengthened regulations, NOV-contaminated shellfish continues to be a problem. The emergence of new NOV strains and more virulent ones, the lack of or the ineffectiveness of some sewage treatments, the prevalence of polluted waters, the lack of sufficient numbers of seafood inspectors and other factors, all combine to make raw or undercooked seafood a game of Russian roulette for *all* consumers.

CHAPTER 10

Rotaviruses and Infant Gastroenteritis

The elderly woman, Vanessa, was very frail but mentally alert. This was a special day for her. It would be the first time she saw her very first great-grandchild, a six-month-old boy. Her granddaughter, Julia, was flying in from the West Coast with the infant for a special visit. A volunteer worker in the long-term health facility helped Vanessa get out of bed and dress. She sat in a chair awaiting the arrival. The visit had been arranged two weeks earlier but had to be postponed. The infant had been vomiting and had diarrhea. Now the symptoms were gone, and the visit was possible.

Vanessa was delighted by the infant and asked to cuddle him as she had done many times earlier with her own children and grandchildren. The infant's mother, Julia, had brought along a bottle of infant feeding formula and the volunteer worker obliged in warming the bottle so that the great-grandmother could feed the infant. While Vanessa held the infant and he drank, she kissed him softly and wiped his runny nose. She reluctantly returned the infant to his mother's arms, sensing that this might be the last time she would see the infant. The visit had been joyous.

The aftermath was not joyous. Several days later, Vanessa began to vomit and have severe diarrheu. She was put on intensive care, rehydrated, and given electrolytes. What Vanessa did not know was that her great-grandson was asymptomatic but shedded a highly contagious virus.

Rotavirus, a highly infectious disease, can affect humans, farm animals such as piglets, poultry, and calves, and wild animals such as rodents and monkeys.

The young are the most susceptible. Human infants between six and twenty-four months of age are most affected, and those from birth to six months of age, less affected. Older children and adults also are at risk, but generally the infection is milder than in infants, except for the elderly and the immunocompromised.

Rotaviral infection is virtually universal in infants, both in developed and in developing countries. Worldwide, it is the most frequent cause of gastroenteritis.

In adults, there is a higher incidence of rotaviral infection than previously recognized, because in adults, the infection is mostly asymptomatic. But a small number of adults do have a similar spectrum of gastroenteritis symptoms as infants.

IDENTIFICATION OF ROTAVIRUS

As early as 1931, seasonal gastroenteritis was noted in young children, but no bacterial agent could be identified. By the 1940s, researchers isolated a filterable agent from children with gastroenteritis during epidemics. They found that the agent could infect calves. Earlier, veterinarians had noted a widespread disease that infected healthy calves or mice with a filterable extract of diseased tissues.

By the late 1940s, Japanese researchers orally inoculated a group of human volunteers with an extract of the filterable agent. The participants became infected. In the same study, another group of volunteers became infected after they were given the same extract, but by other transmission routes: by inhalation, gargling, or being in close contact with diarrheal patients whose infections were from no identified agent.

The infective agent in all these early trials probably was a rotavirus, in the family of *Reoviridae*. The virus is so small that half a billion can fit on the head of a pin. The rotavirus is too small to be seen with an ordinary microscope.

The breakthrough came in 1973, when Ruth F. Bishop and her colleagues in Australia discovered wheel-shaped virus-like particles, by means of electron microscopy, in the intestinal mucosa of infants with gastroenteritis. The agent turned out to be a rotavirus.

After the Australian group made their discovery, the rotavirus was identified in human stools. Once again, the discovery was made by means of electron microscopy, in England, Canada, and the United States. The findings confirmed the identification of the Australian group. Further studies established rotavirus as the leading cause of severe diarrhea in infants and young children.

At the time, the rotavirus could not be grown readily in tissue culture.

Detection of the infection relied solely on stool examination by electron microscopy. It was believed that a vaccine was needed, but there were obstacles, including the inability to grow a vaccine efficiently. Meanwhile, the virus was studied for its characteristics, including its pattern of outbreaks.

SEASONAL PEAKING OF ROTAVIRUS

The rotavirus is thought to be the sole viral agent known for its pattern of consistent annual repetition in geographic sequence and the only intestinal pathogen that has winter seasonality. Most diarrheal-associated diseases tend to occur during warm weather.

The yearly seasonal peaking of the rotavirus in the United States occurs from November to May. Outbreaks begin in the southwest region of the United States and in Mexico, then spread systematically across the country during the winter to the northeastern region and to the Maritime Provinces of Canada in spring. In the northwestern part of the United States, the peaking time—from winter to late spring—is more variable than in the other areas. Often, a mixture of common rotaviral strains varies between regions.

The rotavirus may be present in some populations throughout the year. In tropical climates, the virus does not undergo significant seasonal fluctuations. Environmental conditions of low humidity and people crowded indoors are two factors in outbreaks.

MECHANISM OF ACTION OF ROTAVIRUS

The rotavirus penetrates the intestinal wall and produces changes in the wall's structure and enzymes. The virus activates the enteric nervous system. These nerves control the intestine's movements as well as its functions of fluid absorption and secretion. The activated nerves stimulate cells of the intestinal lining to boost water secretion abnormally, which leads to watery diarrhea.

SIGNS AND SYMPTOMS OF ROTAVIRUS

The onset of infant rotaviral infection is sudden, with vomiting followed by watery diarrhea. These symptoms usually last from two to five days. The infant may be fretful and have a low fever. In extreme cases, the vomiting and diarrhea may persist for up to two weeks.

The rotavirus infectivity rate is similar for a breast-fed and a bottle-fed

PATHOGENS AND GASTROENTERITIS

Although the rotavirus is the main cause of diarrhea and is of major importance worldwide, a number of other viral pathogens also cause diarrhea and enteritis. Many, but not all, are food- or waterborne. Other viral agents include hepatitis, norovirus, echovirus, coxsackievirus, and adenovirus.

Many bacterial agents also cause diarrhea and gastroenteritis. Among them are *Salmonella*, *Shigella*, enterotoxigenic *Escherichia*, and vibrios.

Many species of protozoan parasites cause diarrhea and gastroenteritis. Among them are *Entamoeba*, *Giardia lamblia*, and *Trichomonas*.

infant, but the clinical course of gastroenteritis differs. The breast-fed infant displays milder symptoms, and the infection is of shorter duration. Veterinarians have found similar differences with rotavirally has infected piglets. Those who suckle their mothers' milk fare better than those who are given formula. It is thought that lactoferrin, a naturally occurring substance in mammary milk, has protective features.

Severe and persistent diarrhea in an infant can lead to extreme dehydration and electrolyte loss. Unless an infant is rehydrated and supplied with electrolytes, the infant can die. Worldwide, the lack of adequate medical attention to infants with severe rotaviral infections is a major cause of infant deaths.

The initial rotaviral infection buffers against the severity of subsequent bouts with rotoviral infections. Adults who have been infected early in life, if reinfected, usually have mild cases, or may be asymptomatic. The early infection(s) has (have) bestowed some immunity.

ROTAVIRAL TRANSMISSIONS

The rotavirus is spread by the fecal-oral route. Infected children can spread the infection to other children and/or to adults, especially those closely associated with ill children such as parents, caregivers, medical personnel in pediatric wards, and staff members in child day-care centers. The infection can be spread from an infant who is vomiting, sneezing, has a runny nose, or has contaminated fomites such as a drinking cup or a toy. Anyone who changes an infant's diapers can become infected from the great amount of rotavirus shed in stools.

Elderly patients in health-care facilities, in contact with an infected person, are at high risk due to the immunocompromised status of many of the elderly. An epidemic of viral gastroenteritis occurred in a long-term care facility during 1991. More than a hundred patients and staff members were affected. Some cases were from rotavirus; others from adenovirus; and some from a combination of both these viral infections.

The rotavirus can be spread in food and water by infected food handlers. Poor handwashing practices have been responsible for the spread of rotaviral infections in child day-care centers, especially if staff members change diapers of toddlers and also prepare food.

Laboratory studies showed that handwashing with ordinary soap was ineffective in eliminating rotaviral particles from hands. Volunteers allowed rotaviral-contaminated matter to be placed on the palm surface of their left hands. They air-dried their hands for twenty minutes. Then, liquid soap, plain water, or isopropanol (alcohol) was poured onto the contaminated area of their palms. The participants rubbed their hands together for ten seconds in the usual manner of handwashing. Then, they rinsed their hands in running tap water and dried them with paper towels. Of those who washed with liquid soap, 2.4 percent of the original rotaviral-contaminated matter was still present on their left hands and 0.43 percent was present on the originally uncontaminated right hands; and with tap water, 5.3 percent and 1.0 percent, respectively. The rotaviral-contaminated matter was virtually undetectable on the hands treated with isopropanol.

Raw milk can be a vehicle for rotaviral transmission. Sylvanie Tache and her colleagues in Toulouse, France, reported on an improved method to detect rotavirus in raw milk. Having established that the major inhibitors of foodborne rotavirus were G immunoglobulins, Tache and her team designed a fast and inexpensive method requiring the action of two agents (hydrochloric acid and dithiothreitol) for ten minutes with a 1-milliliter sample of milk. Using this method, the detection of rotavirus present in milk was improved a thousandfold over earlier techniques, and the recovery of the rotavirus was increased about three hundredfold (*Journal of Food Protection*, Apr 1995).

ROTAVIRAL OUTBREAKS

Foodborne rotaviral outbreaks are less common than with other foodborne pathogens, but they do occur. One outbreak was reported among students on a college campus in Washington, D.C., during March and

April 2000. More than a hundred students were sickened. Most of them reported vomiting and diarrhea, abdominal pain or discomfort, loss of appetite, nausea, fatigue, headache, chills, low-grade fever, and myalgia. In addition to these symptoms, a few students reported sore throat, cough, and/or congestion. The duration of their illnesses ranged from one to eight days, averaging four days. A few were extremely dehydrated and required rehydration.

Laboratory analysis identified rotavirus in the stools of some students and kitchen employees. Two line cooks reported that they had symptoms of gastroenteritis before the outbreak. One deli server on campus reported no illness, but he might have been infected, yet asymptomatic. Some of the suspected foods, tuna and chicken salad sandwiches, were items that he might have prepared.

Because of the rarity of foodborne outbreaks from rotavirus, this pathogen may not be suspected. Outbreak investigators need to consider this virus as a possibility in foodborne outbreaks as one of many causes of acute gastroenteritis.

QUEST FOR A VACCINE

After the rotavirus finally was identified, epidemiologists in the United States and elsewhere began to gather statistics about the pathogen. Although the virus was found to infect infants globally, the incidence of the infection and its mortality differ strikingly in developed and developing countries.

By the 2000s, it was estimated that more than 3 million America infants are infected by rotavirus yearly. Some 55,000 to 70,000 require hospitalization. These figures represent one-third of all children under five years of age who are hospitalized for extreme diarrhea due to various causes. Most of the rotaviral-infected cases are children under two years of age. The infection results in 75 to 125 deaths of American infants every year. The estimated medical costs are more than $500 million, and the total costs, more than $1 billion yearly.

As devastating as these statistics are, they pale by comparison to global numbers, especially in developing countries. It is estimated that each year, some 18 million infants are infected with rotavirus, resulting in nearly 900,000 deaths. Mortality is due to lack of medical attention, dehydration, and electrolyte loss. Some public health officials consider that even these staggering figures are gross underestimations. The illness is compounded by other infections and general malnutrition. Obviously something needed to be done about this global public health problem. Logically, the development of an effective vaccine might prevent, or at least reduce, this scourge.

Rotaviral Vaccine: Development and Consequences

Drs. Robert Chanock and Albert Kapikian led a team of researchers at the National Institute of Allergy and Infectious Diseases in Bethesda, Maryland, in an attempt to develop a rotaviral vaccine for infants. By 1985, they succeeded, and patented the vaccine as RRV-TV. After trials, the vaccine was approved and licensed in 1998 to Wyeth-Ayerst Laboratories, a division of American Home Products. The company planned to name the product RotaShield.

The vaccine seemed promising. RotaShield contained a rotaviral strain that infects rhesus monkeys, plus genes from the four most common human rotaviral strains. Another investigational vaccine, RRV-S1, had a single serotype strain. Both vaccines appeared to be protective against rotavirus serotype 1, but RotaShield proteins offered protection against other strains of the disease to infants two years of age, who had gained natural immunity by having earlier rotaviral infection(s).

At the end of August 1998, the Food and Drug Administration (FDA) approved RotaShield, the first rotaviral vaccine ever approved. Three doses of the vaccine were to be given orally to infants; at the age of two, four, and six months.

The vaccine was deemed inappropriate for certain infants: those who had received transfusions of blood cells; those who had liver or kidney transplants; those who had leukemia, HIV infection, lymphoma, or other malignancies; and those who had been given immune-suppressive drugs or therapies.

The RotaShield was launched in the United States shortly after licensing. Soon, the Vaccine Adverse Events Reporting System began to receive notification of infants who, after being given RotaShield, had developed intussusception. This is a type of bowel obstruction that occurs when the bowel folds in on itself. It is a serious condition and often requires surgery. If uncorrected, this condition can lead to death. The Centers for Disease Control and Prevention (CDC) suspected that the number of cases actually was substantially greater than the fifteen cases reported.

On the basis of these reports, in July 1999, the CDC recommended that health-care providers and parents postpone use of the RotaShield. By October 1999, the Advisory Committee on Immunization Practices (ACIP) reviewed the scientific data. Intussusception had occurred with significantly increased frequency in the first to second week after the initial dose of RotaShield had been given. ACIP concluded that it could no longer recommend the vaccine in the United States, and withdrew its previous recommendation. The vaccine's use had not extended outside the United States.

By 2001, studies suggested that the risk-benefit estimates made in 1999 might not have been accurate. The calculations had been that RotaShield would cause one case of intussusception in every 4,670 to 9,474 infants. If used routinely with all American children, between 361 and 732 cases of vaccine-caused intussusception might occur each year. This incidence rate was unacceptable. In 2001, the figures were challenged, and a lively scientific debate followed.

The researchers at the National Institutes of Health (NIH), where the vaccine had been developed and patented, defended the vaccine. They suggested that the vaccine's approval should be restored so that infants in developing countries could receive its benefits.

The NIH's sister institution, the CDC, which had uncovered the problem with the vaccine, had a cautious approach. The possibility of using the vaccine in developing countries, while at the same time prohibiting its use in the United States, posed an ethical dilemma. As one critic remarked, the perception "would be devastating."

Meanwhile, two large pharmaceutical companies had been working to develop rotaviral vaccines that differed from the RotaShield.

A virologist, H. Fred Clark, at the Children's Hospital in Philadelphia, Pennsylvania, funded by Merck Company in Whitehouse Station, New Jersey, led a team that was attempting to develop a vaccine composed of

THE GENOME OF ROTAVIRUSES

The genome of rotaviruses was found to consist of eleven segments of double-stranded RNA. Each one codes for a viral protein. The gene-coding arrangements and function of most of these proteins have been determined.

bovine rotavirus, plus a human strain isolated from sick infants in Philadelphia. In a process known as attenuation, different strains exchange genes. Out of the mix, the researchers selected several viruses that were genetically less than 10 percent human, but displayed a protein on their surfaces to which the human immune system could respond. Eventually, Clark's team created five hybrid viruses. Each was designed to confer immunity against a different common strain of human rotavirus. The strains were blended into an oral vaccine that Merck intended to name RotaTeq.

Concomitantly, Richard L. Ward and his colleagues at the Cincinnati Children's Hospital Medical Center in Ohio, sponsored by GlaxoSmith-Kline Biologicals in Belgium, were attempting to develop a rotaviral vaccine from a human strain. GlaxoSmithKline intended to name the vaccine Rotarix.

Trials Continue

Both RotaTeq and Rotarix underwent safety tests with large numbers of infants. To ensure safety, the tests were described as "the most massive and expensive clinical trials ever undertaken."

Merck's trials involved 60,000 or more infants. They were mostly from the United States and Finland, with smaller numbers from nine other countries.

GlaxoSmithKline's trials involved 63,000 infants, exclusively outside the United States, from eleven Latin American countries and Finland.

By 2008, the FDA approved both vaccines. RotaTeq and Rotarix differ biologically from RotaShield. Neither of these vaccines appears to cause the mild effects, such as fever and some vomiting, associated with RotaShield. Rotaviral vaccine development has evolved. As Roger I. Glass, a pioneer in its development, noted, "the pathway toward a commercial vaccine has proved torturous."

CHAPTER 11

Vibrios: Resurgence of an Old Scourge with New Strains

The biology teacher, Henry, and his wife, Norma, signed up for an alumni trip from the university to travel to Peru. There would be twenty-three participants, plus one alumnus, and a history teacher, who volunteered to lead the group. The itinerary consisted of ten days in Lima, including some day trips to the environs of the city, and then five days in Cuzco with a side trip to Machu Picchu.

The travel group was congenial. After arriving at the Lima hotel, the group gathered for a social hour before supper in order to become acquainted. Henry observed that many allowed ice to be added to their alcoholic or soft drinks. Someone remarked that the alcohol would make the ice safe. Henry raised his eyebrows.

At supper, several in the group ordered ceviche, a popular regional raw fish dish. Henry and Norma ordered baked fish. A member of the group at the table jokingly said that the chili peppers seasoning the ceviche were hot enough to make anything safe to eat. Henry was dubious.

The hotel manager assured the group that the tap water in their rooms was safe to drink. Henry was skeptical. Henry and Norma carried their unfinished bottles of carbonated water from the dinner table back to their room. They used the bottled water for brushing teeth and drinking.

The next morning, a few members of the group did not appear at breakfast. They sent word that they were "indisposed." The rest of the group planned a walking tour in Lima. As they strolled, some bought and ate fruits attractively arranged in the marketplace. Henry winced. The fruits were raw, unwashed, and could not be peeled.

For lunch, the group was free to eat wherever they wished. Some bought foods from street vendors. Henry and Norma found a modest cafe. The place looked clean and so did the food server. Henry and Norma enjoyed piping hot chicken soup accented with a strong garlicky flavor. Before handling the accompanying bread, Henry and Norma used hand-wipes brought from home.

By dinnertime, a few more of the group failed to appear at the table. They sent word that they felt queasy.

At breakfast, fewer of the group appeared. Even the group leader was missing. Some of the group suffered from bouts of vomiting and extreme diarrhea. They were seeking medical help.

By the end of the week in Lima, the group ready to depart for Cuzco had dwindled to six persons. Henry and Norma were among them. In earlier years, Henry had traveled to Latin American countries in field-work. He was well aware that cholera was endemic in the region.

Vibrios are normal inhabitants in marine and estuarine waters. Most cold-water vibrios are harmless. But warm-water species, including *Vibrio cholerae*, *V. vulnificus*, and *V. parahaemolyticus*, can cause human disease. Formerly, enteric bacteria were found to be the major cause of bacterial diseases from molluscan fish. Now, vibrios have become more important. Most of the reported vibrio infections in the United States have involved oysters grown in the warm-water regions of the Gulf of Mexico and the southeastern Atlantic Coast, especially off Florida. The vibrios occur naturally in these areas, and can grow rapidly if there is poor temperature control of shellfish during harvesting and shipping. Vibrios are destroyed by heat, even mild heat. Infection is inflicted only if the shellfish are eaten raw or undercooked. Unfortunately, many Americans prefer to eat raw shellfish, which public health officials regard as "an intrinsically dangerous practice."

VIBRIO CHOLERAE

There is evidence that global warming may lead to climate changes that promote new strains of old diseases such as cholera. For example, a new strain, *V. cholerae* O139 Bengal suddenly appeared in India and Bangladesh in late 1992 and early 1993.

Worldwide, marine ecosystems have increased coastal algae blooms, resulting from the rise in ocean temperature associated with global warming and nitrogen-rich wastewaters, fertilizers, acid rain, and run-off soils. Vibrios have an affinity for algae and weeds. These substances may stimulate vibrios to increase, and to mutate into new forms in these "hot systems."

CHOLERA GAINS VIRULENCE IN THE GUT

The hydrochloric acid produced in the human stomach is strong enough in its acidity to kill many harmful microbes. This has been a survival tool for people over many generations. However, some bacteria, including *V. cholerae,* are not deactivated by hydrochloric acid. Once *V. cholerae* invades the human digestive tract, the bacterium transforms itself into a virulent pathogen, hundreds of times more infectious than the *V. cholerae* living in ponds and rivers.

Formerly, when medical scientists tested cholera in laboratories, the microbes they used typically were those grown from samples collected from ponds and rivers. Tests from the 1970s showed puzzling results. It was difficult for such laboratory-grown cholera to infect human volunteers. By 2002, the reason became clear. Andrew Camilli, a microbiologist at Tufts University School of Medicine in Boston, led a team of researchers who investigated whether cholera bacteria cultured in the laboratory differed from those in the stools of Bangladesh cholera patients. The researchers fed mice *V. cholerae* either from the laboratory-grown or infected patients, and then examined the small intestines of the animals. Passage through the gut increased the strength of *V. cholerae* infectivity.

On average, the *V. cholerae* from infected people produced ten to one hundred times as many microbes in each mouse's gut as the laboratory-grown bacterium. In some animals, the difference was as much as seven hundredfold.

Suspecting that certain genes turn on or off in bacteria exposed to an individual human digestive tract, Camilli and his colleagues examined the DNA of two isolates. Each of the microbe samples had a distinctive pattern of gene activity. In the highly infective microbes, the genes activated were those known to function in iron acquisition and protein manufacture. Both are needed for bacterial growth. Other genes were found that encode proteins that might cause the bacterium to loosen its grip on the intestinal wall and exit from the body. These findings demonstrated that *V. cholerae* may go through a dramatic change during its passage through the human digestive tract.

SOURCES OF *V. CHOLERAE* CONTAMINATION

Some sources of *V. cholerae* are traditional ones: sewage; person-to-person contamination with fecal matter; foods handled by infected persons; crops irrigated by contaminated water; vended street food, especially in developing countries; and contaminated fresh produce eaten unwashed and raw. In addition, some distinctive sources are attributable to *V. cholerae*.

Ballast Water as a Source of *V. cholerae*

Ballast water is taken on board empty ships so that the ships can be deeper in the water and have improved stability. The water is discharged when the ship reaches the port where it boards or unloads cargo. Ballast water, taken from shallow water, often contains large amounts of sediment, home to marine and estuarine organisms, including *V. cholerae*.

In 1991, Tasmania and Australia reported problems. Strains of *V. cholerae* were identified in three ships that previously had docked at ports on the eastern seacoast of the United States. The Food and Drug Administration (FDA) asked districts to sample water for *V. cholerae* from the ballasts and holding tanks of vessels originated from, or having their last port of call, at a number of Central and South American countries experiencing cholera epidemics.

The testing was prompted by confirmation of *V. cholerae* in water samples of the ballasts, holding tanks, and fire mains of freighters from Brazil and Colombia, docked in Mobile, Alabama. *V. cholerae* strains had been found in oysters in Mobile Bay that matched strains from South America. To minimize risks, the U.S. Coast Guard ordered ships entering seaside ports to dump ballast water twice while still at sea. Most freshwater, estuarine, and inshore coastal organisms cannot survive in the ocean.

Ballast water was known to be responsible for other undesired invasions in U.S. waters, and elsewhere. The Asian clam had appeared in the San Francisco Bay area in 1986, likely from ballast tanks of a freighter. The invader threatened to outcompete native clams. Zebra mussels had invaded the Great Lakes. In the Pacific Northwest, some 367 different marine species had been introduced inadvertently, including jellyfish, snails, flatworms, and a variety of microscopic life forms. Earlier, in the 1980s, the North American comb jellyfish rode a freighter into the Sea of Azov, a semi-enclosed body of water in the northern area of the Black Sea, and virtually wiped out the anchovy fishing industry in the region.

Seaweed as a Source of *V. cholerae*

Seaweed, contaminated with *V. cholerae*, caused an outbreak of gastrointestinal illness in seven persons attending a picnic in Hawaii in 1994. Frequently, seaweed is served as a side dish at meals in the Pacific Islands, and is a common component in the diet of many persons living in the Pacific Rim. Often seaweed is harvested at beaches, gathered in nearshore waters, or purchased at local markets. It is served either raw or cooked and commonly prepared with salt and/or spices and herbs. Previous to the 1994 outbreak, reports documented a toxic illness associated with seaweed harvested in some locations in the Pacific. In 1991, thirteen people became ill, and three of them died after eating seaweed harvested in Guam. The following year, three people became ill after eating seaweed harvested in California, and in 1993, two persons became ill, and one of them died, after eating seaweed in Japan. The Centers for Disease Control and Prevention (CDC) identified vibrio and *Pseudomonas* bacterial organisms in and on the seaweed.

Coconut Milk as a Source of *V. cholerae*

Coconut, contaminated with *V. cholerae*, caused another outbreak. In 1991, three people were made ill after attending a picnic in Silver Spring, Maryland. One of the three people required hospitalization and rehydration, resulting from severe watery diarrhea and vomiting. None of the three persons had recently traveled outside the United States nor had they eaten raw seafood. However, at the picnic, all three had eaten a homemade Thai-style rice pudding served with a topping made from frozen coconut milk imported from Thailand.

The FDA's Baltimore District Laboratory cultured an unopened package of the same brand of frozen coconut milk from a different shipment. The technicians identified toxigenic *V. cholerae* O1 (another new strain) from one of six bags tested. Also, other foodborne pathogens were present. The distributor voluntarily recalled the product.

Commercial coconut milk is marketed mostly for home use. Usually it is consumed well-cooked in ethnic curries and desserts. In this outbreak the coconut milk may not have been heated sufficiently to kill the cholera organisms (and possibly other pathogens). Prolonged holding time at room temperature allowed the *V. cholerae* to multiply and reach infectious levels. Canned coconut milk is deemed safe because the heat treatment during the standard canning process is high enough to kill any vibrios that may be present.

Other Sources of *V. cholerae*

Additional sources of *V. cholerae* infections have come from other imported foods, especially from areas where *V. cholerae* is endemic. Other sources include foods served on airlines and foods eaten while traveling abroad.

In one incident, cholera was associated with food transported from a Central American country to the United States. In 1994, a family in Indiana

A PROTECTIVE GENE AGAINST CHOLERA

A basic tenet in evolutionary biology is that genes survive over thousands of generations only if they confer some advantage to the species. The cystic fibrosis gene appears to be one, because it protects against cholera.

Cystic fibrosis (CF) prevents the normal flow of salts out of the gut and lungs. This leads to the formation of thick mucus that can obstruct the intestine and block breathing in the lungs. However, the CF gene may protect against cholera because it blocks the same molecular pathway used by the disease toxin to cause diarrhea. Cholera kills by causing severe and unrelenting loss of fluid. Most of the disease victims die from dehydration. Some lose up to a pint of fluid each hour from uncontrolled diarrhea.

In tests, led by Sherif E. Gabriel at the University of North Carolina School of Medicine at Chapel Hill, laboratory mice carrying CF genes did not suffer the deadly diarrhea typically caused by cholera. This finding may explain why CF continues to be found as one of the most common gene defects. Usually, a gene that codes for a fatal disorder results in a decrease in the numbers of affected people. This has not happened with CF. Gabriel suggested that in the great cholera epidemics that have struck humans over the centuries, persons who were carriers of the CF gene would have had a better survival chance than those who lacked the CF gene. Because of this, the CF gene was carried forward, from generation to generation, in sufficient numbers to remain in the human gene pool. Similarly, the prevalence of the sickle cell gene may confer some immunity against *Plasmodium falciparum* malaria.

shared a meal comprised of home-canned palm fruit in salt and vinegar, as well as bread, and white cheese. All the items had been brought on a flight from El Salvador. Some of the family members became ill and required medical attention. None of the food items were available for testing, but the palm fruit was suspected. When it was tested, *V. cholerae* O1 was detected. A year earlier, another outbreak had occurred with crabmeat, transported in a suitcase from Ecuador. Both El Salvador and Ecuador were countries experiencing *V. cholerae* epidemics during that period. Public health officials advised that travelers not transport food from cholera-affected areas. At the same time, the FDA stepped up its own efforts to test imported foods from countries experiencing cholera outbreaks. Imported foods from Mexico, for example, were inspected with a focus on certain foods: fresh and frozen seafood products; crabs that had been hand-picked but not retorted (subjected to heat) and labeled "refrigerate"; fresh fruits and vegetables, as well as ice and water used for preservation purposes with fresh seafood, fish, or vegetables.

CHOLERA OUTBREAKS

Natural Disasters and Civil Conflicts

Often, cholera outbreaks accompany disasters such as floods, earthquakes, hurricanes, and other natural occurrences. For example, in 2005, after Hurricanes Rita and Katrina struck, there were cases of toxigenic *V. cholerae* O1 attributed to eating undercooked or contaminated seafood from the area. Eighteen wound-associated vibrio cases were reported in Mississippi and Louisiana individuals, as well as in persons displaced from Hurricane Katrina and relocated in Texas, Arkansas, Arizona, and Florida. Laboratory analyses showed that some of these cases were from *V. cholerae* and others from *V. vulnificus* and *V. parahaemolyticus*. Underlying health problems of the infected individuals might have increased the severity of the illnesses. Some of them already had health problems such as heart disease, diabetes, kidney disease, alcoholism, liver disease, peptic ulcers, immunodeficiency, and malignancy.

Cholera outbreaks often accompany manmade environmental conditions such as those in concentration camps, refugee camps, in civil wars and other wartime settings. In 1997, cholera outbreaks occurred among Rwandan refugees in the Democratic Republic of Congo. In 2003, civil conflict led to a cholera epidemic in Liberia.

Cholera Epidemics of the Past

Cholera epidemics occurred repeatedly in the past. Several were recorded in the 1800s. All began in Asia and then swept through Europe. Some crossed to the Western Hemisphere. Some receded after a few years, but became established as a seasonal endemic disease in Asia and South America.

A cholera epidemic in 1832 claimed 6,000 lives in New Orleans, 3,500 in New York, 900 in Philadelphia, and 800 in Baltimore. The infection rate was high, if one compares the numbers with the total populations of the cities in 1832.

V. cholerae, the bacterium responsible for the epidemic of 1832, had contaminated common water supplies, especially those used by the poor. Medical help, even for those who might have afforded it, offered useless remedies. "Cures" consisted of bleeding the patient, or administering a strong purgative. These treatments only hastened the weakening, and sometimes contributed to hastening the death of patients.

A survey in 1833 of more than a hundred American physicians showed that only one believed that cholera was contagious. The rest attributed the sickness to miasmas—bad air.

John Snow, a British surgeon (1813–1858), was convinced that cholera was caused by an infective microbe. In cholera epidemics in England that followed the 1832 outbreak, Snow had an opportunity to test his belief. In an 1854 cholera epidemic, he knew that in one area of London, water was delivered to homes on each street by competing distributors. The South-wark and Vauxhall Company drew its water supply from the Thames River below major sewer outfalls. The Lambeth Company obtained its water supply from the same river before it flowed through London.

Snow studied official case incidence data. Then, he went house to house in the affected area to learn the source of the supplied water. Snow was able to compare the incidence of people drinking contaminated water with those drinking relatively pure water. He found that the infection rate in households supplied by Southwark and Vauxhall was 8.5 times higher in cholera infection than in households supplied by Lambeth.

As Snow was collecting his data, a serious focal outbreak occurred in his own home neighborhood of Soho, London. He interrupted his investigations of the water supply companies in order to address the Soho outbreak. He interviewed residents and mapped the location of homes with infected people. He concluded that the cause of this outbreak was from people in the area who were drawing water from a common street pump on Broad Street, and the source of the water had been contaminated by diarrheal discharges from infected people. Snow took unprecedented action. He recommended that authorities remove the pump handle, thus cutting off the water supply. Snow was credited for shortening the epidemic in the area. Actually, the outbreak had already peaked and had begun to subside before his intervention. Nevertheless, Snow deserves the accolade as the revered "patron saint" of pioneering epidemiology. His work demonstrated the value of inductive reasoning.

Snow was also an educator. He wrote a pamphlet, advising people not to use water for drinking or food preparation into which drains or sewers were emptied. If these measures were impractical, people should boil the water before using it. Snow also recommended that doctors should wash their hands after having any physical contacts with patients.

Cholera epidemics are not just past occurrences. From the late 1880s to the late 1900s, there was a pause. There were sporadic outbreaks, but no large epidemics. By the 1900s, this old scourge resurged vehemently.

The Widespread Cholera Epidemic of 1991

After a century of quiescence, except for some sporadic outbreaks, a widespread cholera epidemic erupted in 1991. It began in January in Peru, where cholera is endemic, and it grew rapidly. By April, the following year, Peru reported more than 400,000 probable cholera cases, and over 3,300 deaths. Before the epidemic ended, Peru had more than 600,000 cases and thousands of deaths.

The nature of the epidemic was characterized by a study in Peru's second largest city, Trujillo. Water was supplied to the city by a series of interconnected underground wells that formed a distribution system. The water was unchlorinated due to cost, lack of chlorine and chlorinators, and the mistaken belief that deep well water was safe. Illegal connections to the water line broke the system's integrity. Some of the illegal connections to the water system diverted untreated sewage to irrigate crops. Also, low and intermittent water pressure caused back-siphoning of contaminants into the well system. Water was available for only one or two hours each day, so many families stored water at home.

Among patients who sought treatment at Trujillos's largest hospital were those suffering from acute and severe diarrhea. *V. cholerae* was identified in most of the stool cultures. Many of the patients had drunk unboiled water taken from the stored containers in homes. Some had dipped their hands into the containers to wash, or to scoop out water. Some of the patients had attended fiestas or other social events at which they drank beverages prepared by many handlers and kept for long periods at room temperatures. Under such conditions, the beverages became good media for *V. cholerae* to grow rapidly, even in foods or beverages previously cooked.

In addition to contaminated water, other food items were associated with the Peruvian cholera outbreak. Frequently, raw seafood and produce such as cabbages, lettuces, carrots, and melons irrigated with raw sewage water, was eaten raw.

The strain of the 1991 outbreak that began in Peru was identified as *V. cholerae* O1. In an attempt to trace the source of the Peruvian outbreak, Pan American Health Organization officials thought that the vibrio had been carried in the bilge water from a Chinese freighter, and that the water had been discharged into the Lima harbor where it contaminated seafood used to prepare ceviche. Then, consumption of this raw seafood dish led to person-to-person transmission.

The 1991 cholera epidemic spread from Peru throughout most of South America, and affected large numbers of people. There were more than 70,000 cases in Ecuador; 17,000 in Bolivia; 14,000 in Colombia; and 10,000 in Brazil. The epidemic had become pandemic as it spread to Argentina, Chile, Guyana and French Guyana, Paraguay, Surinam, and Venezuela. The pandemic continued onward to Central America. There were more than 11,000 cases in Guatemala; 5,000 in El Salvador; and 4,000 in Mexico. People in Belize, Costa Rica, Honduras, Panama, and Nicaragua were affected, too.

Then, the pandemic spread to Asia. A new strain, *V. cholerae* O139 (mentioned earlier), had emerged. The strain affected at least eleven countries in southern Asia. The two strains *V. cholerae* O1 and *V. cholerae* O139 accounted for more than 100,000 cholera cases in Asian countries.

By 1993, when the Latin American and Asian outbreaks were waning, twenty-two cholera cases were reported in the United States. In the following year, forty-seven cases were reported. Of the total of these two years—sixty-nine cases—sixty-five were associated with foreign travel to countries where cholera outbreaks were occurring.

The CDC issued a warning to travelers planning to travel to cholera-affected areas. Among the recommendations, the CDC advised Americans to eat only well-cooked foods, especially fish and shellfish. Travelers should drink only bottled carbonated beverages or water that had been boiled or chlorinated. The CDC cautioned that the licensed parenteral (injected) cholera vaccine available, provided only limited and brief protection against *V. cholerae* O1 and might not provide any protection against *V. cholerae* O139. Therefore, the CDC could not recommend the vaccine for travelers. The new oral vaccine being developed at the time provided more reliable protection, but the CDC cautioned that none of the vaccines had attained a combination of high effectiveness, lengthy protection, easy administration, or low cost.

The CDC advised health professionals to consider the possibility of cholera in any patient with watery diarrhea who had returned within a week from a cholera-affected country. Doctors were told to report cases immediately to local and state health departments. Doctors should administer fluid and electrolyte replacement and antibiotic therapy to affected patients.

TRADITIONAL SUBSTANCES USED AGAINST CHOLERA

Aside from the quest for an effective vaccine to prevent cholera infection, Peruvians used some traditional methods. In the Amazon headwater region of Peru, the toronja fruit grows abundantly. "Toronja" is Spanish for grapefuit. People in the area found that they were somewhat protected against cholera infection by drinking the acidic juice of the toronja.

Lemon juice added to water also appeared to make the water safe to drink. This popular practice was tested. A 2 percent solution of lemon juice was added to water from an underground source. After thirty minutes, the lemon juice made potable water safe. The researchers recommended about two tablespoons of lemon juice per one liter of water. If the water source was very alkaline the amount of lemon juice needed to be increased.

Garlic has played a traditional role in Latin American cuisine. Allicin, a naturally occurring substance in garlic, has antimicrobial activity. Garlic extract has been shown to inhibit the growth of *V. cholerae*, as well as *Staphylococcus aureus*, *Salmonella typhosa*, and *Streptococcus viridans*.

A common phrase of wise advice given to travelers to avoid all types of diarrhea is applicable for cholera prevention. "Boil it, cook it, peel it, or forget it."

Cholera outbreaks will continue. Outbreaks anywhere threaten people everywhere. In the 1980s, Paul Blake, an enteric disease specialist at the CDC, wrote, "Up until about ten years ago we thought we could eradicate cholera. However, formerly we believed the organism lived only in humans. Now we recognize it can survive environmentally. We do not think it can be eradicated . . . What we have to aim for is control."

VIBRIO VULNIFICUS

Vibrio vulnificus, like *V. cholerae*, is a naturally present bacterium in estuarine waters worldwide. In the United States, it is commonly found in coastal waters in the Gulf of Mexico where it may contaminate shellfish. The most common transmission along the Gulf is with raw or lightly cooked oysters. Infectivity occurs mostly in warm weather, but it may occur throughout the year. Regardless of the source of the oysters, however, the potential for *V. vulnificus* infection exists wherever raw oysters are harvested and consumed. Most cases of infectivity involve raw oysters that have been in a distribution chain for more than one day, not from those freshly harvested and promptly consumed. This suggests that the toxicity of the pathogen increases over time, after the oysters are harvested and shipped, and during distribution without refrigeration.

V. vulnificus has been recognized as a pathogen since 1979. By 1994, at least eleven species of vibrios were known to be capable of causing serious human illness. In the United States, *V. vulnificus* emerged as the leading cause of death from foodborne illness in some areas of the country. *V. vulnificus* is a far more virulent vibrio than *V. cholerae*. Yet contamination does not change the appearance, taste, or odor of affected oysters.

HEALTH CONSEQUENCES OF *V. VULNIFICUS* INFECTION

Ingestion of *V. vulnificus*-contaminated raw or undercooked oysters can lead to fever, chills, nausea, abdominal pain and vomiting. It can result in gastroenteritis.

Often *V. vulnificus* is called "terror of the deep" because it has the highest fatality rate of any known foodborne bacterium or virus. Otherwise healthy individuals can be made seriously ill from *V. vulnificus* infection.

For persons with underlying health problems who are infected with *V. vulnificus*, the health risks are far greater. It is estimated that such persons are about 30 percent more susceptible to *V. vulnificus* infection than healthy individuals, and are 200 times more likely to die from the infection. From 50 to 60 percent of them are apt to die from primary septicemia (blood poisoning).

PERSONS AT HIGH RISK FOR *V. VULNIFICUS* INFECTION

Persons with liver disease are at increased risk for *V. vulnificus* infection and death. Such people are susceptible to all bacterial infections because of poor nutrition and defective blood-cell functions, including decreased bactericidal activity. Individuals with alcohol-related and other liver diseases, including iron overload disorders such as thalassemia major and hemochromatosis, also are at high risk for *V. vulnificus* infection.

People with compromised immune systems are at increased risk for *V. vulnificus* infection and death. These include people with AIDS and AIDS-related illnesses, chronic renal (kidney) insufficiency, cancer, diabetes, and steroid-dependent asthma accompanied by long-term treatment with systematic corticosteroid drugs.

People with chronic gastrointestinal diseases, including gastroenteritis and achlorhydria, are at high risk. Achlorhydria is the absence of hydrochloric acid in gastric secretions, and in those with therapeutically induced low gastric juices.

V. vulnificus can cause infection directly in otherwise healthy individuals by contaminating puncture wounds inflicted during shucking of contaminated raw oysters, or in removing contaminated raw lobster meat from their shells. Or, people with open wounds may become infected with *V. vulnificus* by exposure to seawater in swimming or in other marine activities. *V. vulnificus* that enters the body through open wounds can cause blistering tissue damage, or even death. The more virulent form of the bacterium has filamentous (threadlike) appendages that can adhere to human epithelial cells. (Several other bacteria, including *E. coli* have similar appendages to anchor themselves to their host's cells.)

V. VULNIFICUS OUTBREAKS AND ADVISORIES

There have been numerous *V. vulnificus* outbreaks in the United States, especially from raw or undercooked oysters harvested along the Gulf Coast. States along that coast maintain surveillance systems. Most of the

CAN SPICY HOT SAUCES
PROTECT AGAINST *V. VULNIFICUS*?

It was thought that the main ingredients in a traditional New Orleans cocktail sauce used with raw oysters were able to kill *V. vulnificus*. At least, the ingredients showed activity in laboratory experiments. Charles V. Sanders, leading a team from the Medical Center of Louisiana State University in New Orleans, tried to verify this belief by investigating the ingredients. The team was unable to attribute the lethal effect on *V. vulnificus* (as well as on *V. cholerae*) to any ingredient in the sauce. Whatever the ingredient was, it was more effective than other components in cocktail sauces such as horseradish, lemon, or ketchup. The research was conducted in a laboratory setting by adding Louisiana hot sauce to cultures of *V. vulnificus* grown in test tubes.

The investigation was pursued further, by Yi Sun and James D. Oliver, from the Department of Biology at the University of North Carolina at Charlotte. Sun and Oliver put either Tabasco brand hot sauce or horseradish-based seafood cocktail sauce on freshly shucked oysters on the half shell that previously had been incubated with *V. vulnificus* for ten minutes. The Tabasco sauce, but not the horseradish sauce, was highly effective in reducing the number of *V. vulnificus* bacteria on the oyster surfaces, but little reduction within the oysters. The researchers concluded that hot sauces are *not* capable of overall reduction of *V. vulnificus* to a safe level with raw oysters. Because of the strong infectivity of *V. vulnificus,* many public health officials believe that *the only safe level of the pathogen is zero.*

deaths have occurred in individuals with underlying health problems.

In 1991, after the death of an Oklahoma man from *V. vulnificus*-contaminated oysters, the Interstate Shellfish Sanitation Conference (ISSC) urged the FDA to mandate a federal label, warning consumers of the dangers associated with eating raw shellfish. The ISSC is a voluntary organization governed by an executive board that consists, in part, of the shellfish industry.

The FDA would not endorse any point-of-sale advisory. According to Thomas Billy, director of FDA's Office of Seafood, such an advisory might be unnecessary. Billy suggested that harvesting and handling controls, coupled with the FDA's educational brochures, might be sufficient measures to prevent illness. Groups such as the restaurant trade associations and oyster harvesters opposed any advisories, and pressured the FDA. The affected industry worried that advisories would shatter consumer confidence and lead to a drop in business.

Despite the FDA's reluctance, some states and local communities took actions on their own. In California, for example, state health officials were successful in having legislation pass in 1991 to require restaurants and grocery stores to post signs warning patrons and shoppers of the risks associated with eating raw oysters from the Gulf Coast states of Texas, Mississippi, Louisiana, Alabama, and Florida. The posted sign read: "Eating raw oysters may cause severe illness and even death in persons who have liver disease, cancer, or other chronic illnesses that weaken the immune system. If you eat raw oysters and become ill, you should seek immediate medical attention. If you are unsure if you are at risk, you should consult your physician."

The California regulations also required handlers and distributors to tag sacks of oysters, label containers, and keep records to facilitate prompt identification of the source, in the event of outbreaks of illness. These measures were to correct a broken traceback system. Nationwide, only about 40 percent of contaminated oysters could be traced back, due to faulty record keeping. Also, tags were missing or merely "tossed in a shoebox" by food preparers in many restaurants.

Florida followed suit by requiring posted warnings of possible risks, at all points of raw oyster sales. Louisiana required a warning that raw oysters, raw clams, and raw mussels can cause serious illness in persons with liver, stomach, blood, or immune disorders. Other Gulf Coast states took similar actions. Some states advised doctors to issue strong warnings to patients with liver disease about the potential for illnesses and death from

TEMPERATURE CONTROL

Pathogenic vibrios, including *V. vulnificus*, are found in 5 to 10 percent of all marketed raw shellfish. In addition to being present when shellfish is harvested, *V. vulnificus* may grow at temperatures higher than 41°F, whereas temperatures below 39.2°F appear to retard its growth. Cooked seafood is best stored at 39.2°F, or lower temperatures.

V. vulnificus as an infection secondary to eating raw oysters even when oysters are legally harvested and properly handled. The best measure is thorough cooking.

Despite all the advisories, medical advice, and the FDA's attempts to educate the public by issuance of brochures, these efforts appear ineffective. Many people continue to engage in the risky practice of consuming raw or undercooked oysters and other shellfish. Outbreaks, illnesses, and deaths continue from *V. vulnificus* infections. Caroline Ryan, a medical epidemiologist in the Enterics Branch of the CDC remarked, "I think eating raw oysters is the next best thing to going to the Third World."

VIBRIO PARAHAEMOLYTICUS

Vibrio parahaemolyticus is another vibrio associated with shellfish infection. It is a halophilic organism, which means that it requires sodium for growth. For this reason, it is distributed widely in marine environments, but rarely is associated with freshwater environments such as rivers and ponds. Frequently, *V. parahaemolyticus* is present in shellfish in estuaries and inshore coastal waters.

The highest concentrations of *V. parahaemolyticus* occur during warm weather. The pathogen is able to survive colder winter temperatures because of its affinity to chitinous materials (discarded shells from dead shellfish) and plankton. Both sink to the bottom of estuaries during the winter and provide nourishment for the *V. parahaemolyticus*. Then, as temperatures rise the following year, the *V. parahaemolyticus* reappear from the sediment and rise into the water.

In 1950, Japanese investigators were the first to identify *V. parahaemolyticus* as a foodborne pathogen present in shellfish. Later, the organism became recognized worldwide as a health hazard in seafood. It can cause gastroenteritis, and in some cases, septicemia and death. However, it is less virulent than *V. vulnificus*.

Cases of *V. parahaemolyticus* are less common than *V. vulnificus*, but the infections are believed to be underreported and underestimated. For example, in the United States, not all states require the reporting of this disease.

V. PARAHAEMOLYTICUS OUTBREAKS IN THE UNITED STATES

V. parahaemolyticus-associated epidemics with shellfish began to appear in the mid-1990s. The number of episodes kept increasing, and spreading.

At least one new strain emerged: *V. parahaemolyticus* O3:K6. Outbreaks appeared in India, the southeastern area of Japan, and by 1996, infection with the new strain became pandemic in Asia. The outbreaks reached parts of Europe (France and Spain) and South America (Chile), and by 1997 and 1998 three regions in the United States experienced multistate outbreaks, with more than 500 people made ill.

The Northwest outbreaks encompassed California, Oregon, and Washington, as well as contiguous British Columbia, Canada. More than 200 people were made ill, and one person died. The Canadians took swift action. After twenty people were sickened, and one made critically ill, a medical officer, John Blathewick ordered all restaurants in Vancouver and neighboring Richland to stop serving raw or undercooked oysters. On the U.S. side of the border, federal action was weak. The FDA merely advised consumers in the Pacific Northwest to practice caution when choosing fresh oysters. The term "fresh" was used, rather than "raw" possibly not to discourage sales at restaurants with oyster bars.

The Washington State Department of Health closed three oysterbed areas: Hood Canal, Totten Inlet (including Skookum Inlet), and Samish Bay to harvesting oysters intended for retail sale.

Another region struck was Long Island, New York. It was the first reported outbreak, ever, in the New York waters and the Northeast Atlantic Coast for *V. parahaemolyticus.* In the Northeast outbreak, more than 200 people were sickened and one died. The multistate outbreak affected people in New York, New Jersey and Connecticut.

The third region hit was Galveston Bay, Texas. In a multistate outbreak, *V. parahaemolyticus*-infected oysters had been shipped to California, Colorado, Florida, and Louisiana. The oysters had probably reached other states, in secondary distributions. The outbreak was blamed for at least 128 cases of illness, and led to a massive oyster recall. The entire Galveston Bay was closed to oyster harvesting.

Risk Assessment of *V. parahaemolyticus*

After these three regional outbreaks in the United States, federal authorities admitted that they lacked information about *V. parahaemolyticus* to make a risk assessment of its potential health impact. There were numerous data gaps. The FDA requested scientific data on the frequency of occurrences of pathogenic strains of *V. parahaemolyticus* in shellfish waters. The agency also sought information about the parameters, such as water temperature, salinity, turbidity, and nutrient profiles, to use as indicators for the presence of the bacterium in waters. The agency wanted to determine the numbers of viable pathogenic cells present in contaminated shellfish at the time of their consumption. Evidence from outbreaks showed that levels as low as 100 to 1,000 cells per gram of food had caused illness. Yet in the risk assessment, completed in 2001, 10,000 or fewer cells per gram of food were deemed acceptable. A heated argument followed, pitting consumers against the affected industry. The former wanted stringent regulations; the latter, more relaxed ones.

In 2001, the General Accountability Office (formerly the General Accounting Office—GAO), an investigative branch of the U.S. Congress, conducted its own investigation on the safety of shellfish. By then, more than 100,000 people in the United States were being made ill each year from contaminated shellfish from various infective agents.

The GAO learned that the FDA collected so little information on the safety of shellfish that the agency could not determine whether its efforts to improve inspections and reduce illnesses yielded any significant results. Instead, the FDA relied on the states to conduct inspection of processing plants and to identify contaminants. The FDA did little to check on the states, or on the patrolling of coasts to stop the practice of dumping waste from boats in waters inhabited by shellfish. Instead of reviewing state reports, the FDA measured compliance with the rules by visiting as little as 5 percent of shellfish processors in some states—a rate deemed by the GAO and some lawmakers as wholly inadequate. In reaction to this GAO information, Senator Tom Harkin (D-IA) asked, "How can consumers have confidence in a food safety agency that does not even know how well it is doing?"

The specter of vibrios and other infections eroded confidence in raw shellfish. Many seafood restaurants and stores nationwide discontinued offering them, fearing liability suits.

In 2001, Red Lobster, the nation's largest seafood chain, chose another approach. The only raw oysters from the Gulf Coast that the chain served were treated first to kill the bacteria.

Costco, a wholesaler, began selling only oysters that had been treated. R. Craig Wilson, vice president for food safety at Costco, reported, "Before that, I refused to allow anyone to buy them."

V. PARAHAEMOLYTICUS IS STILL WITH US

V. parahaemolyticus-infected raw shellfish is not merely a problem of the past. It is still with us. As recently as 2006, there was another multistate outbreak in the East, in New York City, and in the West, in Oregon and Washington. Both regions experienced repeats from the late 1990s.

The numbers of people affected in New York City in the 2006 outbreak were much higher than expected, and were greater than the yearly averages for the entire United States, between the years of 2000 and 2004.

Traceback investigations in the Washington-Oregon outbreak in 2006 associated it with contaminated oysters and clams harvested in the state of Washington and in British Columbia, Canada. Shellfish from those sources were distributed nationwide to seafood markets and restaurants.

It is likely that *V. parahaemolyticus*, as well as other vibrio-contaminated shellfish, will continue to be a health risk. All pathogenic vibrios are found in 5 to 10 percent of the total marketed raw shellfish. In addition to being present when shellfish is harvested, as mentioned earlier, the vibrios increase in the shellfish over time, especially at warm temperatures. Sufficiently cold temperatures retard the growth. Shellfish needs to be kept cold, not only before cooking but also if stored after cooking. Shellfish should be eaten promptly. From the above discussion, it should be apparent that for safety, shellfish should be well cooked, and not eaten raw.

CHAPTER 12

Yersinia: From Gastroenteritis to Septicemia

In 1982, a woman in Arkansas gave her three-year-old child some milk she had bought from the local grocery store. She had been buying the same brand for years, and liked it. The milk had been pasteurized in a dairy in Memphis, Tennessee.

On this occasion, her child became ill after drinking the milk. He had diarrhea, abdominal pain, and fever. The next day, he had a sore throat and felt achy all over. The child was hospitalized and underwent an appendectomy. The surgery was unnecessary, due to misdiagnosis of the child's ailment. Actually, he was suffering from yersiniosis from contaminated milk.

Yersinia *enterocolitica* is a foodborne bacterium of growing concern to public health officials, federal regulatory agencies, food processors, and the consuming public. Like *Listeria* (see Chapter 8), *Y. enterocolitica* is a psychrotroph that continues to grow in foods held at temperatures as low as 32°F. It can reach infectious levels within four days of refrigerated storage. Often *Y. enterocolitica* is found in the digestive tract of animals. It can contaminate raw and cooked foods from animal sources, and foods such as pork, beef, lamb, poultry, both raw and pasteurized milk, and shellfish such as crab, oyster, and shrimp. However, with the exception of pork, the isolates from most foods of animal sources are not pathogenic to humans. Pork is the exception. Pathogenic strains of *Y. enterocolitica* have been identified in the oral cavities and tongues of pigs; in raw or under-cooked pork; and even in processed pork products.

CHARACTERISTICS OF *YERSINIA*

The genus *Yersinia* is comprised of three species of bacteria that cause human diseases. *Y. enterocolitica* inflicts a range of classic food-poisoning symptoms, usually of limited duration, but also can inflict chronic health disorders. Only some serotypes cause disease. *Y. pseudotuberculosis* causes diarrhea and emaciation. It can be fatal. *Y. pestis*, the most virulent species, causes plague. In previous centuries, it killed a significant portion of the world's population. It was the infamous "black plague" of the fifteenth century, which reduced the European population by some 23 million. However, plague is not a long-eradicated infection of the past. Recent sporadic cases have occurred in the United States and elsewhere.

In recent times, *Y. enterocolitica* (serotype O:3) has become a major cause of food poisoning in Europe, especially in cool regions. Outbreaks have occurred in Belgium, the Netherlands, Finland, Sweden, Germany, Ireland, and Italy. Elsewhere, outbreaks have occurred in Australia, Japan, and Canada. In many countries, *Y. enterocolitica* has surpassed a major foodborne disease, *Shigella*, and rivals *Salmonella* as a cause of acute gastroenteritis.

In a case-controlled study, Robert V. Tauxe and his colleagues from the Centers for Disease Control and Prevention (CDC) attempted to determine the risk factors of yersiniosis in Belgium, where the incidence of the infection is high. The researchers found that the onset of the disease was associated strongly with raw pork consumption two weeks earlier.

To date, *Y. enterocolitica* has not been as severe in the United States as elsewhere. But the true incidence of *Y. enterocolitica* is unknown. It is suspected that the infection is underreported. The predominant European serotype O:3 of *Yersinia* has emerged on the East Coast of the United States, where there have been a few large food-associated outbreaks and some sporadic cases.

Y. enterocolitica was identified as a human pathogen in 1939, but was unrecognized as a foodborne pathogen until the mid-1970s. We now know that, in addition to foods from animal sources, other sources of *Y. enterocolitica* contamination include untreated water. Additional sources are ethnic dishes, such as chitterlings and brawn (both to be discussed shortly). Vehicles for *Yersinia* transmission include blood transfusions, infected companion animals, flies, and dirt.

Yersiniosis shows seasonal variation. Most cases occur in the autumn and wintertime. Different serotypes are found in various regions of the world. In the United States, sporadic cases are associated with several serotypes, but the most commonly reported one associated with outbreaks is *Y. enterocolitica* O:8.

SOME HEALTH CONSEQUENCES OF YERSINIOSIS

Although yersiniosis is not among the main foodborne infections in the United States, its consequences can be grave. The severity of the acute infection may be exacerbated in persons with iron overload, and can result in septicemia (blood poisoning), which can be fatal.

Arthritis has been identified as an infrequent but significant consequence of yersiniosis. Reactive arthritis (ReA) especially may be involved. This condition usually is initiated by an infection in a genetically predisposed individual. Typically, it is characterized by recurrences of arthritis, conjunctivitis, and urethritis. (See Chapter 2.)

Within a year of *Yersinia* infection, people were at increased risk of developing ReA according to the findings of Anders Ternhag and associates at the Karolinska Institute in Stockholm, Sweden. The group found that an episode of acute enteric infection, such as *Yersinia*, involving extraintestinal organs (apart from the gastrointestinal tract), can lead to complications and trigger chronic diseases. The complications include ReA, as well as irritable bowel syndrome (IBS), hemolytic uremic syndrome (HUS, described in Chapter 2), and Guillain-Barré syndrome (GBS, described in Chapter 5). The researchers suggested that there may be other late effects of acute enteric infections, perhaps unusual and less documented, such as inflammatory bowel disease (IBD). In Sweden (and in the United States) there is no active followup on reported cases of bacterial enteric infection, in terms of disease outcome or long-term complications.

"Certain individuals may suffer chronic joint diseases, such as reactive arthritis, after being infected with bacteria ingested with food," reported James L. Smith, formerly at the U.S. Department of Agriculture's (USDA) Agricultural Research Service (ARS), Eastern Regional Research Center at Wyndmoor, Pennsylvania, where for years he had studied the relationship of foodborne bacteria and arthritis. Then, as a collaborator and microbiologist emeritus at the Center's Microbial Food Safety Research Unit, in 1996, he announced his findings that *Y. enterocolitica*, as well as *Campylobacter, Salmonella*, and *Shigella*, may lead to ReA. Such pathogens can lead to inflammation of an organ or joint that is far removed from the infection site.

Smith explained, "When we think of bacterially induced arthritis, it's usually the septic type in which the infecting organism is present in the joint. As it grows there, it can cause inflammation and destruction of joint tissue. In reactive arthritis (ReA), organisms are not present in the joint.

Antigenic components of the infecting bacteria are there, but visible, living organisms are not."

Smith continued, "Genetic makeup may predispose individuals to reactive arthritis. No one knows why, but individuals carrying the gene responsible for producing the human leucocyte antigen HLA-B27 are more susceptible to arthritis. We do know that the molecular structure of antigens from these particular foodborne bacteria mimic the HLA antigens. It has been suggested that this antigen mimicry could be a mechanism for causing arthritis."

The HLA-B27 gene is found in about 10 percent of healthy Caucasians, 1 percent of Japanese, and up to 4 percent of African Americans, but is absent from Africans and African Australians. Only about 2 percent of people who suffer from food poisoning develop arthritis, but about 20 percent of those infected develop arthritis if they also have the HLA-B27 gene. "For most people, an infection from foodborne bacteria just means

MECHANISM OF *YERSINIA* AND ITS VIRULENCE

The *Yersinia* bacteria first invade the ileum's mucosa, and then the pathogens multiply within Peyer's patches. These are large oval patches of closely aggregated lymph follicles in the walls of the small intestines, especially in the ileum. The patches disappear partially or fully in advanced age. In certain infections, such as typhoid fever, they become a targeted place for ulceration, which may perforate the intestines. (Sometimes, Peyer's patches are called the Peyerian glands, named after Johann K. Peyer, an early eighteeth-century physician and anatomist.) The *Yersinia* then migrate to lymph nodes and can become a systemic infection. As soon as the *Yersiniae* penetrate the intestinal epithelium, they are enveloped by phagocyte cells such as macrophages. The organisms recede within vacuoles of these cells and multiply within them. Vacuoles are small cavities in the cytoplasm of cells. They are bound by single membranes and contain water, nourishment, and metabolic waste.

The virulence of *Yersinia* depends on a certain plasmid (40-48MD) that encodes for several virulence-related antigens. There are two types of virulent *Y. enterocolitica* strains: O.8 and O.21. Given orally to laboratory mice, both produce fatal infections. Strains O:3, O:5,27, and O:9 colonize in the intestines of laboratory mice and lead to chronic diarrhea and death.

feeling rotten for a day or so. But for the unfortunate few, it can mean the severe hardship of arthritis," Smith observed.

In addition to ReA, yersiniosis has been associated with pneumonia, and inflammations of vertebrae, lymphatic glands, liver, and spleen. Also, yersiniosis has been linked to inflammations in various parts of the body, including the intestines, skin, and brain.

Y. enterocolitica O:3 may be responsible for a phenomenon known as "molecular mimicry" (described earlier on page 11) that can trigger autoimmune thyroid disorders, especially Graves' disease. Some evidence suggests that *Y. enterocolitica* can mimic the effects of the body's own thyroid-stimulating hormone, influence the autoimmune system, and cause suppressor-cell dysfunction.

SOURCES OF *Y. ENTEROCOLITICA* CONTAMINATION

Pigs are regarded as the major reservoir for *Y. enterocolitica.* Many investigators believe that the pathogenic strains of the organism are normal residents of pigs, and that these animals play a major role in the epidemiology of human yersiniosis. Indirectly, rats also may be involved. Rats residing in slaughterhouses may carry virulent strains of *Yersinia* from pig wastes. Foods in contact with contaminated raw pork or swine waste are likely vehicles for sporadic human yersiniosis cases by cross-contamination.

In an investigation, more than nine of ten lots of swine ready for market contained one pig with *Y. enterocolitica*, according to the findings of researchers from the College of Veterinary Medicine at the University of Illinois (*Journal of Food Protection*, June 1999). It is thought that too little attention has been given to this problem in the United States, even though yersiniosis is thought to cause from 3,000 to 20,000 cases of human disease annually in this country.

Chitterlings as a Source of Yersiniosis

Chitterlings (or chitlins) are a favored ethnic dish for some African Americans. They are served at holidays such as Thanksgiving, Christmas, and the New Year. Chitterlings are prepared by boiling the large intestines of pigs after fat and fecal matter are removed. Because chitterlings traditionally are boiled thoroughly, the final cooked product is unlikely to be contaminated bacterially. The preparation process, however, involves substantial handling of large amounts of a potentially contaminated product, and the risk is high for infants exposed to this process.

From November 1988 to January 1989, fourteen African-American infants averaging three months of age, and one young boy fourteen years of age, were made ill at the time that their mothers were preparing chitterlings in Atlanta, Georgia. All the children had diarrhea and fever. Some had small streaks of blood in their stools. They vomited and were irritable. The illnesses lasted from three to twenty-eight days. Seven children required hospitalization.

The mothers had prepared the chitterlings two weeks before the onset of illness in the children. The infants had not been in direct contact with raw chitterlings. But some of the women who prepared the dish remembered later that they had touched the children while cleaning the chitterlings. On one occasion, the mother of the fourteen-year-old boy remembered that he had touched the raw chitterlings as she was cleaning them, and he had not washed his hands afterward.

After this outbreak, raw chitterlings were tested from several regions of the United States. More than half of them contained *Y. enterocolitica* O:3. This finding suggested that recently this serotype had become widespread in the American swine population. The appearance of an animal reservoir, and the occurrence of the outbreak, probably signified that *Y. enterocolitica* O:3 was an important emerging enteric pathogen in the United States.

In 2002, another outbreak of *Y. enterocolitica* associated with chitterlings occurred with infants in Chicago. The following year, there was a similar outbreak in Tennessee. An investigation found that infants were roaming freely in walkers in the room where women were cleaning chitterlings. Water used to clean the chitterlings splashed on clean dishes and on baby bottles. Also, the baby bottles were washed in a sink not thoroughly cleaned after washing chitterlings. Contamination also resulted by handing a pacifier to an infant during the cleaning or preparation of chitterlings.

The CDC launched an educational program through the WIC program (Women, Infants, and Children) on feeding. However, the CDC noted that "Attempts to educate the public and change traditional methods of preparation have been unsuccessful in preventing chitterling-associated outbreaks, and vulnerable 'innocent bystanders' continue to be affected by the disease."

Brawn as a Source of Yersiniosis

Another pork-based ethnic dish has been associated with yersiniosis. Christmas brawn ("julesylte") is a Norwegian specialty prepared by layering precooked head muscles of pork and veal, with lard and spices in a mold. After cooking the mixture, it is removed from the mold. Commercial brawn may be vacuum-packed for sale. *Y. enterocolitica* can survive in MAP (modified atmosphere packaging). Usually the brawn is whole, but sometimes it is sliced. At some delicatessens, the packages are opened, and the product is sold in slices. This dish is also prepared in homes.

Correct cooking of brawn should eliminate *Y. enterocolitica*, but microbiologic analyses have shown that bacteria can survive in the interior of the molded food. Lard, with its high-fat content, can enhance the bacteria's chance of survival. Cross-contamination can occur if strict hygiene procedures are not observed when the brawn is removed from the mold before packing. Slicing can spread any organisms present throughout the product. *Yersinia's ability to grow at refrigerated temperatures may further compound the problem.* There have been yersiniosis outbreaks from contaminated brawn. The most recent one occurred in 2007 in Norway.

Milk as a Source of Yersiniosis

The frequent presence of *Y. enterocolitica* in raw milk, and the ability of the organism to survive and replicate at refrigerated temperatures, make milk a potential vehicle for yersiniosis. This is especially true if the milk is pasteurized inadequately or mishandled after pasteurization.

In the 1970s, *Y. enterocolitica* outbreaks began to appear in milk, both raw and pasteurized. In 1974, children who drank raw milk in Montreal developed yersiniosis. The pathogen was identified in outbreaks in the United States in 1974 and 1979 with pasteurized milk, but no illnesses were associated with the outbreaks. Generally, *Y. enterocolitica* does not survive standard pasteurization, but it may survive pasteurization if the pathogen is present in large numbers.

In 1976, a yersiniosis outbreak occurred in New York State from contaminated chocolate-flavored milk. The cause was probably the addition of ingredients to the milk after pasteurization.

Although yersiniosis rarely has been associated with pasteurized milk in the United States, a large multistate outbreak occurred in 1982, and affected people in Arkansas, Tennessee, Missouri, and Mississippi. The source of the outbreak was a dairy plant in Memphis. At least 148 persons developed enteric infections with diarrhea and/or abdominal pains, accompanied by fever. Twenty-four of these persons had additional infections in the throat, blood, urinary tract, central nervous system, and wounds. Almost half the cases were children younger than five years of age. Most of the affected people required hospitalization. Seventeen of the patients were misdiagnosed and underwent needless appendectomies. Investigators of the outbreak thought that the likely cause of yersiniosis was cross-contamination. The source was pig-manure crates used to deliver outdated pasteurized milk to a pig farm. The same vehicle was used to deliver fresh pasteurized milk for human consumption to stores.

Because of the psychrophilic nature of *Yersinia* species, dairy-plant coolers and freezers must be sanitized to prevent colonization and proliferation of the pathogen. Todd Pritchard and his colleagues at the University of Vermont in Burlington surveyed dairy processing plants. Twenty of the 357 sites investigated showed one or more *Yersinia* strains present. Half the contaminated samples were from coolers and entrances to freezers. The researchers noted that "a very real possibility" exists for post-pasteurization contamination with *Yersinia*.

Eggs as a Source of Yersiniosis

Mohammed K. Amin and Frances A. Draugton at the Department of Food Science and Technology of the University of Tennessee, Knoxville, found that "*Yersinia* contaminates eggs in a manner analogous to common egg spoilage microorganisms and species of *Salmonella*. *Yersinia* can penetrate egg shells and subsequently infect egg contents due to improper washing, storage, or handling conditions."

Yersinia can penetrate the shell of an egg and infect its contents. If contaminated eggs are eaten raw, as in uncooked eggnog, uncooked mayonnaise, or Caesar salad; or undercooked as in "runny" eggs where the whites are not set firmly, as with lightly scrambled eggs or meringues, the result may be yersiniosis.

Water as a Source of Yersiniosis

Contaminated spring water and stream water were identified as sources of yersiniosis. Contaminated water was the vehicle in a large 1982 outbreak in the United States. Tofu was packed in untreated spring water, contaminated with *Y. enterocolitica* O:8. The outbreak occurred in the state of Washington. Eighty-seven persons were made ill after eating the tofu. Many had fever, abdominal pain, diarrhea, nausea, vomiting, bloody stools, joint pains, and skin rashes. The symptoms lasted from one day to four weeks. Two patients were ill for more than two months. Seventeen of them required hospitalization for two to seven days. Two of the hospitalized patients, misdiagnosed, underwent appendectomies, and a third, also misdiagnosed, underwent a partial colectomy (excision of part of the colon). Two patients suffered from other foodborne infections as well. In addition to yersiniosis, one had salmonellosis from *Salmonella* Typhimurium and the other, a rotaviral infection.

Investigation of this outbreak of locally produced tofu found that the water supply used to pack the tofu came from an untreated nearby stream. Inspection of the plant disclosed unsanitary conditions, including dirty equipment, use of an outdoor privy, and poor personal hygiene.

In another outbreak, commercial bean sprouts had been rinsed in contaminated water.

Blood as a Source of Yersiniosis

People can carry *Y. enterocolitica* asymptomatically. This feature has led to clinically normal people donating blood that has caused septicemia in recipient patients given transfusions. From 1985 to 1997, there were at least twelve deaths in the United States attributed to *Y. enterocolitica*-contaminated blood transfusions.

TESTS TO DETECT *Y. ENTEROCOLITICA*

Until the early 1990s, testing for *Y. enterocolitica* required days to complete. The testing was cumbersome, unreliable, and inconclusive. This changed in 1991, when a USDA molecular biologist, Saumya Bhaduri, developed and patented a test that could detect *Y. enterocolitica* accurately within minutes, and distinguish between harmful and harmless strains of the pathogen. Bhaduri used a crystal violet dye to bind the disease-causing strains of the pathogen. The technique did not allow for further testing because it killed the pathogen. However, the rapid detection made the test useful for investigators of infective outbreaks to identify the pathogen.

Another patented test uses Congo red dye. This test proves to be especially helpful when it is essential to isolate the organism but keep it alive for more detailed study. This test is useful in field laboratories of food processing plants, hospitals, and sewage treatment facilities.

In 1991, bacteremia (bacteria in the blood) and endotoxin shock were associated with *Yersinia*-contaminated blood, and resulted in serious adverse reactions, including deaths.

In the United States, it was found that all units of the blood that caused fatalities had been stored for more than twenty-five days. A Food and Drug Administration (FDA) advisory committee, in discussions about possible measures to reduce adverse reactions, recommended against reducing the blood storage time, fearing shortages. Instead, they suggested continuation of a program of publicizing information about the possibility of bacteremia due to blood transfusions. Additionally, physicians were urged to report cases of transfusion-associated *Y. enterocolitica* infections to the CDC through state health departments. However, reporting was not mandatory.

With heightened public awareness of the potential risks for transfusion-transmitted diseases, both patients and physicians became more knowledgeable about the benefits of autologous donations (blood drawn from individuals and then used for their transfusions). However, even this practice carries risks.

In 1991, a seventy-four-year-old man with a four-year history of osteoarthritis donated four units of his own blood in anticipation of its use during an operation for a total knee replacement. Prior to the operation, a registered nurse took a complete medical history, which indicated no bacterial infection. The man's blood was drawn four times, and stored refrigerated. For the first transfusion, the oldest unit of blood was administered. It had been stored for forty-one days. The patient became confused and cyanotic (lacking an adequate amount of oxygen in the blood). He experienced respiratory distress, with wheezing, shortness of breath, and severe shaking chills. Further transfusions for him were drawn from donor blood, and the patient experienced no further incidents. As follow-up, the stored patient's blood units were cultured, and found to contain *Y. enterocolitica*. This was the first reported case of *Yersinia* transmission by an autologous unit of blood.

CHAPTER 13

Hepatitis: A Virus Linked to Liver Disorders

In 1999, a thirty-eight-year-old man, his wife, and two daughters ordered food at a popular Mexican-style restaurant. Several weeks later, the man thought that he had the flu. He felt achy and nauseous. Over-the-counter medication and rest failed to help. He was taken to the University of Pittsburgh Medical Center. He was suffering from acute liver failure, and his other organs were shutting down. Surgeons transplanted a liver, flown from California, but the man died. His liver failure was caused by hepatitis A virus infection. He was the first of three persons to die, and many more made ill, in what federal health officials designated as the largest foodborne outbreak, to date, in the United States, from foodborne hepatitis A virus infection. The source of the contamination was traced to scallions served in the restaurant.

Hepatitis is a viral disease that infects the liver. Different forms of hepatitis are attributed to different genuses.

Hepatitis A virus is food- and waterborne. Hepatitis viruses B and C are spread by contact with infected blood and other body fluids from people who are infected, through sex of men with men, needle sharing, hemodialysis, or (rarely) a blood transfusion. Health workers exposed to infected patients are at high risk.

Hepatitis viruses A, B, and C lead to acute and chronic liver diseases worldwide.

Non-A and non-B hepatitis are caused by at least two distinct viral agents, transmitted by the fecal-oral route, person to person, or by inadequate sewage disposal.

Hepatitis D acts in combination with hepatitis B. It is found especially in Italy, Eastern Europe and Russia, and among drug addicts in the United Kingdom.

Hepatitis E is unrelated to other hepatitis viruses. It is food- and waterborne, and is transmitted from raw sewage.

Several new or mutant hepatitis strains were discovered in the early to mid-1990s. One international research team reported finding another hepatitis virus, which they named hepatitis F. The identification requires confirmation. During the same period, other researchers identified a cluster of viruses associated with hepatitis. Among scientists, they are known as the hepatitis G viruses.

Both hepatitis A and hepatitis E viruses are listed as "severe hazards" in the Food and Drug Administration's (FDA) Food Code, Appendix V (1995). This chapter will focus on hepatitis A and hepatitis E.

HEPATITIS A

The hepatitis A virus (HAV) became recognized in the 1940s. The first association was with shellfish outbreaks from oysters in Sweden. By the mid-1950s, the virus was recognized worldwide. Initially, the virus was called "epidemic jaundice" and later "infectious hepatitis."

Most foodborne viral diseases are caused by HAV, and by Norwalk-like viruses, or small round structured viruses (SRSV), now renamed noroviruses (see Chapter 9). Public health officials regard HAV of such importance that medical practitioners in all states are required to report it. This action is not mandatory for other viral diseases.

PRE-EXPOSURE AND POST-EXPOSURE PROTECTION

The CDC recommends routine vaccination of children as the most effective measure to reduce hepatitis A incidence nationwide over time for the entire population. Because most children with HAV infection are asymptomatic, they play an important role in HAV transmission to other people. The vaccination also provides pre-exposure protection for adults and for those who are at high risk for infections, such as persons with chronic liver disease.

Individuals who travel to countries where HAV is endemic are advised to have immune globulin administered as a preventive measure, or to have it administered as a protective post-exposure measure.

It is thought that HAV is responsible for more foodborne illnesses than many better-known bacterial foodborne pathogens. In compiled data, the Centers for Disease Control and Prevention (CDC) found HAV to be the fourth leading cause of foodborne infections.

THE RESILIENCE OF HAV

HAV is resistant to freezing, drying, acid-treatment, various solvents, and irradiation. When researchers wish to store HAV samples for future study, they freeze the virus because it survives freezing, and can be studied at a later date. HAV has been found to survive drying in the environment for at least a month.

Harsher treatment is required. HAV is destroyed in food by high heat. HAV is inactivated on contaminated surfaces by household bleach.

In 1999, Israel had instituted a universal immunization program against HAV. By 2006, the incidence of the infection declined. In the United States, a similar decline was noted in several states after implementing childhood vaccination programs against HAV.

Despite the decline, every year about a hundred people die in the United States from acute liver failure due to HAV. In addition, persons with chronic liver disease, if infected with HAV, are at greater risk of developing fulminating hepatitis, a condition that occurs suddenly and with great intensity.

SIGNS AND SYMPTOMS OF HAV INFECTION

The HAV infection displays many of the signs and symptoms of other food- and waterborne infections, but also has some signs and symptoms that are characteristic of HAV.

The infection can be symptomatic or asymptomatic. In children under six years of age, some 70 percent may be asymptomatic. Usually, such children do not show signs of jaundice, which is one of the characteristic signs of the infection.

In older children and adults, more than 70 percent are symptomatic, and show signs of jaundice. This condition is characterized by yellowish discoloration of skin, sclerae (whites of the eyes), and mucous membranes. The discoloration is caused by bile salts being deposited in these tissues because the liver has lost its normal ability to process the bile. The discoloration extends to certain body fluids, and the excreted urine may be dark in color. All these discolorations signify a liver disorder.

The signs and symptoms of HAV infection manifest themselves long after the infection actually occurs. The lag time may be from fifteen to fifty days after the infection, and usually averages four weeks. Yet, it is during this asymptomatic phase that the infection is most contagious. Infected persons are capable of transmitting the infection to many other people long before they realize that they, themselves, are ill.

The onset of signs and symptoms may be abrupt but similar to those that accompany many foodborne infections: diarrhea, vomiting, nausea, abdominal pain, loss of appetite, and fever. After a few days, the signs of jaundice appear. The HAV replicate in the liver, excrete in the bile, and shed in the stool. The peak of infectivity is within two weeks before the onset of symptoms and jaundice or an elevation of liver enzymes, when the virus is concentrated at its highest amount in the stool. Within a week after the onset of symptoms and when jaundice appears, the concentration of the virus declines in the stool.

The symptoms can be severe, especially in people with liver disease. The infection can cause permanent impairment of liver functions. This feature is important, because the liver has numerous functions in the body. (To learn more about these functions, see the inset opposite.)

HEPATITIS E

Hepatitis E virus (HEV), a food- and waterborne infection, is transmitted from raw sewage. In the past, it rarely had been experienced in developed countries, but had been common in developing countries, and endemic in Pakistan, India, Central and Southeast Asia, the Middle East, Africa, China, and Mexico.

The incubation period of HEV is from two to nine weeks. Those at highest risk are persons from fifteen to forty years of age, and pregnant women. It causes intrauterine infections, and can result in the death of up to 20 percent of pregnant women. Also, their offspring may suffer illnesses or death.

The fecal shedding in patients can last for as long as seven weeks, and may contribute to the contamination of water supplies, and result in water- and foodborne contamination. HEV is considered to be a major health risk.

Researchers discovered a new strain of HEV in the United States in 1997. It is known as HEV-US-1. It is only the third known HEV strain in the world. HEV is a major contributor to fulminating hepatitis and liver failure in developing countries, and it is especially devastating to pregnant women.

SOURCES OF HAV INFECTION

Shellfish, including clams, cockles, mussels, and oysters, can transmit viruses to humans when the waters in which they grow are contaminated with raw sewage. Produce can be contaminated when the crops are irri-

THE LIVER: AN IMPORTANT ORGAN

Because the liver is so strongly affected by hepatitis infections it is important to understand its functions and how they can be impaired. One of the liver's key roles is to synthesize and store important molecules such as blood, proteins, sugars, fats, vitamins, and minerals. The liver regulates the blood level of many of these nutrients. Another important role of the liver is to act as the body's main detoxification mechanism. Virtually everything that enters the body passes through the liver, where it is subjected to transformation by the liver's detoxification processes. If these substances are not soluble, the liver makes them soluble, so that they can be excreted readily in the urine or bile. In its detoxification role, the liver attempts to eliminate potential poisons from the body before they can do harm.

Currently, it is estimated that we are exposed to more than 100,000 xenobiotics (substances foreign to the body, such as chemical compounds and pesticides) in our environment, in addition to prescription and over-the-counter drugs. The liver must transform all these substances after they have entered the body, and eliminate them. In addition, many microorganisms in the gut produce toxins and enzymes that create toxic molecules from other molecules that undergo enterohepatic (involving the intestine and the liver) recirculation. When pathogens enter the gut, the beneficial microbes present play an important role in detoxification. The gut is responsible for the "first pass" metabolism of xenobiotics that enter through the digestive tract. Detoxification takes place at the tips of microvilli of the small intestine. When the gut mucosa is healthy, detoxification is efficient, and lessens the demands on the liver for detoxification. The detoxification functions of the liver, as well as the gut, work best when these organs are healthy.

gated with contaminated water. Any food can become tainted with HAV by infected handlers, all along the food chain, from farm to table.

Even when food is suspected of HAV contamination, it is difficult to detect because of the small quantity of virus relative to the size of the food sample. Also, for identification, HAV does not grow well in cell culture.

PERSONS AT HIGH RISK FOR HAV INFECTION

International travelers are at high risk, especially if they travel to areas of the world where HAV is endemic. Other persons at high risk for infection are those with clotting-factor disorders such as hemophiliacs, users of injected drugs, and on rare occasions, those who require blood transfusions. Other individuals at high risk are men who have sex with other men, persons working with primates born in the wild, and those with chronic liver disease, which can lead to fulminating hepatitis.

HIGH-RISK SETTINGS FOR HAV INFECTION

Certain environmental settings place persons at high risk for HAV infection. Day-care centers are high-risk areas. Young toddlers frequently are sources of transmissions. Numerous outbreaks of HAV infections at such facilities led the CDC to collect surveillance data. The findings showed that from 13 to 15 percent of all reported cases of HAV infection were of children in day-care centers. In turn, infected children infected other children as well as workers at the facilities. The CDC found that diapered children, under three years of age, were the most likely to be infected. The CDC noted that some diaper-changing facilities in the centers were inadequate, and inappropriate containers held soiled diapers. Frequently, adults who changed diapers also served as food preparers. Often, there was no routine daily cleaning of furniture, surfaces, or objects such as toys that young children might lick, or attempt to put into their mouths. Some infected children and workers attended such centers, even though they should have remained at home. Some infected workers who attended the centers spread the infection to children and other workers. Some apparently non-infected children were transferred to other centers. Yet, they may have been infected but were asymptomatic. The CDC recommended changes in day-care center procedures. In addition, the CDC suggested that for six weeks after the last recognized case of infection at a day-care center, new admissions of children should be suspended, or the new children should be required to receive immune globulin.

Another environmental setting that places people at high risk for HAV infection is restaurants. Just one infected food handler can infect large numbers of people. This feature is demonstrated in recent outbreaks that will be discussed shortly. Other environmental settings include health-care institutions and places for those with developmental disabilities, schools, and sewage facilities.

LARGE OUTBREAKS OF HAV INFECTION

As part of the U.S. Department of Agriculture's (USDA) school lunch program, any foods distributed to schools must be grown in the United States. The reason for this policy is twofold. First, use of surplus domestic commodities helps support American farmers. (The choice of surplus crops may be unrelated to the nutritional needs of children.) Second, limiting the choices to domestic crops is a tacit admission that domestic crops have a somewhat better record of safety than their imported counterparts. Against this background, in 1997 the USDA distributed frozen strawberries to schools in many states as part of the school lunch program.

A Case of Tainted Illegal Berries

In March 1997, more than 200 children and teachers were made ill from HAV infection in Calhoun County, Michigan. Soon, more children and teachers were affected in other states including Maine, Wisconsin, Louisiana, and California. The infection was transmitted by frozen strawberries served in the schools.

Investigators of the outbreaks learned that the strawberries had *not* been grown domestically, but had been imported from Mexico. They had been certified falsely. The company had used three unwitting food brokers in New York and California to disguise the fact that the strawberries were foreign grown. A false certification of origin had been submitted to the USDA as "100 percent grown domestically."

During a U.S. House of Representatives subcommittee hearing in the aftermath of the outbreaks, it was revealed that the USDA's Agricultural Marketing Service (AMS) had heard rumors in January 1997 that the strawberries were Mexican, but Ken Clayton, from AMS admitted that the division failed to investigate the rumor before the March "events did overtake us." The AMS is in charge of inspection of school lunch contractors for quality standards and basic sanitation. However, it is not responsible for detecting foodborne diseases. If any are suspected, the division refers the case to the FDA.

Representative Sonny Bono (R-CA) raised the issue on the floor of the House of Representatives after the strawberry outbreak. "Almost every product is clearly labeled 'made in China' or 'made in Mexico' except the produce we eat. Every other type of food is labeled. Why not the produce?"

Three-dozen lawmakers joined a coalition of U.S. growers, processors, and farm groups to urge the U.S. Customs Service to require that the front panel of packages of frozen produce list the source of the country. Packages of frozen produce are supposed to carry a country-of-origin stamp, but the coalition, American Alliance for Honest Labeling, reported that often the rule is ignored and that compliance is minimal. Imported produce is supposed to meet the same standards as domestically grown produce.

Fred Shank, director of the FDA's Center for Food Safety and Applied Nutrition (CFSAN) testified at the subcommittee hearing that the FDA had inspected the Mexican berry farms after the outbreaks and found a situation conducive to the spread of HAV, with "open unlined pit privies, immediately adjacent to the fields," too few sanitation facilities, and no handwashing stations. In the aftermath, Mary Ellen Camire, from the University of Maine, also had inspected the Mexican strawberry farms, and testified that workers "relieved themselves, then went right back to work using their bare hands to twist the caps off the strawberries."

The federal government quarantined millions of pounds of frozen strawberries in fifteen states and the District of Columbia. Some seventy lawsuits were filed. At least one adult remained hospitalized, and several children were unable to return to school.

VULNERABLE TO CONTAMINATION

Strawberries, as well as other berries, come into contact with many sets of hands, with water from many sources, and with many different locations in the food chain. All these factors combine to produce some degree of risk. Because the edible portion of the strawberries is close to the ground, the berries are more subject to contamination than tree-grown fruits.

After the outbreaks, the USDA strengthened certification procedures for processors who supply produce to the school lunch program. Formerly, a signature attested to United States origin. The USDA now requires that processors supply packing dates, lot numbers, and country-of-origin information.

A Case of Contaminated Deli Food

Schlotzsky's is a franchise of fast-food delis that serve pizzas, sandwiches, soups, and salads. The company has more than 750 franchises throughout the United States. In 1999, twenty-five people sued a deli franchised by Schlotzsky's for having been infected two years earlier from contaminated vegetarian pizza and turkey sandwiches in Marietta, Georgia. The plaintiffs claimed that the food was contaminated with HAV by an infected food handler, and that Schlotzsky's "demonstrated a reckless indifference and disregard of the consequences of its actions." Some of the infected plaintiffs had required hospitalization, and one required a liver transplant.

According to the plaintiffs, the infected employee was "visibly sick," failed to wear gloves when handling food, and did not wash his hands after coughing or putting his hands in his pockets. The lawsuit claimed that Schlotzsky's "did nothing to discipline or reprimand" the infected employee for his unsanitary work habits, even after an outside consultant told managers about the employee's illness, as well as unsanitary conditions of the deli.

A Case of Contaminated Scallions

In 1999, the FDA began testing domestic and imported produce for three microbial pathogens other than HAV. One of the investigators, V. Dato, noted that scallions (green onions) "may be particularly susceptible to contamination because plant surfaces are particularly complex or adherent to viral or fecal particles."

Four years later, Dato's observations were confirmed. In September 2003, patrons at restaurants in Tennessee, North Carolina, and Georgia were made ill. In late October and early November 2003, additional restaurant patrons were made ill in Pennsylvania. By then, more than 500 people were sickened, and three had died. The outbreaks were traced to raw or lightly cooked scallions, and the infective agent was HAV. A traceback identified the scallions from four farms in Mexico. Inspectors found unsanitary conditions such as "inadequate handwashing facilities, questions about worker health and hygiene, the quality of the water used in the fields, packing sheds, and the making of ice."

The restaurant responsible for one of the deaths was a Chi Chi's restaurant located in Beaver Valley Mall in Pennsylvania. Chi Chi's, based in Louisville, Kentucky, was considered to be the first restaurant chain to introduce standardized Mexican fare to American diners. The company claimed that it had taken "extraordinary" voluntary measures to ensure safety of its foods, including removal of green onions from all its hundred restaurants after the outbreaks, and had instituted a procedure to have employees sign wellness statements. The Beaver Valley Mall restaurant had received high scores (90 percent or higher) and one perfect score (100 percent) in its previous four health inspections prior to the outbreaks. The case demonstrates that even when a restaurant has high sanitary standards, it may suffer from earlier negligence in the food chain, and beyond its control.

Beth Bell, an expert on viral hepatitis at the CDC, noted that scallions are handled extensively in food harvesting. "At the place of harvest if there is a person around who is excreting hepatitis A [virus] in the stool, and that person handles the onions [scallions] . . . strip[s] the outside layers off, and wraps them in rubber bands—that person can contaminate a few bunches." A few bunches can lead to outbreaks.

A Case of Contaminated Orange Juice

HAV is highly endemic in Egypt. In 2004, an outbreak of HAV infection occurred in a hotel in the Red Sea resort of Hurghada. Orange juice served at a breakfast buffet sickened 251 tourists from nine different European countries. Inspectors examined the hygienic conditions under which the juice was processed in Egypt. They found that during its manufacture, an infected worker with poor hand hygiene, and/or by contact of the fruit or machinery with sewage-contaminated water, were the likely causes. As noted earlier, HAV is quite resistant to acid. It is likely to survive for prolonged periods in acidic orange juice.

HAV OUTBREAKS LIKELY TO CONTINUE

The three large HAV outbreaks attributed to contaminated strawberries, scallions, and orange juice are only a few among numerous outbreaks resulting from contamination by this pathogen. Such outbreaks are likely to continue. Foodborne illness from produce is sharply on the rise. In 2000, the last year for which information is complete, there were almost as many reported cases of food poisoning from produce as there were from beef, poultry, fish, and eggs combined.

"It's a huge problem and not one easy to solve," observed Glen Morris, chairman of the Department of Epidemiology and Preventive Medicine at the University of Maryland School of Medicine, and a former Agriculture Department official. "Produce is emerging as an important cause of food-borne illness in this country."

The sharp rise in contaminated produce is attributed to several trends. People are eating more fresh produce. People desire to have more fresh produce available year-round. In turn, this leads to an increase of imported produce, some from countries with poor sanitary standards. Because only a miniscule amount of imported produce is inspected, much contaminated produce enters the country. When the FDA tested 1,003 samples of fresh produce imported from twenty-one countries in 1999 and 2000, 4.4 percent were found to be contaminated with pathogens. In contrast, of 959 samples of domestic produce, 1.3 percent were contaminated.

CDC epidemiologist Robert V. Tauxe reported, "The American diet has really shifted, and we are eating more that is minimally processed and getting it from a broader variety of different sources. There has been an increase in the volume of production, so when something goes wrong it goes wrong on a bigger scale. It's a difficult trade-off if you want to have fresh produce in the off-season."

CHAPTER 14

Cyclospora: Emerging Food- and Waterborne Parasites

The young couple hoped for a perfect wedding ceremony and reception banquet. They had completed arrangements at the church, with the florist, printer, and musicians. They had reserved an elegant ballroom in an upscale hotel for the reception, and were working with the maître d'hôtel to plan the food and beverages for the banquet of more than a hundred guests. The hotel was renowned for its excellent cuisine.

Among the suggestions for the menu, the maître d'hôtel had suggested French pâté, cheeses, chanterelles, champagne and wines, New Zealand lamb, Scottish smoked salmon, Russian beluga caviar, out-of-season fresh Guatemalan raspberries, Ethiopian demi-tasse, and Belgian chocolate favors.

The wedding and the reception banquet were joyous occasions, and up to expectations. The food and drinks were presented beautifully and were delectable. Indeed, it seemed to be perfect—except the aftermath. Most of the guests became ill, and suffered from severe bouts of diarrhea. Some developed inflammations in several body organs.

In June 1996, health officials in the United States and Canada were mystified by the spread of an intestinal infection caused by an "exotic" microbe that had insinuated itself into the food supply. During the month, several hundred infections were reported in the states of Florida, Illinois, Massachusetts, New York, Ohio, Pennsylvania, and Texas, as well as in Toronto, Canada. The reports were of multiple, clustered (at social events), and sporadic outbreaks. Additional suspected cases were reported in five more eastern states. By the end of the month, more than 1,400 cases had been reported. Some people required hospitalization.

CHARACTERISTICS OF THE MYSTERIOUS INFECTION

The people who became infected reported a "flu-like illness." After an incubation period of about a week, the infection inflicted explosive watery diarrhea with frequent bowel movements, stomach cramps, bloating, flatus, vomiting, loss of appetite, weight loss, fatigue, and low-grade fever. These symptoms lasted for up to three weeks. Even after these unpleasant symptoms subsided, many people experienced relapses. Although the acute infection targeted the small intestine, the protracted chronic effects experienced by some individuals were a pattern known as Reiter's syndrome, or reactive arthritis (ReA). The syndrome is characterized by inflammation of several organs of the body, conjunctivitis in the eyes, urethritis in the urethra, and oligoarthritis. ReA can be triggered, as well, by other foodborne infections, including *Cryptosporidium, Salmonella, Shigella, Yersinia,* and *Campylobacter.* (See discussion on foodborne infections and joint diseases in Chapter 2.)

Guillain-Barré syndrome is another health problem experienced by some persons in these outbreaks. (See Chapter 5 on *Campylobacter.*)

The mysterious outbreaks appeared to be associated with fresh imported berries, mainly strawberries and possibly raspberries.

THE 1996 *CYCLOSPORA* OUTBREAKS

Although the species of *Cyclospora* had been described and classified only three years prior to its 1996 outbreaks, the microbe was known. Until 1996, however, the incidence was low among industrialized populations in temperate climates. Cases were thought to have been acquired during travel to endemic areas, such as tropical and subtropical coastal regions of Peru, and in Guatemala and Nepal. The pathogen was reported first in patients in New Guinea in 1977. The report received little medical attention. Then, the infection was described in 1985 in New York City and in Peru. The first reported outbreak of diarrheal illness associated with *Cyclospora* in the United States was 1990. Tap water from a physicians' dormitory in a hospital was implicated. During the summer of 1995 one outbreak occurred in New York, attributed to contaminated water, and another outbreak, in Florida, attributed to fresh produce. Then came the massive outbreak in 1996. *Cyclospora* was emerging as a serious public health problem in developed as well as developing countries.

An Uncanny Resemblance

Cyclospora (not to be confused with the drug, cyclosporine) has many characteristics similar to *Cryptosporidia*, which is discussed in the following chapter. Both pathogens:

- Early on were given little attention and were regarded to be of little significance to human health
- Are one-celled protozoan parasites, with similar forms and structures that sporulate and form oocysts (eggs)
- Shed oocysts in feces, which may survive for extended periods of time in the environment
- Require few oocysts to infect people
- Infect a range of creatures, including humans
- Are transmitted through food and water
- Resist ordinary chlorine disinfection, and even irradiation
- Induce diarrheal disease in humans, and mainly affect the intestines
- Display similar features in infected individuals with symptoms that last for weeks, and are intermittent and protracted
- May have long-term health consequences

Because of the uncanny resemblance of the two pathogens, it is suspected that many cases of diarrheal illness—formerly attributed to *Cryptosporidia*—were caused possibly by *Cyclospora*.

IDENTIFICATION AND CLASSIFICATION

Ultimately, the incriminating pathogen was identified as a newly emerging protozoan parasite now known as *Cyclospora*. It had been known earlier, and identified in reptiles, rodents, myriapods (for example, centipedes) and insectivores (small mammals such as moles and shrews that feed mainly on insects). However, if these creatures are infected, the *Cyclospora* oocysts differ in size from the oocysts found in *Cyclospora*-infected humans, which are from a different species known as *Cyclospora cayetanensis*. This species was first recognized as a cause of human illness in 1977, but it had not yet been named.

After taxonomists deliberated, they first designated the microbes as "*Cyanobacterium* or *Coccidia*-like bodies" (CLBs). Also, they tentatively considered the microbe to be blue-green algae. In 1993, taxonomists named the pathogen *Cyclospora cayetanensis*, and defined it as a protozoan parasite.

THE MECHANISM OF *CYCLOSPORA*

To be infectious, the tiny spherical oocysts—sized from 8 to 10 micrograms—must sporulate in the environment. This process requires several days. When the oocysts are examined microscopically under ultraviolet light, they fluoresce. Like *Cryptosporidia*, in being stained, *Cyclospora* usually is acid-fast.

The Food and Drug Administration (FDA) has exercised no control at the point of origin at farms. It does not test the water used for irrigation, or to mix pesticidal sprays. It does not examine the cleanliness of the food handlers, to learn if workers lack toilet facilities. It does not determine if domestic or wild animals roam through fields where food crops are grown. Yet other countries, notably Japan, exercise control at the point of origin of imported foods. Our recent experiences with contaminated foods, feeds, and other consumer goods from China and elsewhere demonstrate the necessity to strengthen surveillance at the point of origin. Long overdue, the FDA has begun to institute changes. In contrast, the U.S. Department of Agriculture's (USDA) Animal and Plant Health Inspection Service (APHIS) inspects *every imported shipment* of produce for plant diseases and insect pests in an effort to protect U.S. crops. However, this concern to protect U.S. crops does not extend to testing for contamination that may affect human health; this is the domain of the FDA.

THE CAUSE OF THE 1996 OUTBREAKS IDENTIFIED

Ultimately, the 1996 outbreaks were linked to contaminated fresh raspberries from Guatemala. The investigators found the illnesses to be in "clusters" (associated with events, such as receptions and banquets to time-place related exposures, such as meals at the same restaurant on the same day) and in "sporadic" cases (not associated with events) attributed to recent travel outside the country, and on a cruise ship that departed from Florida. Fresh raspberries from Guatemala had been served at nineteen of the twenty-one events, and were the sole food common to all nineteen events. The investigators learned that the raspberries had been rinsed in water at some, but not all, of the events. However, washing fails to remove all *Cyclospora* oocysts.

After the 1996 outbreak, the Guatemalan Berry Commission (GBC), in consultation with the FDA and the CDC, voluntarily implemented a system of Hazard Analysis and Critical Control Point (HACCP), and improved water quality and sanitary conditions on individual farms. Despite the implementation of this system, outbreaks continued in 1997 with imported fresh Guatemalan raspberries. Some of the farms may not have implemented the control measures fully, or the contamination was from a source against which the control measures were not directed. To learn more about how HACCP strengthens food safety, see the inset on the opposite page.

At the FDA's request on May 30, 1997, the government of Guatemala and the GBC voluntarily suspended the temporary export of their fresh raspberries to the United States. The following year, the Guatemalan government lobbied the FDA all winter to lift the ban in time for the U.S. spring berry import season. The FDA was unconvinced, and the ban was effective from mid-March to mid-August—the period when Guatemala usually exported the berries.

By 1998, the FDA found Guatemalan farms in compliance, in a program called Model Plan for Excellence (MPE), developed jointly by Guatemala and the United States. Despite this development, another outbreak from Guatemalan raspberries occurred in 1998, this time in Canada. The Canadian Food Inspection Agency had been allowing imports of fresh raspberries from "low-risk" Guatemalan farms. The Canadian government changed its policy to allow imports solely from those farms that met the conditions set out in Guatemala's MPE. Also, Canada instituted a "border look-out" program for Guatemalan raspberries so that customs officials could ensure that raspberries were from farms that met the emblem of MPE.

DESPITE A TRACEBACK SYSTEM, OUTBREAKS CONTINUE

Despite attempts to improve safety measures with fresh imported Guatemalan raspberries, outbreaks continued to occur. In June 1999, several hundred conventioneers at a Palm Beach, Florida, hotel were made

HACCP: A PROGRAM TO STRENGTHEN FOOD SAFETY

The program known as Hazard Analysis and Critical Control Point (HACCP, pronounced as "has-sip") has been used by many food companies as early as 1959, and extended through the food-handling chain. Originally, the program was conceived and developed by the National Aeronautics and Space Administration (NASA). The organization wanted to provide a very high level of confidence in the safety of foods eaten by the astronauts. After all, it is no joking matter if astronauts, up in space, in a closely confined unit, develop diarrhea and vomit from foodborne illness.

HACCP is a scientifically based systematic plan to monitor the microbiological, chemical, and physical safety of prepared foods, based on seven principles to:

1. Assess the hazards and risks associated with the growing and harvesting of raw materials, added ingredients, processing, manufacturing, distributing, marketing, preparing, and consuming of food
2. Determine the critical control points (CCPs)
3. Control identified hazards
4. Establish critical limits for each identified CCP
5. Establish procedures to monitor the CCP's corrective actions
6. Establish effective record keeping, and
7. Establish procedures for verifications of the records

ill, and Guatemalan raspberries were suspected. Investigators conducted a traceback on items served in a fruit plate. Both Guatemalan raspberries and blackberries, and Chilean fruits, and some U.S. grown fruits were in the medley, making the traceback quite complicated.

The problems with fresh produce imported from Guatemala continued into more recent years. In the summer of 2002, a foodborne outbreak in Pennsylvania was traced to raw produce imported from Guatemala. Once again, the infectious agent was *Cyclospora*. This time, it was not raspberries, but snow peas. Some fifty people who were residents, staff members, and volunteers in a residential facility were sickened after eating raw snow peas from Guatemala that had been washed and added to salad.

Salad greens have also been a problem with other *Cyclospora* outbreaks. In 1998, domestically grown mesclun greens (also known as "spring mix," "field greens," or "baby greens") were found to be contaminated with *Cyclospora*. This type of product, consisting of various types of baby lettuce leaves, had become popular as a convenience item. The outbreak occurred in Florida, where another mesclun outbreak had occurred a year earlier. The investigators were thwarted by the same problem that had hindered other *Cyclospora* investigations. It was difficult to find contaminated samples of a perishable product that had sickened people weeks, or even months, before the investigation had begun. In one of the outbreaks with mesclun, the people had consumed the contaminated greens on December 3, but the traceback did not begin until January 28. The time lag was due to the number of days needed to gather and ship samples, perform tests, and confirm analyses. Due to the elapsed time, none of the suspected mesclun was available.

Ultimately, the traceback showed that the greens had been shipped from RDI Industries, a processor in St. Cloud, Minnesota. The greens were from Florida, California, and Peru (a country where *Cyclopora* is endemic). By the time the greens had arrived from Florida, they had experienced quite some travel for so-called fresh greens. In Florida, the investigators of the previous outbreak of *Cyclospora*-contaminated mesclun had been able only to trace the greens back to a Miami distributor who had obtained the greens from a number of different sources. Florida officials had been unable to ascertain precisely where and when the contamination had occurred.

In 2000, the first foodborne cyclosporiasis outbreak was reported in central Europe. Thirty-four out of forty persons were made ill after attending a luncheon at a restaurant in southern Germany. The *Cyclospora* was traced to salads prepared from lettuces imported from southern Europe and spiced with fresh green leafy herbs. The salad green ("mixsalat" in German) consisted of lollo rossa, lollo bianco, oak leaf, and romaine lettuces, plus red and white cabbages, carrots, cucumbers, and celery. The leafy herbs were dill, chive, parsley, and green onion. The investigators of the outbreak found that the various lettuces were grown in southern France, and the province of Bari in southern Italy. The dill, parsley, and green onions were grown in Naples and Eboli in southern Italy, and the chive, in a greenhouse in Germany. The investigators found that the *Cyclospora* oocyst isolates from the lettuce were traced back to

Peru, Egypt, and Nepal. The most likely sources of the outbreak were attributed to crops being fertilized with human waste or contaminated water used to irrigate the crops, to prepare pesticides, or to clean the produce. Another possible factor was contamination by migrant field workers who had no access to proper sanitary facilities. Like other foodborne outbreaks, the contamination of salad in Germany reflected the difficulties of traceback of multiple foods from numerous sources.

There had been another instance of a complicated traceback. In 1997, an outbreak of cyclosporiasis occurred in northern Virginia, Washington, D.C., and Baltimore, Maryland, from basil-pesto pasta salad served cold. The basil had been supplied by a chain-store company. Its stores carried eighty-eight items made with basil or basil pesto. The basil had been grown in Costa Rica, Egypt, Israel, and Mexico, as well as in California, Maryland, and Pennsylvania.

USING MODERN TECHNOLOGY FOR IMPROVED TRACEBACKS

Consider the comparative ease of traceback used by one olive oil company, Colavita, in Italy. On the back of the food label of each bottle of its oil there is a code indicating the production year, and the history of each bottle of oil. There is a statement of the country of origin (100 percent Italian). This statement was initiated by Colavita because many olive oils are imported into Italy from other countries, and a statement "packed by" slyly evades the information about where the olives used for the oil were grown. The label gives coded information about the individual farm in Italy where the olives were grown, the pressing mill used, the date of the pressing, and the date of the bottling.

Surely in this age of high technology, including computers, better methods can be devised for traceback of fresh produce such as raspberries, snow peas, mesclun, and other items. An improved system would provide ready information for investigators needing to conduct tracebacks after outbreaks. Such tracebacks are incorporated in current HACCP programs, but apparently are not functioning efficiently.

CHAPTER 15

Cryptosporidia: Emerging Food- and Waterborne Parasites

Jason, a young man, woke up to another workday. He began his usual routine of pull-ups and then drew water from the kitchen tap to make tea for his mother, Gladys. Although she was housebound, she enjoyed reasonably good health.

Jason took his usual jog through the streets of Milwaukee, stopping now and then to take sips of water from the bottle he filled that morning. He was health conscious and knew the importance of hydration.

Jason returned home, showered, shaved, and prepared a healthy breakfast for his mother and himself. Gladys would have more tea. Jason had never acquired a taste for caffeinated drinks, and he would have some tap water as he swallowed his vitamin pills. He packed his lunch, with a thermos of water. He shunned the soft drinks available in the vending machine in the hall outside the office. He preferred to have his thermos of water at his desk, and avoid the chitchat around the water cooler.

Jason left home, assured that the neighbor would bring some hot homemade soup as she did each day, and that his mother enjoyed.

Later, the day seemed like all other workdays. However, it would end differently. Jason began to have abdominal pain, cramps, fever, and diarrhea. Gladys felt well. But Jason would be joined by more than 400,000 other Milwaukee residents in what they termed 'the waterworks flu.'

"Cryptosporidium must be one of the most successful and adaptable parasites known," remarked Saul Tzipori, a parasitologist at Tufts University in Boston who has investigated this pathogen.

Doubtless, *Cryptosporidia* have been in our environment for a long time, yet they have risen from relative obscurity as protozoan parasites to substantial public health importance only within the last twenty-five years.

Cryptosporidium was identified in the stomach of a mouse in 1907 by parasitologist E. E. Tyzzer. The pathogen was not described in livestock until 1971. It received no attention from the medical community until 1976, when it was identified in a child with diarrhea. The parasite was judged to be a rare infective organism of little or no consequence until 1982, when the AIDS epidemic emerged. *Cryptosporidium* became recognized as a life-threatening organism by inflicting debilitating diarrhea in already weakened AIDS patients, as well as for others with impaired immune systems. It was estimated that cryptosporidiosis was killing nearly 20 percent of AIDS patients.

CHARACTERISTICS OF *CRYPTOSPORIDIUM*

The parasite infects the entire bowel, but most commonly, the lower small intestine, where extensive mucosal changes occur. The infection gained recognition as an important cause of gastroenteritis in hospitalized patients, which indicated that the infection was common even in patients with *normal* immune systems. *Cryptosporidium* became recognized, too, as an important cause of enterocolitis (inflammation of the small intestine and colon) and diarrhea in a number of mammalian species. The infection was found to be an important cause of childhood diarrhea, especially in day-care centers.

Subsequently, hundreds of studies demonstrated that *Cryptosporidia* are the leading cause of diarrhea due to protozoal infections worldwide, both in developed and developing countries.

Formerly, it was thought that *Cryptosporidia* were species-specific, meaning that infected creatures could transmit the infection only to their own kind. Now we know that these parasites can be transmitted from some species to a wide variety of other species, with or without causing illness. Thus, infected humans, calves, goats, lambs, and deer readily infect other species. But there were some strange discoveries, too. Infection may cause diarrhea in pigs, yet not cause apparent illness in mice, rats, guinea pigs, chickens, or foals. Isolates from infected humans readily infect adult mice, but not baby mice. They are infected more readily with isolates from other species.

Cryptosporidia's characteristic lack of host specificity is uncommon among other infective organisms in the same family of enteric coccidia. *Cryptosporidia* are considered to be zoonotic, transmitting infection from

animals to humans, as well as to other creatures. *Cryptosporidia* have been
detected in food animals as well as in wild animals. The list includes pigs,
lambs, goats, foals, calves, rabbits, birds (such as chicken, turkey, goose,
pheasant, guinea fowl, quail, and parrot), reptiles, cats, raccoons, squir-
rels, and mice. *Cryptosporidia* have been found to infect the trachea and
other organs in birds, the stomach in mice and snakes, and the bile ducts
of monkey and immune-deficient foals.

UNDERSTANDING *CRYPTOSPORIDIA* BETTER

Researchers gained insight into *Cryptosporidia's* chemical structure by isolating one of its enzymes. They were able to define the enzyme, dihydrofolate
reductase-thymidylate synthase (DHFR-TS), by taking DNA from *Cryptosporidia* and cloning it to the fast-grown bacteria, *E. coli,* in order to harvest large amounts of the enzyme. Then, the *E. coli* were broken open to
release all the *Cryptosporidia* proteins. The proteins were mixed with beads
or tags, which pulled out only the DHFR-TS enzyme. After the enzyme had
been isolated, it was collected, concentrated, and crystallized. The crystals,
which are an ordered array of enzyme molecules, were subjected to a powerful x-ray beam. Diffracted x-rays emerged and were imprinted on film.
The researchers used mathematical algorithms to interpret the x-ray data,
which eventually revealed the protein's structure.

The study contributed to the understanding of *Cryptosporidia,* as well as
to related parasites in the same family: *Toxoplasma,* the organisms that
cause central nervous system disorders, and *Plasmodia,* the organisms that
cause malaria.

—Journal of Biological Chemistry, Dec 26, 2003

THE LIFE CYCLE OF *CRYPTOSPORIDIUM*

Cryptosporidium parvum, the major strain that affects humans from fecal-
infected water and food, completes its life cycle on the mucosal lining of
the small intestine by adhering to the brush border of enterocytes. (The
brush border forms along epithelial membranes, and is associated with
nutrient absorption.) This action causes partial atrophy, fusion, and distortion of the villi, which results in maldigestion in the brush border, and
malabsorption of nutrients.

C. parvum completes its life cycle on the intestinal and respiratory surface epithelium of mammals. It lives in the intestines of cattle and other animals and is excreted in feces. The oocysts of *C. parvum* are infective as soon as they are passed in the stool. In a moist environment, they can remain infective outside the body from two to six months.

Oocysts present in water or food remain dormant until they are swallowed. Digestive juices dissolve the thick wall of the oocysts, and trigger a growth cycle that ends in reproduction. The tiny protozoans attach themselves to intestinal walls and grow. It is thought that while they are attached, they exude some irritating toxin, causing the host organism to expel the oocysts produced by the adult organism through diarrhea and vomit.

C. PARVUM'S MODE OF TRANSMISSION

C. parvum is transmitted by ingestion of oocysts excreted by animals or persons to other persons, ingestion of contaminated water or food, or contact with fecally contaminated environmental surfaces. An infected person may produce some hundred million oocysts daily. Although the usual location of the infection is the intestines, cryptosporidiosis also has been found to infect biliary (bile ducts or the gallbladder), conjunctival (membrane lining the eyelid and covering the eyeball), gastric, and respiratory sites. Cryptosporidiosis resists many drugs that have been used successfully for treatment against other protozoan infections.

Based on experiments with healthy people, the cryptosporidiosis infective dose appears to be about 500 or fewer oocysts. Some people become infected with as few as thirty oocysts. Based on mathematical algorithmic modeling, some individuals would become infected with as few as one oocyst.

SYMPTOMS OF CRYPTOSPORIDIOSIS INFECTION

The most common symptom of cryptosporidiosis is watery, foul-smelling foamy stools, with as many bowel movements as twenty-five per day. The diarrhea may be profuse, with as much output as 17 liters daily. The diarrhea may be accompanied by vomiting, nausea, flatulence, abdominal pain, headache, fever, and mild to severe dehydration, for at least three days, but lasting as long as two weeks, in otherwise healthy individuals. There may be malaise and anorexia. The symptoms tend to come and go, but cease in immunologically healthy people after two to four weeks. Due to the severe dehydration, ample rehydration and electrolyte replacement are essential. The oocysts may continue to be excreted as long as two months after symptoms have ceased in immunocompromised individuals.

WATER AS A VEHICLE FOR *CRYPTOSPORIDIUM* OOCYSTS

Cryptosporidium oocysts can contaminate water, such as rivers, streams, and ponds, with feces from farm or wild animals, or from humans. The oocysts are present in 65 to 97 percent of all surface waters sampled. High numbers of oocysts have been found both in raw and treated sewage effluence. Water rafters as well as swimmers, who inadvertently swallow water, can become infected. Weather conditions, such as drought, heavy rainfall, floods, invasion of seawater, and climate change, are factors that increase the infectivity risk.

In North America, *Cryptosporidia* peak during the summer and early fall, due to recreational water uses. There may be person-to-person transmission of fecal matter in community, hotel, or private swimming pools. Expansion of recreational water facilities now include wading pools for toddlers, water-wave pools, water sprinkler fountains, interactive water fountains at beaches, hot tubs, and whirlpool baths. Cryptosporidiosis outbreaks have occurred in all these water environments.

As a public health issue, infected tap water from municipal water supplies pose even greater threats because so many people can be affected. In 1987, a waterborne cryptosporidiosis outbreak in western Georgia made 13,000 people ill. However, the largest waterborne outbreak to date from cryptosporidiosis occurred in late March and early April 1993 in Milwaukee, Wisconsin. More than 400,000 people were made ill, and more than a hundred people died. The outbreak represented the largest epidemic of diarrheal disease ever recorded due to a parasitic infection.

Milwaukee is a modern city, with its tap water supplied by a municipal water system. How could such a massive outbreak occur?

Investigation showed that the municipal water system's filtration system was inadequate, and permitted the tiny parasitic oocysts—invisible to the naked eye—to enter the water supply. The chlorination, used commonly as a disinfectant in municipal water systems, is effective against many waterborne infective organisms but is *ineffective* against the hard-encased oocysts of *C. parvum*.

Further investigation led health officials to conclude that the contamination probably occurred from a high runoff level into Lake Michigan, the source of the water, from area dairy farms or slaughterhouses near the water plant's intake pipes. A former Sara Lee Corporation affiliate, the Peck Meat Packing Corporation, was charged with negligence in dumping animal waste contaminated with *C. parvum* into a public sewer. Sara Lee proposed a $250,000 settlement to release itself of any liability in the outbreak, but denied any wrongdoing.

Public health officials concluded that current standards of public water supplies might not be able to prevent *C. parvum* contamination of drinking water. After the Milwaukee outbreak, additional ones have occurred, repeatedly, on smaller scales, up to the present in the United States and elsewhere.

Because any body of water can be contaminated with *C. parvum* oocysts, it is not surprising to learn that bivalve mollusks, such as oysters and mussels, acquire *C. parvum* oocysts from fecally contaminated estuarine water in which the mollusks live. In one study, many species of migratory and residential waterfowl, amphibians, reptiles, and numerous mammals inhabited the drainage areas of sites from which oysters were collected. Only bovine and human genotypes of *C. parvum* were identified in the oysters.

In 1999, a study identified *C. parvum* in oysters found in commercial harvesting sites in the Chesapeake Bay. Of forty-three sites, seven were tested for the presence of *C. parvum* oocysts, during three collecting periods. *C. parvum* oocysts were identified in oysters collected in all seven sites.

These findings indicated that animal or human feces in water at these sites contaminated the oysters. The oocysts can be rendered noninfective by heating the raw oysters to a boiling temperature. Researchers as well as health officials recommend that oysters be cooked before being eaten, especially by persons with impaired immune systems. The oysters also can be made noninfective by freezing at 24.8°F (–20°C) for twenty-four hours. However, viral or other pathogens, in addition to *C. parvum* also may infect oysters from water contaminated with feces, which are able to survive freezing. Therefore, adequate cooking is safer than freezing.

ENVIRONMENTS AT HIGH RISK FOR CRYPTOSPORIDIOSIS

The emergence and spread of *C. parvum* and other waterborne diseases has developed as a result of human activity. There has been increased international travel and commerce, and changes in technology, demographics, and human behavior. There has been microbial evolution, and a breakdown of public health systems. Global freshwater consumption increased sixfold between 1900 and 1995—throughout the twentieth century and beyond—placing more stress on available drinking water reserves, and with water sources more highly contaminated.

Health-care settings are high-risk sites as sources of waterborne *C. parvum* infections. Water can be a reservoir for discharged hospital wastes containing pathogens from rinse water; hydrotherapy pools; water bathing, including infant bathing; irrigation therapy in burn units; water baths used to warm up dialysis fluids, fresh frozen plasma, and albumin; and holy water used in last rites. After the Milwaukee outbreak, it was recommended that the incidence of diarrhea should be monitored in nursing homes because of *C. parvum*.

Day-care centers, too, have become recognized as high-risk sites as sources of waterborne *C. parvum* infection. Some children with diarrhea infect other attending children. Diaper changing offers an opportunity to infect other children and caregivers, surfaces of furniture and toys, or as cross-contamination with foods. Contamination with *C. parvum* is similar to contamination by other pathogens at day-care centers.

Farms are high-risk environments for cryptosporidiosis. In 2005, Agricultural Research Service (ARS) zoologist, Ronald Fayer, and his colleagues collected data from fifteen dairy farms in seven states, to determine the prevalence of *Cryptosporidia* species in preweaned and postweaned calves. Fecal samples taken from 971 calves showed that 345 were infected with *Cryptosporidia*. More preweaned calves than postweaned calves were affected by several species, including *C. parvum*, the only known species that infects humans. *C. parvum* caused 85 percent of the cryptosporidiosis infections in preweaned calves, but only 1 percent in postweaned ones.

Using molecular techniques, the researchers found that what previously was thought to be *C. parvum* in postweaned calves are different species altogether, and not infective to humans, but infective to cattle and sheep. This finding indicated that people handling or otherwise exposed to calves older than two months are less at risk for *C. parvum* infections than those exposed to younger calves.

The problem of airborne cryptosporidiosis in agricultural settings has been largely unexplored. Yet respiratory cryptosporidiosis has been reported in animals and in humans. Scientists suggest that workers in animal processing plants probably inhale viable airborne *C. parvum* oocysts.

At an annual ARS-Food Safety Research Program Planning Workshop held in 1993, *Cryptosporidium* was a topic of great interest. A study conducted by the USDA's Animal Plant Health Inspection Service (APHIS) found that 60 percent of farms and 22 percent of calves were exposed to bovine cryptosporidiosis.

Fayer, mentioned above, reported that 78 percent of food plants that followed safe water treatment rules, nevertheless, were found to have water contaminated by *C. parvum*.

According to another ARS researcher, Jim Harp, cattle are likely to be responsible for many, if not all, *C. parvum* outbreaks. Harp reported that cattle can secrete 10^{10} oocysts (10 trillion) daily "enough to infect everyone in the world once, if not twice."

Frequently, *C. parvum* oocysts are identified in calves and adult cows. Poor udder hygiene can lead to milk contamination. Proper pasteurization kills the oocysts.

A *C. parvum* outbreak occurred in England due to improperly pasteurized milk. Forty-eight school children developed diarrheal illness, traced to milk served at school. The milk had come from a local farm where the pasteurization equipment had not been functioning properly.

POTENTIAL FOOD SOURCES OF *C. PARVUM*

A USDA survey in the early 1990s found that *C. parvum* was present in more than 90 percent of all dairy farms. It was found virtually in all large- and medium-sized milking herds. Other possible sources include: raw produce, raw seafood, sausages, tripe (intended for pet foods), and processed animal carcasses; direct contact with feces from infected calves by immunocompromised farm workers; veterinarians and veterinarian students caring for infected calves; and infected farm workers who transmit *C. parvum* oocysts to family members and others.

PERSONS AT HIGH RISK FOR CRYPTOSPORIDIOSIS

Individuals at high risk for *C. parvum* infection include individuals with impaired immune systems, congenital immunodeficiency, undergoing chemotherapy with immunosuppressive drugs, concurrently infected with another organism (for example, *Toxoplasma gondii*, and travelers who have acquired traveler's diarrhea. The young of all species are at high risk, including human infants and animals, such as calves and foals. Workers at child-care centers and health-care facilities are at high risk. Individuals who are exposed to human feces by sexual contact, and those with extensive animal contact, such as veterinarians and animal handlers, also are at high risk.

FOOD AS A VEHICLE FOR *CRYPTOSPORIDIUM* OOCYSTS

With water as a vehicle for *Cryptosporidium* oocysts, it is inevitable that contaminated water in contact with food at any stage can result in infection. By 1991, *C. parvum* was described as an "undiagnosed food industry problem," and "an emerging concern for the food industry" by researchers Jonathan C. Hoskin and R. Eugene Wright at Clemson University in South Carolina. The pathogen is a concern with fresh and refrigerated foods, which are not subjected further to heat or drying—two controllers of *C. parvum*.

Food processing plants that rely on municipal water in order to make products without further treatment are vulnerable to *C. parvum* infection. After the Milwaukee water outbreak in 1993, more than one hundred food items either were recalled or withheld from the market due to concern that they might have been contaminated. Most of the items were salads, including fruit salads and pasta salads. Also, there were artificially flavored fruit drinks made from powder and dissolved in municipal water. There were "party foods" including different kinds of cottage cheese; hard-boiled pickled eggs packed in vinegar brine; herring party bites in wine sauce or in sour cream; and herring rollmops in wine sauce. No illnesses had been linked directly to contaminated foods in the Milwaukee outbreak.

Although *C. parvum* resists chemical treatment such as chlorination, the oocysts are killed by heat. Milwaukee residents had been advised to boil the tap water.

Food and beverage processors had been led to believe that freezing automatically killed the oocysts, but research conducted by the U.S. Department of Agriculture (USDA) demonstrated that the oocysts can survive for at least six hours, and perhaps longer, at freezing temperatures. After the Milwaukee outbreak, George Jackson, then acting director of the Food and Drug Administration's (FDA) Office of Special Research Skills, advised processors to freeze foods and beverages for twenty-four hours at 24.8°F (–20°C) to ensure the killing of *C. parvum* in products made with water or ice.

Kenneth J. Patten and Joan Rose at the University of South Florida, in Tampa, conducted laboratory research on the longevity of *C. parvum* oocysts in various beverages. They found that the oocysts died off quickly in beverages with a low pH and high carbonation, such as beer and colas. They reported on their results at the annual meeting of the Institute of Food Technologists in 1994.

A disturbing finding was that in liquid foods containing fats, such as infant-feeding formulas, the oocyst populations not only survived, but also even could proliferate. The researchers cautioned that the ability of the parasite to survive in infant-feeding formulas, coupled with the vulnerability of infants to become infected with *C. parvum* makes it imperative to boil the water used to prepare infant-feeding formulas.

FOODBORNE OUTBREAKS OF CRYPTOSPORIDIOSIS

In 1993, an outbreak of cryptosporidiosis occurred with fresh-pressed apple cider. Students and staff attending a school agricultural fair in Maine were affected. Oocysts were detected in the cider, on the cider press, and in the stool specimen of a calf on the apple farm. Oocysts were identified, also, in the stools of the people affected. The outbreak was the first large-scale one in which foodborne transmission was documented. It underscored the need for agricultural producers to take measures to avoid food contamination by infective agents such a *C. parvum*, common on farms.

Another foodborne outbreak of cryptosporidiosis occurred in the state of Washington in 1997, attributed to green onions as the likely source. Some fifty-four people were made ill at a banquet in Spokane. The onions had not been washed before their delivery to the restaurant. The food preparers reported that they had not washed all the onions consistently before preparing them. Two of the food preparers tested positive for *C. parvum* Another worker later admitted that he had worked while he had diarrhea, but could not remember the dates precisely. This outbreak highlights features common in many outbreaks. People with *C. parvum* infection may remain infected for as long as two months, and continue to shed oocysts in their stools. Asymptomatic infected workers probably shed oocysts, too. Food preparers need to be meticulous about washing their hands thoroughly before handling foods, especially those that may be served raw. The FDA's Food Code prohibits barehanded contact with fruits and vegetables after being washed, if the produce is intended for ready-to-eat foods.

SOME LONG-RANGE EFFECTS OF *C. PARVUM* INFECTION

The infection from C. *parvum* may be brief in healthy individuals, but those who are immunologically deficient may suffer prolonged illnesses. In one report, two children, each six years of age with congenital immunoglobulin deficiency, and also infected with C. *parvum*, had persistent diarrhea. In one child, the diarrhea lasted for three years; in the other, six years and culminated in death.

In another study, infected patients, also with impaired humoral (fluids) and cellular immunity resulting from immunosuppressive chemotherapy, suffered from persistent diarrhea. Death resulted in one, reported to have resulted from severe malabsorption due to C. *parvum* infection in the small intestine for two years.

In biopsies of some patients, there were mucosal changes in the intestines. These included partial atrophy of villi, lengthening of the crypt, low carboidal surface epithelium, and cellular infiltration of the lamina propria of the jejunum and ileum.

In a study of long-term effects of early childhood diarrhea from C. *parvum*, researchers found impaired physical fitness and poor cognitive function, four to seven years after the infection. The children studied were from a poor urban community in northeast Brazil. The researchers suggested that the findings have major implications for estimating global disability-adjusted life years (cases of premature death, disability, and days of infirmity due to illness from a specific disease or condition), and for the potential cost effectiveness of targeting intervention for early childhood infections and diarrhea.

CHAPTER 16

T. spiralis (Trichinosis): Knocked Down, But Not Yet Out

In 1931, a man in Detroit suffered a violent seizure after eating a piece of bread. To butter the bread, he used an unwashed knife, previously used to slice raw pork sausage.

There is a dirty little secret unknown to many Americans. People know that many countries will not import our meat from livestock treated with growth hormones, or buy our genetically modified foods. What is not well publicized is that many countries do not permit the importation of our pork. The United Stated has been dubbed as the 'trichinosis capital of the industrialized world.' This unsavory reputation has been earned due to lax farm and slaughterhouse practices and surveillance; regulations that call for voluntary rather than mandatory compliance; and an undue burden placed on hapless consumers. In other industrialized countries, vigilant surveillance and mandatory compliance have assured a pork supply that is nearly trichinosis free.

Trichinosis is a foodborne infection caused by the cysts of a roundworm, *Trichinella spiralis*. Domesticated swine and wild animals are reservoirs for *T. spiralis*. Pigs on a farm may ingest the larvae of *T. spiralis* by eating rodents on the farm or invading animals, such as raccoon, skunk, fox, and opossum. Wild game animals, such as bear, wild boar, walrus, and cougar, also are reservoirs for *T. spiralis*. An important former source of infection for swine was the practice of feeding them raw garbage. The practice has been banned.

A human, consuming any of these contaminated animals in a raw or undercooked state, becomes infected with the larvae (trichella), which grow to adult worms in the human intestine. There, new larvae are released that are able to pass through the intestinal wall, travel through the bloodstream, and reach muscle tissue. There, the larvae encyst themselves in protective sacs in the striated muscles of the human.

PUZZLING SIGNS AND SYMPTOMS OF TRICHINOSIS

The initial symptoms of trichinosis are similar to those of many other foodborne illnesses. Within the first week, the individual may suffer from diarrhea, vomiting, constipation, abnormal pain, and low-grade fever. However, the classical trichinosis symptoms may appear several weeks later as the larvae encyst in the muscles. The symptoms include a high white blood count, swelling of the eyelids and face, headaches, myalgia (muscle pain), intermittent fever, pruritus (itching), rashes, and coughing.

Trichinosis has a wide range of effects. At one end, it can be asymptomatic. At the other end, it can be fatal, if there are neurologic and myocardial complications. As the larvae go through their life cycle, new cysts continue to form in the muscles. The condition becomes chronic.

Many cases of trichinois infection are asymptomatic. It has been termed 'a common infection, not a rare disease.' An autopsy study, done in 1943, at a time when *T. spiralis* infections were more common, found trichinae cysts in over 16 percent of more than 5,000 randomly selected human diaphragms. By the late 1960s, only about 4 percent of more than 8,000 diaphragms contained the cysts. Many physicians have little or no experience with the infection and have difficulty diagnosing it. This is especially true when infected individuals are asymptomatic. Some people acquire trichinosis (as well as many other food- or waterborne infections) in travel to developing countries.

In order to confirm a diagnosis of trichinosis, it is essential for the doctor to take a muscle biopsy. If trichella larvae or their cysts are present, trichinosis is confirmed. Also, there should be testing for serum antibodies. Such assays are available through state health or commercial diagnostic laboratories.

The Centers for Disease Control and Prevention (CDC) advises physicians to include trichinosis on their checklist whenever they face puzzling diagnoses, especially in patients with high white blood cell counts. Also, physicians should include trichinosis and other food- and waterborne diseases in pre-travel counseling of patients.

A BRIEF HISTORY OF TRICHINOSIS

T. spiralis was identified in 1835. For about 100 years, it was believed that the infection was caused by a single species. Later, DNA fingerprinting and other biochemical and statistical technologies of *T. spiralis*-infected animal samples taken worldwide showed at least five species in the genus of *Trichinella*.

The species that infects domestic pigs is the same as the one that infects wildlife coming in contact with farm pigs. This causes the wildlife to become reservoirs for reinfection of the farm pigs. Other species and genetic types of the parasite that are found commonly in wildlife have a very low infectivity for farm pigs.

FREE-RANGE PIGS AND TRICHINOSIS

Is pork from a free-ranging pig safer to eat than pork from a conventionally raised one? This question was addressed in a 2008 study sampling more than 600 pigs in North Carolina, Ohio, and Wisconsin. Two free-range pigs carried trichinae; confined pigs, none. The free-range pigs also had higher rates of *Salmonella* and *Toxoplasma gondii* than the confined pigs. In freely ranging, animals are more likely to interact with rodents and other wildlife, and domesticated cats. All these creatures can carry transmissible infections. Also, free-range pigs may be in contact with moist soil, an environment conducive for pathogens to survive and thrive.

The Trichinosis Experience in Germany

In Germany, pork has long been a favored meat. In the mid-1880s, trichinosis was so widespread there that a butcher was jailed for a month because he had violated local regulations of meat inspection. Around the same time, a harsher punishment was meted out to a German meat inspector. He spent six months in jail for his failure to identify pork that had caused trichinosis in consumers.

Understanding the risk of eating pork in Germany was reflected in a legend. Rudolf Virchow, a pioneering parasitologist (1822–1902), encouraged public education about health. Also, he was a feisty, outspoken member of the German parliament. He was challenged to a duel by Prussia's famous "Iron Chancellor" Bismarck. As the story goes, Virchow proposed fighting the duel with pork sausages. One would be *Trichinella*-contaminated. Each of the combatants would eat a sausage, with Bismarck having the first choice. Bismarck declined. The proposal was too risky. Although the story may be mere fantasy, it underscores the impact of the parasite in human history.

In Germany, a policy of strong regulations and vigilant surveillance was instituted to assure trichinae-free pork. In the summer of 1880, Germany banned the import of U.S. ground pork and sausage due to our high rate of trichinae-infected pork. Later, Germany expanded the ban to *all* U.S. pork. One reason was the health risk. Another reason, charged the affected industry, was economic. Europeans did not appreciate having their markets flooded with cheap, abundant, American pork.

The German bans led to a protracted squabble with the United States. Germany wanted certification that American pork was trichinae free. The bans made the United States threaten retaliation by proposing mandatory certification of imported German wine. The U.S. Secretary of Agriculture argued irrationally that "certified American meats are as wholesome as foreign wines."

Attempts to Strengthen Safety

Perhaps the economic incentive to sell more food abroad was a greater incentive than protecting American health. Gradually, federal regulations were strengthened somewhat, but insufficiently. There was resistance to a recommended practice that all pork be inspected microscopically to detect *T. spiralis*. This practice had been instituted in other industrialized countries, and proved to be highly effective. But industry lobbied, and persuaded federal authorities that microscopic examination would be too laborious and costly. Instead, the Food Safety and Inspection Service (FSIS), a department of the U.S. Department of Agriculture (USDA), embarked on an education program to encourage consumers to cook pork and pork products thoroughly. Thus, if trichinosis occurred, it was the fault of the food preparer. Farmers, slaughterers, and pork processors would be blameless and not held accountable. National reporting of trichinosis was initiated in 1947.

Many consumers did learn to cook pork thoroughly, but found it to lose flavor and texture. The decline in food quality was a tradeoff for safety.

THE RISE AFTER THE DECLINE IN TRICHINOSIS

Gradually, there was a decline in trichinosis outbreaks in the United States. The decline was attributed to the prohibition of feeding raw garbage to pigs, greater use of home freezers, and the practice of cooking pork thoroughly.

Unfortunately, the pattern changed. Several factors were involved in the rise in trichinosis outbreaks.

The Microwave Oven and Trichinosis Risk

Extensive use of microwave ovens presented a new hazard in cooking pork thoroughly. The appliance cooks food from the exterior to the interior. As a result, even though a cooked pork roast might appear to be fully cooked, sections in its interior might still be undercooked.

This problem was addressed in a press release issued by the FSIS in 1981. The FSIS advised consumers who used microwave ovens to cook pork roasts so that the internal temperature of the meat would reach 170°F, and allow standing time after cooking to assure even heat distribution. Were the USDA's recommendations adequate to assure safety? Not from findings published two years later.

Researchers cooked pork roasts intentionally infected with *T. spiralis* by twenty-nine different methods, using the USDA's recommendations, and instructions recommended by several industrial groups and microwave oven manufacturers. The researchers found viable infective *T. spiralis* still present in fifty out of 189 pork roasts after cooking. Five different temperature readings were above the USDA's recommendation of 170°F; forty-eight of the infected roasts did not meet the temperature recommendations that were more stringent than those of the USDA. Furthermore, a single temperature reading from the mid-point of the roast after cooking presented a risk. Suggestions for how to thoroughly cook pork and pork-containing foods in a microwave are given in the inset on the following page.

Regional Preferences for Pork and Trichinosis Risk

The mid-Atlantic region of the United States has the highest prevalence of trichinosis cases in the country. Small slaughterhouses buy hogs from brokers rather than from producers. The brokers may have purchased the hogs from other brokers, or at auctions. Processors have little control or knowledge about the way the hogs have been raised. This arrangement makes the problem of traceback quite different from former times, when contaminated pork from a small butcher shop could be traced back to a specific farm in the same vicinity.

People in the mid-Atlantic region of the United States favor pork products, including ethnic-style sausages, chops, hams, pickled pigs' feet, and smoked pork. Some of these pork products come directly from farms, but most are from large commercial sources.

Ethnic Pork Dishes and Trichinosis Risk

Another factor in the rise of trichinosis outbreaks in the United States is cultural. Many immigrants from Italy, Poland, and other East European countries, as well as those from South Asia and elsewhere, had been accustomed to eating dishes containing raw pork, because raw pork had been safe in their homelands.

Two large outbreaks of trichinosis occurred in 1990. Both outbreaks were related to cultural practices of ethnic groups.

AT WHAT TEMPERATURE IS *T. SPIRALIS* KILLED?

It would appear that a straightforward answer could be given to the question: "At what temperature is *T. spiralis* killed?" It turns out that the answer is not clear-cut.

Freezing pork at 5°F (-15°C) for twenty-one days or longer should kill any *T. spiralis* present. However, if the meat is .5-inches thick (1.5 centimeters) or more, longer freezing is necessary. Also, freezing wild game may require lower temperatures and/or longer periods of freezing.

Cooking, too, has many qualifiers. At different times, the USDA has made different recommendations. For years, the recommendation was to cook pork to an internal temperature of 165°F in conventional ovens. Then, with the widespread use of microwave ovens, the recommendation was upped to an internal temperature of 170°F. In 1986, the FSIS recommended 160°F for the internal temperature for medium- to well-done pork. This recommendation was continued, even though a number of health professionals considered it "an unacceptable risk" according to Kenneth N. Hall, in the Department of Nutritional Sciences at the University of Connecticut in Storrs.

It had been established as early as 1939 that most *T. spiralis* are destroyed at 131°F (55°C), but the results are not valid for rapid cooking methods.

By 1992, the USDA regulations specified a thermal death point at

In Iowa, three prior trichinosis outbreaks had occurred among its 900,000-immigrant population. In 1990, a wedding was held in Des Moines, attended by Southeast Asians. Of 250 people in attendance, 90 developed trichinosis. The outbreak was traced to uncooked pork sausage used in a traditional dish. The pork had been purchased from a commercial supplier.

Another trichinosis outbreak occurred in 1990, in Staunton, Virginia. Uncooked sausages were implicated. The meat was bought in bulk at local stores, and made available from a local processing plant. Fifteen people, mostly from East European extraction, developed trichinosis. Nine of them required hospitalization. One of the infected individuals had not actually eaten the pork, but had been a meat handler in the plant traced to the infected meat.

137°F for trichinae in ready-to-eat pork products in federally inspected plants, when slow-cooking methods are used. This allows sufficient time to destroy the parasites. However, a temperature of 165°F was considered to offer a reasonable margin of safety when fresh pork is cooked in homes by more rapid methods. In microwave ovens, cooking pork to an internal temperature of 160°F would kill any bacteria present, as well as the *T. spiralis.*

The microwave oven was a new factor to be considered. In the *Journal of Food Science,* a team of researchers led by W. J. Zimmerman offered five suggestions to minimize the risk of trichinosis from microwave-undercooked pork:

1. Cook roast using low wattage (50 percent or less power).

2. Use roasts with bone-in or bone-less, weighing 4.4 pounds (2 kilograms) or less.

3. Allow roasts to stand covered with foil, or hold with oven temperature probe inserted and set for 170°F (76.7°C) for ten minutes or longer.

4. Measure the temperature of the roast at several locations including center, ends, and near the bones; if any temperature is below 170°F (76.7°C), recook until all temperature measures reach 170°F (76.7°C).

5. Make visual observation of cut-up products; if any pink or red meat is evident, cook longer.

Additional Trichinosis Outbreaks

In the same year of the two dramatic outbreaks of trichinosis in Iowa and in Virginia, yet another occurrence was associated with this parasitic pathogen. France banned all imports of horsemeat from the United States due to a trichinosis outbreak in a human, traced back to infected horsemeat intended for human consumption. The ban lasted several years.

The European Union (EU) banned all horsemeat from the United States to its member countries. The EU ban was lifted in 1994, but required the USDA to certify that the meat had been tested and found negative for *T. spiralis*.

The following year, a Wisconsin trichinosis outbreak was the largest experienced in that state for a decade. There were twenty-two probable cases and five more suspected cases of trichinosis linked to mettwurst, an ethnic sausage sold in specialty meat stores in Germantown, Wisconsin.

Interest in Exotic Game Meats and Trichinosis Risk

Another factor in the rise of trichinosis cases in recent years is an increased interest in exotic game meat. As segments of the American population have become more affluent, they either engage in game hunting or purchase game meats. As a result, trichinosis outbreaks now occur with the consumption of meat from animals, such as the black bear, grizzly bear, polar bear, wild boar, walrus, and cougar.

Until 1995, wild boar had not even been considered as a potential reservoir for *T. spiralis* transmissible to humans or domestic animals. The infection had been found only in woodland animals such as raccoons, foxes, and tiger cats, and in birds such as tawny eagles and rooks. Also, the infections of these creatures were found in remote regions, such as the Caucasus, Kazakhstan, and Tasmania. In 1995, the parasite was detected in wildlife in the United States, in domestic and cohabitating animals and humans in Russia, and in humans in Thailand.

A trichinosis incident in 1995 occurred in Idaho, involving cougar meat. The meat had first been frozen and made into homemade meat jerky. The CDC reported that most species of *T. spiralis* are killed by freezing. CDC investigators were surprised to learn that the cougar meat sample isolate was freeze resistant. Two freeze-resistant strains of *Trichinella* are known, and one of the strains was identified in the cougar. The meat jerky had been brined and then smoked. However, the smoker appliance never achieved real heat, only mild warmth. The cougar jerky had been eaten by fifteen people. Ten of them suffered from myalgia, fever, rashes, weakness, and arthralgia (pain in one or more joints).

In 1999, in France, four people were infected with trichinosis after eating barbecued wild boar. It is difficult to cook foods evenly on grills, and in this instance, the boar meat was undercooked.

An outbreak of trichinosis in Canada was attributed to uncooked smoked boar meat. The meat had been cold-smoked for twenty-four hours, without any temperature monitoring. The case led to new Canadian requirements. All wild boar submitted for slaughter must be tested for *T. spiralis*. Inspectors must make sure that smokehouses, drying rooms, and freezers used to destroy trichinae must have automatic recording thermometers.

The FSIS recommended that wild game be cooked to an internal temperature of 160°F. Although the trichinae are killed at a lower temperature (137°F), the higher temperature assures that other pathogens, which might also be present in the meat, will be killed.

Other Food Practices That Add to Trichinosis Risk

Certain food practices account for some cases of trichinosis. When butchers were still functioning operators in food stores, they might fail to clean the meat grinders thoroughly after grinding raw pork. The subsequent batch of meat being ground might be beef. Some of the raw pork, mixed with the beef, would not be apparent to the shopper. At home, the beef patties might be cooked insufficiently to be safe for the pork. Or, butchers might deliberately add ground pork to "all-beef" ground meat for a greater profit, because pork generally sells at a lower price per pound than beef. This practice was not only an economic fraud and illegal adulteration, but also it posed a hidden health risk for unwary consumers.

In homes, some food preparers intentionally blend some pork with beef for flavorsome patties or meatloaves. However, food preparers have been alerted to the need for thorough cooking of pork-containing foods.

In recent years, pork has been incorporated into some poultry products. In 1992, the FSIS amended regulations to provide that poultry products, to which pork has been added, are subject to the same trichinae treatment requirements as meat products containing pork.

Another factor in the rise of trichinosis outbreaks is due to changes that have developed in food selections. More and more processed foods, prepared away from home, have been introduced into the food supply. Some are minimally cooked to conserve food quality. Others are lacking in some preservatives that formerly had assured safety. Among these food products are ready-to-eat pork products, including dry sausages and dry-cured hams. The techniques used to create these ready-to-eat convenience foods do not always assure safety. Techniques vary for brining, smoking, and curing these pork products.

TRICHINAE-TESTED PORK—HOW SAFE?

It is necessary to examine the details of the FSIS's role in attempting to standardize these techniques in order to comprehend the weakness of the measures taken, purportedly to strengthen safety. There had been several incidents in which so-called trichinae-tested, ready-to-eat pork products still were contaminated with other viable pathogens. The FSIS noted that earlier, sausage manufacturers "accidentally permitted the growth of tox-ogenic *Staphylococcus aureus* during the [trichinae treatment] process, and more recently, *Salmonella* was found to have survived in a fully treated dry-cured ham. These incidents indicate that some manufacturers may not recognize that the trichinae treatment does not preclude adulteration by bacterial pathogens." The FSIS proposed to insert a warning in the reg-ulations that would alert processors that they "may need to use addition-al heating, acidification, fermentation, salting, or drying to inhibit and destroy pathogenic bacteria."

The emphasis that had been given solely on trichinae-control instead of on total pathogen destruction in pork products was criticized by Edward L. Menning of the National Association of Federal Veterinarians. Men-ning condemned the USDA-sanctioned label for "trichinae-tested" pork as giving consumers "the false idea that the meat, eaten rare or raw, is safe, whereas in reality, trichinae still may be present in more than 30 per-cent of raw pork."

WEAK FEDERAL REGULATIONS

The FSIS's new recommendations allowed economic concerns to override safety concerns. The FSIS proposed two different methods that processors could use. One treatment would extend the drying time of the pork to a full 150 days at 55°F, combined with a curing period of 206 days. The other treatment would have a brief drying period of only four days, at a higher heat of 110°F, combined with a curing period of at least thirty-four days. The brining process of such products is an important aspect of safety for such pork products. Yet, the FSIS yielded to the processors' pressures to allow them "the freedom to vary and lessen the amount of salt" to be used in these products. The FSIS agreed to allow processors to vary the salt content in the brine. A minimal concentration of 6 percent salt would need to be in the internal brine.

By the summer of 2000, the USDA instituted a two-year pilot program to certify pork trichinae-free, based on good farm management. It was hoped that this program would serve as a model for control of other food-borne pathogens at the source of infections. Pork producers were recruited to volunteer for certification by having their operations audited for good management practices, such as preventing the pigs from exposure to infected rodents or wildlife, or to raw garbage. By 2008, the USDA final-ized the rule for a trichinae certification program. The agency would certi-fy pork produced under certain prescribed practices. However, the program does not serve the public because it remains voluntary, not mandatory.

STRONG REGULATIONS ELSEWHERE

In Germany, trichinosis screening of all pork was mandated as early as 1937. As a result, the country has an extremely low prevalence—three or fewer infected pigs identified out of approximately 40 million pigs slaughtered each year in Germany.

Italy, too, has achieved a low incidence of trichinosis, after obligatory screening of all slaughtered swine was instituted in 1959. The rare incidents of infection have been mainly with game animals, such as foxes, wolves, and wild boar. There have been some trichinosis cases with infected horse-meat. A popular myth in some areas attributes the consumption of raw horsemeat or wild boar to an improvement of blood and body strength.

When rare trichinosis outbreaks occur in Europe, typically, they are caused by meat or meat products distributed locally from a single infect-ed animal. This is in sharp contrast to large outbreaks in the United States where contamination is difficult to trace back through large-scale opera-tions, brokers, and auctions.

A mandated rather than voluntary program is in effect in all country members of the EU. Each pig carcass is tested for the presence of trichinae. The EU expects its trading partners to do the same. U.S. packers claim that carcass testing is too costly, and cumbersome. Thus, in the United States, we are still at square one: relieve producers and processors of responsibility, shift responsibility to consumers, and tell them to cook pork thoroughly.

CHAPTER 17

C. botulinum (Botulism):
An Infection Long with Us,
But from New Causes

The patty melt sandwich on the restaurant menu was a popular item. In order to save time in preparing the dish, the chef cut up the onions, added seasoning, and sautéed them in a large amount of margarine. He placed the mixture on a corner of a warm stove where the onions, smothered by the margarine, were handy for use.

Twenty-eight people who ate the patty melt sandwiches were hospitalized. One person died. Others were incapacitated for months.

After five years, half of the patients became easily fatigued, and some complained of muscle weakness, headache, and blurred vision.

Many people regard botulism as a problem of former years, resulting mainly from improper home canning. Unfortunately, botulism is still with us, but resulting from other causes such as changes in plant breeding, introduction of minimally processed foods, new techniques in food packaging, and innovations in restaurants. Botulism outbreaks in homes are still a problem, but not necessarily due to home canning. Botulism outbreaks in restaurants, where greater numbers of people can be affected, account for some incidents. Ethnic foods, prepared in nontraditional ways, are responsible for other outbreaks. Both farm animals and wildlife, as well as humans, can suffer botulism toxicity. Indeed, botulism should not be viewed as a problem of the past, but rather one that continues to be a problem of concern. Often, when botulism strikes, it is fatal. When not fatal, it can result in long-term health problems.

Botulism is one of the oldest recorded foodborne infections. The first designated cases of botulism were recorded in 1735 in Europe, resulting from German sausages. *Botulus* is the Latin word for sausage.

Botulism is caused by *Clostridium botulinum*, a bacterium capable of producing several very powerful poisons. They are termed collectively as

234

botulinum toxin. The lethal dose of the toxin is approximately 1 nanogram, an amount too small to be seen and too small to be weighed. To appreciate its size, compare it with salt. A grain of salt is about 1 milligram, and 1 nanogram is about one-millionth of a grain of salt. Yet the fatal dose of the botulinum toxin is 100-billionths of a gram. Botulinum toxin is considered to be among the most, if not *the* most lethal biological toxin known. Some researchers estimate that 1 milligram of the toxin would kill more than 10 billion laboratory mice, and approximately 20 grams of purified toxin would kill all humans on earth.

BOTULINUM TOXIN AS AN AGENT IN BIOLOGICAL WARFARE

In World War II, several countries produced botulinum toxin as a potential biological weapon. Fortunately, it was never used. However, at a later date, it was reported that the toxin had been used in a test, and sprayed over an area of Canadian wilderness. It was reported that all animals in the area died within six hours.

In August 1991, Iraq officials admitted to a United Nations' inspection team that it had performed research on the offensive use of botulinum toxins in a period prior to the Persian Gulf War. Additional information supplied in 1995 revealed that Iraq had filled and deployed more than a hundred munitions containing botulinum toxin. This toxin, inhaled, as well as ingested, can be lethal. An aerosol attack would be the most likely scenario for the use of botulinum toxin. The toxin also might be used to sabotage food supplies.

C. BOTULINUM'S MODE OF ACTION

C. botulinum is an anaerobic, spore-forming bacterium that commonly inhabits the soil. As an anaerobe, it is unable to grow in the presence of atmospheric oxygen. As a spore-forming microbe, it produces highly resistant spores, which can survive in the presence of oxygen, such as in the soil, or elsewhere, for extended periods. The spores are quite heat resistant, and can survive in boiling water for two hours.

The spore is a resting form of the microbe, which neither reproduces nor feeds, but merely hibernates under adverse conditions such as in the presence of oxygen, until it finds a suitable environment. People are likely to ingest some of these dormant spores. In a healthy individual, colonized with normal gut flora, ingestion of the dormant spores does not present any health problems. The spores simply pass through the digestive tract. However, when *C. botulinum* spores find their way into a suitable anaerobic environment that lacks competing bacteria, they convert themselves into vegetative bacilli, and begin to multiply. As their numbers increase, they develop into very powerful toxins. Seven types of toxin have been identified, strains A through G. A, B, E, and F strains cause most cases of botulism in humans. The toxin may be proteolytic or nonproteolytic. The former type has enzymes that break down proteins in foods, and release compounds that produce offensive odors such as putrescine and cadaverine. These odors provide us with warnings not to eat the foods. The latter type lack these enzymes, and can grow in a food and make it toxic without spoilage signs in appearance, taste, or odor. This insidious aspect of botulism makes it imperative not to taste any food suspected of having botulinum toxin.

If *C. botulinum* begins to flourish in a food, such as a stew or soup, the food ultimately becomes poisoned. A person who eats the food becomes ill, due not to the bacteria, but to the toxin.

SIGNS AND SYMPTOMS OF BOTULISM POISONING

Within eighteen to thirty-six hours (but sometimes as short as four hours or as long as eight days), the infected person will begin to exhibit signs of marked lethargy, weakness, and dizziness, usually followed by double vision, and progressive difficulty in speaking and swallowing. The tongue becomes very dry and feels furry. Often, there is difficulty in breathing, weakness of muscles, abdominal distension, and constipation.

The toxin binds to nerve endings and prevents the release of the neurotransmitter acetylcholine, which transfers messages from one nerve to the next. The toxin causes paralysis by blocking the motor nerves. The paralysis progresses symmetrically downward, usually starting with the eyes and face, down to the throat, chest, and extremities. When the diaphragm and chest muscles become fully involved, respiration is inhibited, causing asphyxia and death. Throughout the progression of these terrible symptoms, the patient will not have any fever, and will remain mentally clear. If not treated promptly and correctly with antitoxin, the patient mortality rate is between 30 and 75 percent, depending on the specific strains of toxins and other factors. Many physicians have never encountered patients with botulism, and have difficulty in making a proper diagnosis. At times, botulism has been misdiagnosed as stroke or other health disorders. Unless the proper diagnosis is made, and made promptly, improper medication instead of the antitoxin, can be disastrous.

The gravity of botulism is reflected in the fact that in the United States, it is a notifiable disease that must be reported. Even if only one case is identified, it is considered an outbreak. Fortunately, botulism is not a communicable disease, and is not transmissible from one person to another.

SIGNS AND SYMPTOMS OF INFANT BOTULISM

Infant botulism is a life-threatening infection. Unlike conventional botulism acquired by eating foods containing botulinum toxin, infant botulism is caused by a toxin produced in the infant's large intestine.

An infant's digestive system is far less acidic than an adult's. Ingested spores of *C. botulinum* germinate and temporarily become part of the bacterial flora in the infant's intestine where they produce the toxin. The low acidity favors the toxin's survival and multiplication. The toxin does not cause any inflammation within the infant's gastrointestinal tract but is absorbed. It acts irreversibly on the automatic nerve endings by preventing the passage of stimuli from the motor nerves to the muscles. As the disease progresses, more muscles, failing to be stimulated to contract, become paralyzed. Eventually, the respiratory muscles needed for breathing are affected.

Infant botulism was identified in 1976. Before then, its description had never appeared in a medical textbook. Many cases were hidden, no doubt, in a multitude of misdiagnoses, such as sepsis, viral syndrome, failure to thrive, Guillain-Barré syndrome, and myasthenia gravis. Infant botulism has become recognized as a global problem. It occurs in urban and rural settings, among all racial and ethnic groups, and in all social strata.

Botulinum spores are found everywhere in the environment. They are present on the surfaces of raw fruits and vegetables. Although children and adults can ingest these spores without ill effect, young infants are at risk. All raw produce should be washed and peeled before giving them to infants. Because young infants put many objects into their mouths, their fingers, pacifiers, rubber nipples, toys, and other items need to be washed frequently and thoroughly.

By the late 1970s, honey was implicated in infant botulism. It was common practice to sweeten water fed to infants with honey, and to coat pacifiers and rubber nipples with honey to encourage their acceptance.

When tested, from 10 to 15 percent of all commercial honey was found to contain botulinum spores. The spores in the environment can be transferred by bees from flower pollen to the honey stored in the hive. Also, the spores can be carried in the bee's digestive tract. Bee-feed, too, is implicated as a possible source of contamination, and C. botulinum can multiply within dead bee larvae. Commercial honey is heated only slightly for bottling, to kill yeast spores. At higher temperatures, C. botulinum spores might be killed, but the texture and flavor of the honey would be damaged seriously.

Honey is not essential for infants. It is recommended that infants under the age of one year not be fed honey. For older children and adults, honey is safe.

About 98 percent of infants hospitalized with infant botulism have been under thirty-five weeks of age. Typically, the infant is from five to twelve weeks of age, and formerly was well. This unique characteristic sets the disease apart from all other known bacterial infections.

Early signs of infant botulism are not recognized readily because the symptoms are common and nonspecific. At first, the infant may be constipated and lethargic. Within an hour or two, but as long as one or two weeks, neurological symptoms begin to develop. The infant cries feebly; displays poor sucking and feeding ability; has droopy eyelids; shows a slow response of the eye pupils to light; has a flattened facial expression; displays a diminished gag reflex; has poor head control; shows diminished muscle tone; and displays a generalized weakness. An infant who displays such symptoms is described as a "floppy baby." If medical help is delayed, infant botulism can result in sudden respiratory arrest and death.

Medical help needs to be given as soon as possible: the shorter the interval between onset of infant botulism and medical treatment, the more promising the outcome. It has been found that a broad-spectrum antibiotic should *not* be given. Such treatment may be detrimental rather than helpful. The antibiotic may alter the normal intestinal microbiological environment of the infant, and allow the C. botulinum bacteria to thrive and multiply.

SIGNS AND SYMPTOMS OF WOUND BOTULISM

Wound botulism, unrelated to foodborne botulism, is a syndrome of flaccid paralysis that results when spores of *C. botulinum* germinate in a wound and produce botulinum toxin. Wound botulism was first reported in 1943. Wound botulism attributable to injecting drugs was recognized in 1982. A patient with a history of drug abuse was examined due to neurologic and respiratory problems. Since then, cases of wound botulism frequently have been attributed to drug use, especially injected black tar heroin (a variety of heroin produced primarily in Mexico). Treatment for wound botulism is botulinum antitoxin—similar to the treatment of foodborne botulism.

ALERTS, WARNINGS, AND RECALLS

The Food and Drug Administration (FDA) and the U.S. Department of Agriculture (USDA) have several means of warning both industry and the public about a potential botulism hazard. One tool is an Alert. An example of an Alert was when the FDA informed the public about possible underprocessed canned mushrooms imported from Indonesia. A botulism Alert has been described "as dramatic and highly prioritized as a hurricane warning." States also may issue statements to the industry involved as well as to the public, by means of a Warning Letter. An example was in 1992, when the state of California sent a warning letter regarding a vacuum-packaged, uneviscerated (the gut is left inside the fish), dried herring product. It had been air-dried at an ambient temperature for seven to ten days. *C. botulinum* could be present, yet lack any clear indication of product spoilage.

A potent tool is the Recall. The FDA issues recalls of food for various reasons. Among them is the potential hazard of suspected botulism. The agency classifies the hazards as Class I Recalls: clear and imminent dangers; and Class II Recalls: remote but potential danger. (There are additional Classes, concerning issues such as adulteration, mislabeling, etc.)

EXAMPLES OF CLASS I AND II BOTULISM RECALLS

It is instructive to examine recalls concerning botulism for a few representative years. Not all cases involved canning, after other types of packaging were introduced. Some of the Class I Recalls for a single year (1992) included: chili con queso cheese dip from Texas; Szechuan chili sauce from Oregon; undercooked refried beans; chopped garlic in soybean oil;

HOW WELL DO FOOD RECALLS WORK?

Both the USDA and the FDA work informally with companies whenever problems come to their attention. The companies are encouraged to initiate their own voluntary recalls. If this informal approach fails, the USDA and the FDA can take further actions. However, procedures differ between the two agencies.

The USDA can detain a product for up to twenty days. During that time, the agency seeks a court order to seize the food. The USDA has the power to remove its inspectors from a meat or poultry slaughterhouse or packing plant. This action leads to the closing of the plant. It is illegal to ship uninspected meat and poultry from one state to another. However, the USDA rarely uses this power. On the few occasions when the agency has removed inspectors, companies have challenged the action in court. Cases are time-consuming and costly, and the litigation may continue long after the questionable food no longer exists.

The FDA's protocol differs from its sister agency. If a company undertakes a voluntary recall, the FDA district office sends a "24 Hour Alert to Recall Situation," a notification to the relevant center and to the FDA's Division of Emergency and Investigational Operations. The notification describes the product, the recalling company, and the reason for the recall. The FDA also informs state officials about the problem, but the state does not become involved actively with routine recalls.

If this informal approach fails to work, the FDA can issue a formal written request for the company to conduct a voluntary recall. If the company still fails to act, the FDA may take an additional step of persuasion by repeating the request and offering the company one last chance to take action. However, unlike the USDA, the FDA *has no detention authority.* If the company still fails to comply, the FDA can seek a court order for an injunction or a seizure and take other legal action.

After a serious and widespread outbreak of foodborne illness in 1993 from *E. coli* O157:H7 in contaminated beef patties (see Chapter 4) the U.S. Congress proposed a bill to give the USDA the power to mandate meat recalls, and to impose civil fines. Sponsors of the legislation noted that the FDA can mandate prompt recalls of harmful drugs and medical devices, yet lacks the authority to order prompt removal of harmful foods. Delayed recalls can result in such foods continuing to reach the public.

Also, the federal Consumer Product Safety Commission can mandate nationwide recalls of unsafe consumer goods to protect the public. Why not prompt removal of dangerous foods? In 2009, this question, often asked, was considered, among others, in serious deliberations to empower the FDA to strengthen food safety.

Congress's 1993 bill failed to pass. Similar bills introduced in subsequent years, have failed to pass. In 2000, when a similar bill failed to pass, which would have given mandatory recall authority to the USDA and the FDA, members of Congress requested that the General Accountability Office (GAO) study the food recall procedures. The GAO reported that actions were needed by both agencies to ensure that companies carry out food recalls promptly. The GAO reported that the USDA can confirm more readily than the FDA whether contaminated meat and poultry products are removed from distribution. Unlike the FDA, the USDA has access to company distribution records at all points in the distribution chain. Also, USDA inspectors, store employees, and consumers are able to identify recalled canned meat and poultry products because processors *are required* to mark canned products with codes that allow for ready identification and tracing of the production lot.

In contrast, FDA-regulated foods (with the exceptions of infant-formula products and low-acid and acidified foods) *are not required* to have such label coding. FDA officials admitted to the GAO that access to distribution data and product coding would facilitate the agency's recall efforts and help ensure that contaminated foods are removed from food stores expeditiously.

vacuum-packaged smoked milkfish; salt-cured dried uneviscerated fish; smoked pheasant with no label statement that the product should be stored under refrigeration; underprocessed chopped clams; air-dried salt-cured uneviscerated vobla fish in woodcrates from Russia; canned mushrooms and canned water chestnuts from China; and salted frozen uneviscerated yellow corvina fish (croaker) from Korea.

The following year, there were Class I Recalls due to potential botulism risk from canned tuna; garlic spread; and La Choy beef pepper oriental (B-pack) dinner. In that year, the Armour Star company conducted a nationwide voluntary recall of its canned beef stew, due to a concern about a potential botulism problem.

The next year, Class I Recalls due to potential botulism continued, with cheese in vacuum-packed plastic from Texas. There was a voluntary recall of a multipack of plastic-wrapped cans of white tuna in water. The cans may have been dented or punctured during shrink-wrapping of the cans.

The Class I Recalls continued through the years. Mascarpone cheese, a soft cream cheese used in desserts, was packed in plastic tubs, and imported from Italy. Deaths from botulism had already occurred in Italy, traced to mascarpone cheese. There were more recalls for refried beans, Irish stew in defective cans, and Beefaroni (macaroni with beef in tomato sauce). The list continued, year by year.

As recently as July 2007, the FDA issued a Class I Recall of canned hot dog chili sauces, produced by Castlebury's Food Company in Augusta, Georgia, a subsidiary of Bumble Bee Seafoods based in San Diego, California. The recall was issued after a botulism outbreak occurred with four people—two children in Texas, and two adults in Indiana. All required hospitalization after consuming the chili sauce. The company recalled the chili sauce it had produced under ten different brand names, as well as canned corn beef hash, and other canned products. Then, the company recalled more than eighty types of canned chili, beef stew, corned beef hash, and other meat products as well as dog foods, in addition to the brands it had recalled earlier. In total, the company recalled more than 300,000 cans of ninety-one different products from forty-nine states. The problem was traced to anaerobic conditions, an inadequate level of acidity, too little salt/sugar concentrations, and inadequate heat.

During the same time when Class I Recalls were being issued regarding botulism, Class II Recalls were issued as well. These warnings of "remote potential" for botulism included cheesecake; a nonfat pasteurized processed-cheese product; diced pimientos; tea; dried herring imported from the Philippines; and pâté found to be leaking from improperly sealed glass containers.

Over the years, the recalls due to a potential botulism hazard have not lessened. The numbers of recalls issued in 1996 were twenty-five; in 2002, there were one hundred twenty-six; in 2005, fifty-two; and in 2006, thirty-four. The record is still one of concern. In addition to the Castlebury recalls discussed above, the USDA conducted twenty meat-and-poultry product recalls in 2007. Obviously, the potential for botulism still hovers over us.

PRACTICES THAT INCREASE BOTULISM RISK

Botulism has been with us for a long time. However, the contributing factors have changed. Formerly, improper canning of foods was a main cause. Now, newer techniques in preparing, preserving, packaging, and transporting foods are major factors in botulism.

Botulism from Commercially Canned Foods

Considering the astronomical number of commercially canned foods that are processed annually, the industry has had a notable history of safety. There have been a few incidents through the years, mainly due to improper canning procedures and/or sloppy quality control.

Two cases from the 1970s achieved great notoriety. The first demonstrated how poorly monitored surveillance can create conditions for a disaster waiting to occur.

On a hot summer evening in July 1971, a couple in Bedford Village, a suburb of New York City, dined on cold vichyssoise, canned by Bon Vivant, a cannery located in Newark, New Jersey. Subsequently, the man died, and his wife was in serious condition. Investigation identified at least five cans of the soup to be contaminated with botulinum toxin. The cans were found to be defective. The FDA initiated a massive recall of all foods from the cannery, which processed the vichyssoise under some two-dozen different brand names. The cannery also processed some fifty-two varieties of soups, nine types of gourmet sauces, and fourteen other food products. The cannery's total annual production was about 4 million cans of various food products, distributed throughout the United States, and abroad. The USDA also was involved in the recalls, because some of the products included chicken à la king and lamb stew. Products containing poultry and meat are under the purview of the USDA.

Investigation of the cannery revealed inadequate sanitary procedures, careless record keeping, and the majority of its products "not [to be] safe for consumption by man or animal." Irregularities included frequent undercooking of canned soups in sterilizing devices, and cooking records so inaccurate, inconsistent, and incomplete that they were judged by the investigators to be "totally worthless" in any determination of proper product sterilization.

The FDA's role was far from sterling. John Walden, an agency spokesperson, admitted that the FDA's previous investigation of the cannery had shown a large percentage of the company's products on the market consisted of cans that were swollen, or had leaking or defective seams. In one case, 69 percent of the examined cans of the company's spaghetti sauce were found to be defective. Despite this known record, the FDA had not inspected the plant for four years prior to the 1971 outbreak. Walden reported that the agency had only 210 inspectors to cover some 60,000 plants nationally. If this sounds familiar in 2009, it should be. The agency's resources continue to be overstretched and underfunded, and as a result, the consuming public is poorly served.

The other publicized case of botulism poisoning from commercial canning occurred in 1978, and created an international crisis. The outbreak resulted in one of the most far-reaching investigations in the annals of public health. It began in the outskirts of Birmingham, England, where the illness of two adults was traced to salmon from an Alaskan cannery. The FDA's Emergency Command Center, a unit of the Epidemiology and Environmental Health branch, sprang into action with London's Food Hygiene Laboratory. The salmon was found to contain large numbers of gram-positive sporulating rods.

Serum drawn from the patients' blood, injected into mice, produced characteristic botulism symptoms of wheezing and hind legs extended within two and one-half hours. Within four hours, all the mice were dead. Official confirmation of botulism led to prompt administration of antitoxin to the human victims. The can, when examined, had a rusty abraded area on the bottom seam, through which botulism spores might have entered. The investigators reasoned that the food within the can would have clogged the hole and sealed the live spores in an oxygenless environment needed for the spores to produce their deadly toxin. The British Department of Health and Social Security issued warnings to the public not to use or purchase canned Alaskan salmon, nor to open old stock of such products. The British authorities notified the British Embassy in Washington, D.C., and the British Commission in Ottawa, Canada, and the Canadian Department of Health and Welfare. The importer issued a press release urging consumers to return cans with a certain code number. Some 400,000 cans were returned. The retrieved cans were inspected by canning experts at laboratories of the government and of the manufacturer.

Australia also was involved. Australian officials sent the FDA cans of salmon via diplomatic pouches to the U.S. State Department.

An American investigative team flew to Alaska in a single-engine plane with a bush pilot. The plane was buffeted by strong winds and heavy rain, and landed on a flooded airstrip. The investigators slept in sleeping bags on the floor of the cannery. They conducted an on-site investigation of the cannery. They found defective double-seam formations in the cans, with microleaks due to abrasion.

There was extensive communication among Alaska, Washington, D.C., England, Australia, and elsewhere, with three months of investigation. Meanwhile, the two people originally infected, had died.

Botulism from Home-Canned Foods

In former years, improper home canning was the major source of botulism in the United States. A concerted educational effort launched by the USDA's home extension service taught proper canning techniques, and led to a decline in botulism from home-canned foods. People learned that low-acid foods, such as green beans, asparagus, corn, winter squash, pumpkin, beets, peppers, carrots, onions, mushrooms, and meat require higher heat than high-acid foods such as tomatoes, pears, and other fruits. Home canners learned that a pH of 4.6 is critical. Highly acidic foods, below pH 4.6 do not allow *C. botulinum* to thrive and form botulinum toxin, but low-acid foods above pH 4.6 will allow for dangerous growth and production of the toxin. Home canners were also informed never to use any home-canned foods that had leaking jars, nor to taste foods from such jars.

Then, botulism from home-canned foods rose, due to new developments. Tomatoes, always considered a highly acidic food, changed with the advent of mechanical harvesting. Tomatoes were being bred to be less acidic. The pH breakpoint of 4.6 became confusing. Overripe tomatoes often may have a pH slightly higher than 4.6 while less ripe tomatoes will have a pH below 4.6. As a result, commercial processors were faced with a borderline dilemma. By adding a small amount of acid, they could lower the pH below 4.5 and eliminate the possibility of botulinum toxin development. However, home canners who were not always aware of the changes in tomato breeding might not recognize the necessity of adjusting their canning procedures.

Also, home-canning skills declined as more people used freezers for food preservation. With the movement of back-to-the-land and self-sufficiency in the late 1970s, there was a revival in canning interest, but often without adequate knowledge or appropriate equipment. When the interest in home canning had declined, there were fewer canning jars or rubber rings manufactured. The self-sufficient people were faced with a dearth of jars and rings, and at times resorted to unsuitable jars and reused rings for canning. Often, their homes lacked electricity by choice, and the canning operations were conducted on woodstoves, which supply uncontrolled heating temperatures. Precise temperature is critical for proper and safe canning. These combined features were conducive to botulism from home canning, once again.

Botulism from Restaurant Practices

The nation's third worst outbreak of botulism since 1899 occurred in 1983, not in commercial or home canning, but in a restaurant practice. Patty melt sandwiches were popular in a restaurant in Peoria, Illinois. In order to fill orders promptly, the cook decided to cut and sauté the onions in advance to have them ready to fill orders. He sliced a number of onions, seasoned them, and put them into a pan with two one-pound blocks of margarine, and cooked the mixture for ten to fifteen minutes. Then, he transferred the mixture to a steam table tray and placed it on a corner of a warm stove, for ready access. The onions remained, smothered in margarine, ready to use for individual orders.

Twenty-eight people who ate the patty melt sandwiches required hospitalization due to botulism. One person died. Others were incapacitated for months.

Investigators of the outbreak found that the onions had come from a three-state western area known to have botulinum spores in the soil. This finding was not unusual, because botulinum spores are widespread in many soils, and on raw produce, too. The investigators tested the restaurant's supply of onions and found botulinum organisms present on the stems of some of the whole onions. Recreating the cook's procedure in the laboratory, the investigators found that the deadly toxin developed at the temperature of the cooked onions stored on the stove. The temperature was well within the range for incubating the bacteria that cause the botulinum toxin to form. In fact, it was very close to the optimal incubation temperature to produce the toxin. The margarine, which sealed the onions off from outside air, provided an ideal anaerobic environment for the toxin to grow and thrive.

Five years after this outbreak, in 1988, researchers led by Felissa L.

Cohen at the University of Illinois in Chicago, examined the long-term effects of botulism in the twenty-eight individuals who had eaten the patty melt sandwiches in Peoria. The team found that although the patients might appear to be fully recovered after a period of time, actually half of these individuals continued to be easily fatigued. Other chronic effects included muscle weakness, headache, and blurred vision.

Another botulism outbreak in a restaurant involved baked potatoes. In 1984, a woman ate lunch at a local restaurant in Baton Rouge, Louisiana. She ordered a baked potato. Soon after, she became ill and required hospitalization. She had slurred speech, blurred vision, and respiratory problems—all signs of botulism.

Investigation showed that the baked potato had been a leftover from the day before. It had been baked previously in a foil wrap and held overnight at room temperature. The chef had reheated the potato before serving it. These circumstances were favorable to activate botulinum spores. A laboratory analysis of another foil-wrapped baked potato, which had been discarded from the restaurant, was recovered from the restaurant's garbage. When tested, it was positive for the same type of botulinum toxin identified in the hospitalized woman.

Restaurant outbreaks can affect far greater numbers of people than outbreaks in home preparations. For example, between 1976 and 1984, botulism outbreaks from restaurant dining in the United States represented only 4 percent of the total number of outbreaks. However, they accounted for 42 percent of the total number of cases after that period. It may be difficult to trace people who are made ill from restaurant food, if they are visitors in large cities and return to other locations.

Some botulism outbreaks in restaurants have occurred due to the use of home- or in-house canned foods. Some states prohibit this practice, but others do not. Outbreaks of botulism have occurred in restaurants where improperly prepared home-bottled mushrooms or peppers have been served. In 2004, over a hundred people were made ill in Italy after eating at a restaurant where home-preserved green olives were served. Investigation showed that the olives had been held in salt water, with a pH of 6.2, a level far above the pH level needed to prevent botulinum toxin from developing.

Other restaurant practices account for some botulism outbreaks. Potato salad prepared, in part, from leftover baked potatoes resulted in one outbreak. In another, aluminum foil-wrapped baked potatoes were held at room temperature for eighteen hours, and then added to dips. One outbreak was traced to a delicatessen, which served processed cheese sauce in barbecued stuffed potatoes.

The economic costs of botulism outbreaks in restaurants were demonstrated in 1978. Thirty-four people who ate potato salad at a country club in Clovis, New Mexico, developed botulism. All of them required hospitalization; two died. A protracted legal action ended three years later. The cost of the outbreak exceeded $5.8 million, which included investigation, medical care, settlement, and legal charges. The total cost strengthens the rationale for public and private expenditures for foodborne disease prevention, and to improve food safety measures.

In recent years, it has become popular to prepare in restaurants or at home products bottled in oil. They include items such as garlic in oil, chili/garlic in oil, blackbeans in oil, chopped shallots in oil, slices of roasted eggplant in oil. Many of these infusions are stored at room temperature, in restaurants and at home. Unless an acid is added to these products, they are potential candidates for botulinum toxin development.

Outbreaks occurred from oil infusions. Eight persons developed botulism after eating an in-house homemade garlic-and-potato dip that had been served in a restaurant. In another restaurant outbreak, three people developed botulism after eating bread spread with a commercially made garlic-and-oil infusion, but lacking an acidifier.

These occurrences prompted the FDA to inform food manufacturers that to ensure safety of infused oil products, they were required to add a microbial inhibitor or acidifier (phosphoric acid or citric acid) to prevent growth of botulinum toxin. Also, such products needed to be labeled "keep refrigerated."

The FDA also advised consumers regarding home-prepared garlic-in-oil (or butter or margarine) mixes. Such products may spoil faster than commercial ones, which have a protective additive. Even if refrigerated, such home-prepared products should not be stored for extended periods.

Botulism from Improper Food Preparation and Storage

Intact raw eggs have several antimicrobial defenses, but cooked eggs are vulnerable to botulinum development if the eggs are left at room temperature for two to three days. A common practice is to allow boiled eggs to cool in the water in which they have been cooked. A natural contraction of the eggs during cooking creates an air pocket between the albumen (the white) and shell membrane, which produces a vacuum that can draw in bacteria through the shell's pores while the eggs are in the cooling water. Air-cooling of boiled eggs is safer than water-cooling. The boiled eggs should be refrigerated.

The first report of a botulism outbreak with pickled eggs was in 1997 in Illinois. Home-pickled eggs were prepared by peeling hard-boiled eggs, which were punctured and immersed in a commercial mixture of prepared beets, hot peppers and vinegar, and stored in a glass jar. The jar was closed with a metal screw-on lid, and stored at room temperature. Occasionally, the jar was exposed to sunlight. Investigation of the outbreak identified botulinum toxin type B. The toxin was a thousand times greater in the egg yolks than in the pickling liquid. It was undetected in the beets. The pH of the pickling liquid was 3.5, which was sufficiently acidic to prevent botulinum toxin from forming in the liquid. However, egg yolks normally have a pH of 6.8, making them vulnerable to the toxin. Setting the jar in sunlight provided warmth that would facilitate bacterial growth and toxin production.

From time to time, botulism outbreaks occur due to faulty storage of foods left at room temperature for extended periods, instead of refrigerating them promptly. This practice permits botulinum toxin development. Various outbreaks have occurred both in restaurant and home settings, from improperly stored foods. Reported cases have included, among others: black bean dip, potato dip, beef and tomato stew, chicken pot pie, turkey loaf, fresh-filled pasta, and pesto sauce. Many of these foods had been consumed without reheating, or without thorough reheating. Be vigilant in restaurants. For example, if soup is not piping hot when it is served, do not hesitate to send it back to the kitchen for thorough heating.

Botulism from Improper Transportation

A bizarre incident of *C. botulinum* occurred when, in December 1988, a French merchant exported fresh truffles to the United States. He was concerned that the pungent odor of the fungus would attract thieves to his shipment of eleven pounds of truffles, valued at more than $2,000. To keep the truffles' identity secret, he packed the truffles in clear, airtight plastic bags and shipped them unrefrigerated by United Parcel Service from France to the international import hub in Louisville, Kentucky. Normally, shipped truffles are canned. Because canned truffles are a low-acid food, canners must file their processing procedures for each product and each size can. This information appears on invoices and import notices.

An FDA investigator went to inspect the shipment at Louisville, only to learn that the truffles already had been forwarded to a wholesaler in Alexandria, Virginia. The inspector requested that the product be returned to Louisville for inspection. Finally, by the time the truffles were examined, the packing box was bulging. The inspector cut it open, whereupon Styrofoam packaging pieces flew everywhere. The plastic bags were swollen. Dark juice in the bags showed that the truffles had decomposed. Scientists determined that fresh truffles, packed in airtight plastic bags and shipped unrefrigerated, could support the growth of *C. botulinum* bacteria and produce botulinum toxin. The truffles had to be destroyed immediately and handled carefully to ensure that the plastic bags did not explode and emit spray. The truffles were incinerated in February 1989, two months after their inappropriate shipping procedure from France.

INNOVATIVE FOOD PRODUCTS IN NEW TYPES OF PACKAGING THAT INCREASE BOTULISM RISK

As American consumers became aware of quality and flavor, they sought "fresh" foods. Food manufacturers responded by developing "lightly processed" or "minimally processed" fresh foods. In order to retain the "freshness" in such foods, without resorting to preservatives, innovative packaging was needed. The response from packaging manufacturers was to produce new types of packing, including vacuum packaging that excludes oxygen, and packaging from which oxygen is replaced by nitrogen, carbon dioxide, or carbon monoxide.

Botulism and Nanotechnology

Nanotechnology, a rapidly expanding technology, is being applied to food packaging. The technique uses substances at exceedingly low levels. For example, a nanometer is one-billionth of a meter in diameter. (At present, the safety of substances used at such low levels is unknown in the human body, or when they enter wastewater facilities that are unable to filter them.) Substances with known properties and functions at their normal size can function quite differently in nanosize. Using nanotechnology, Honeywell of Morristown, New Jersey, and other companies have tweaked plastic's molecular structure to create a virtually impenetrable barrier through which oxygen molecules cannot enter. Such packaging is intended to keep foods "fresher" for a longer time, but increases the botulism risk.

Botulism and Vacuum-Packaged Foods

Donald A. Kautter from the FDA's Center for Food Safety cautioned food-packaging manufacturers that packaging chilled prepared foods under modified atmosphere packaging (MAP), or vacuum packaging including "sous vide" (to be discussed shortly) to extend shelf life, "limits or inhibits the growth of spoilage flora [molds and yeasts] but not necessarily [the growth of] pathogens."

Kautter had in mind, especially, the major hazard with these types of packaging: botulinum toxin development. Foods, with enough moisture content to allow bacterial growth, placed in an environment that discourages growth of common aerobic spoilage organisms but supports the growth of anaerobes, may look, smell, and taste acceptable, but actually can be toxic due to botulinum toxin development. In MAP and vacuum-packaged foods, where aerobic growth is curtailed and spoilage is not apparent, extended shelf life can provide time for *C. botulinum* to grow and produce toxin. Because nonproteolytic strains of *C. botulinum* produce toxin at refrigerated temperatures, the longer storage time may constitute a significant hazard.

Refrigerated minimally processed foods are designed to appear "fresh," contain no preservatives, and yet maintain their freshness from four to six weeks. These qualities appeal to many consumers. But are they safe? This question was studied by researchers, led by S. Notermans at the National Institute of Public Health and Environmental Protection at Bilthoven, the Netherlands. The researchers conducted a series of studies and their findings raised serious questions about the potential hazard in these products. Nonproteolytic strains of *C. botulinum* grow at temperatures as low as 3.3°C, which is well below the temperatures of the more common proteolytic strains at 10°C. The pasteurization type of heat treatment used to prepare these convenience foods is not always adequate to kill botulinum spores. Also, there are opportunities for recontamination during processing. Further, tests showed that these products, stored at temperatures at which chilled foods commonly are stored in retail stores and in home refrigerators, could result in the nonproteolytic strains producing botulinum toxin within three weeks. Ordinary heating of the product before its consumption was insufficient to kill the toxin.

The advent of vacuum packaging led to numerous types of foods packaged in MAP, including raw meats, fish, and produce. The USDA determined that vacuum-packaged raw steaks were as perishable as raw chicken. Some states had already begun to prohibit the practice of vacuum packaging of meats. Food scientists at Utah University in Logan expressed concern, by noting that some large food stores were selling vacuum-packaged meats. The scientists considered the practice "a time bomb just waiting to explode."

Regarding the hazards of vacuum-packaged foods, Wilfried Kernbach, president of Better Marketing Company, in a 1995 letter to processors, suggested that ready-to-eat foods could be made safe by putting some oxygen back into the packaging. Robert Buchanan, the USDA's deputy administrator of science and technology at the Food Safety and Inspection Service (FSIS), sent a warning letter to processors that vacuum-packaged ready-to-eat meats were safe only under certain conditions. They required constant refrigeration, salt, nitrite, and an appropriate pH level that would not permit botulinum toxin to develop.

Studies conducted with various products intentionally inoculated with botulinum toxin and nitrogen, vacuum-packaged, and then held at room temperature, were analyzed. Hamburger samples were toxic. Five sausage samples, incubated for seven days, *appeared* to be somewhat acceptable yet three were toxic. Similar studies were conducted with vacuum-packaged smoked fish. The products *appeared* to be acceptable five to eighteen days after the samples were inoculated, yet eleven of forty-five samples were toxic. People might eat the food that appeared to be safe.

A research team led by Anne D. Lambert from McGill University and the Canadian Bureau of Microbial Hazards, Health and Welfare investigated the effect of different types of modified atmosphere packaging with fresh pork. They tested different levels of radiation doses and at different storage temperatures in fresh pork intentionally inoculated with *C. botulinum*. Temperature was found to be the most critical factor. All products stored at higher temperatures eventually produced botulinum toxin. The presence of oxygen in the headspace of the packaging was not protective. Irradiation was of value only under anaerobic conditions.

An outbreak of botulism, affecting eleven persons in Argentina, occurred in 1999, as a result of vacuum-packaged meat roll (*matambre*). The meat was cooked in water for four hours, and then sealed in heat-shrink plastic wrap. Refrigeration did not cool the product adequately.

Investigation showed that the cooking time and temperature were insufficient to keep the vacuum-packaged meat safe.

Many raw or smoked fish are vacuum-packaged with MAP. In laboratory studies with salmon, cod, and whiting fillets, intentionally inoculated with *C. botulinum* spores, and stored in a carbon dioxide atmosphere, the fishes developed botulinum toxin.

In 1999, the FDA issued a warning letter about food safety problems of *C. botulinum* with vacuum-packed hot-smoked salmon, trout, halibut, and smoked salmon spreads. The smoking of fish may mask dangers, by killing spoilage flora, but that allow botulinum toxin (and *Listeria* bacteria) to continue flourishing.

Another study showed that there was no margin of safety if MAP-packaged catfish fillets were temperature abused. The toxin could not be detected prior to spoilage detection.

According to Kathleen A. Glass and Michael P. Doyle from the University of Georgia at Griffin, very few studies have been conducted regarding the microbiological safety of refrigerated vacuum-packaged convenience foods. Fresh pasta, for example, has a potential for botulinum toxin development. The water activity in fresh pasta is the principal factor in preventing botulinum toxin development under conditions of temperature abuse. More than half the samples of filled pastas (with meat or cheese ravioli, and meat or cheese tortellini) had conditions, including pH values, that were conducive to toxin formation.

Water-packed tofu came under USDA scrutiny. The agency identified *C. botulinum* as well as *Salmonella* and other pathogens as potential microbial contaminants in these products. Because pasteurization is performed after the tofu is packaged, heat-resistant spore-forming bacteria can remain viable, and grow if the tofu is not refrigerated properly, or if it is kept refrigerated too long.

MAP-wrapped, fresh-cut produce has become a popular convenience for many consumers. Its safety was the subject at a 1997 conference sponsored by the International Fresh-cut Produce Association (IFPA). Speaker after speaker warned that cases of botulism could wreck the market for ready-to-eat salads, mini-carrots, and other fresh-cut produce. Rather than trying to eliminate all bacteria—a procedure that could have disastrous consequences—the industry must accept a high level of "friendly" flora. High numbers of harmless bacteria contribute to healthy microbiological diversity. Misguided efforts to reduce bacterial counts in packaged fresh-cut produce could create perfect conditions for *C. botulinum* growth. Participants at the conference were addressed by Larry Bell of Fresh Express, a major company in fresh-cut produce. He said, "people think that because we're not canning, we don't need to worry about botulism." Bell continued, "the reason lettuce doesn't have a botulism problem is that it has a high level of beneficial organisms and spoilage organisms." Attempts by processors to "sterilize their products removes beneficial microbes such as spoilage bacteria, which render produce grossly inedible long before enough botulinum toxin is produced to harm humans. Without spoilage bacteria, consumers have no way to recognize that the product is contaminated."

In 1996, the FDA cautioned about MAP-packaged vegetables. Studies showed a low overall incidence rate of *C. botulinum* spores in precut fresh vegetables packaged in MAP, but a potential hazard if the products were mishandled, or relied heavily on refrigeration for safety. Studies with samples of Italian salad mix, shredded cabbage, chopped green peppers, and escarole all tested positive for *C. botulinum* spores types A or B. (Many foods may contain viable spores. Their presence does not always indicate a hazard unless other factors such as a high pH or temperature abuse are involved.)

In 1999, FDA's Bob Buchanan (mentioned earlier) addressed the American Society for Microbiology. He predicted, "We're just about due for a new botulism problem. We're all basically waiting to see what form it takes."

In September 2006, Buchanan's prediction materialized. There were four botulism outbreaks, in Georgia and in Florida, linked to fresh carrot juice in plastic bottles. In at least two of the outbreaks, it was suspected that the bottles were temperature-abused either in transit or in storage, even before consumers purchased them. The carrot juice had been processed by Bolthouse Farms in Bakersfield, California, under different brand names, with a "best if used by [date]" on the labels. *C. botulinum* type A was identified in the carrot juice. The FDA issued a warning to consumers not to drink the product with certain dates on labels, and advised consumers about the critical need to keep such raw juices, as well as pasteurized juices, refrigerated at all times.

Another concern was the sale of vacuum-packaging equipment to households for home use. Unless such procedure is done with meticulous care, it can be hazardous.

Sous Vide Packaging

Vacuum packaging was expanded to yet another application. "Sous vide" (French for "under pressure") is a food-processing technique developed in France in the 1970s and later introduced in the United States and elsewhere. Fresh foods are vacuum sealed in impermeable plastic pouches, and slowly cooked at a low temperature in circulating water. Then, they are chilled and held at refrigerated temperature for up to three weeks, before being reheated and served. Such foods are subjected to less processing than foods that are frozen or canned. Although sous vide foods maintain high qualities of flavor, texture, aroma, and nutrition, there is concern about their microbiological safety. With no preservatives, it is vital to maintain strict sanitation along the entire chain of food preparation, storage, distribution, and cooking processes. As with other vacuum-packaged foods, sous vide may kill many microorganisms that cause readily detectable spoilage, but does not kill pathogens such as *C. botulinum*.

Sous vide is attractive to upscale restaurants. Such foods permit restaurants to have a large selection of main entrées made with gourmet ingredients, yet require no preparation other than reheating. Restaurants that depend largely on sous vide entrées no longer need to pay highly skilled staff trained in culinary schools. The restaurants need not invest in expensive kitchen equipment. All that is required is adequate refrigeration and cooking facilities. Although the cost of sous vide items is higher than most ready-to-serve items prepared off premises, they have a far higher price on menus, and are far more profitable. What is offered is a television dinner, disguised as a gourmet entrée—and one with some risk.

ETHNIC TRADITIONS THAT INCREASE BOTULISM RISK

Alaskan natives have the world's highest incidence of botulism, according to Jeffrey Rhodehamel, a research biologist at the FDA's Center for Food Safety and Applied Nutrition (CFSAN). Traditional foods include home-processed blubber (fat) from fish or sea mammals such as whale or seal. The methods of preparation foster contamination or growth of *C. botulinum*.

In the early 1900s, whalers and explorers noted that whole families of Alaskan natives sometimes died, and the cause was thought to be botulism.

Their traditional methods of preparing and storing seafoods promote *C. botulinum* contamination and growth. Animals are slaughtered on

CHECKLIST TO DETECT DEFECTIVE PACKAGING

If you detect any of the following signs of defective packaging in the items below, avoid even tasting the contents:

Metal cans with . . .

- A swollen top and/or bottom
- A bulging side
- Dents (some dented cans are sound)
- A leak
- An obvious opening underneath the double seam on its top or bottom
- A fracture on the double seam
- A pinhole or puncture
- An unwelded portion on the side seam

Glass jars with . . .

- A pop-top that fails to pop when opened, indicating a loss of the vacuum seal
- A damaged seal
- A crack in the glass of the jar
- A chip in the rim of the jar
- Any leakage

Plastic cans with . . .

- Any opening or nonbonding of the seam
- A break in the plastic
- A fractured lid
- Swelling or dents

Paperboard boxes with . . . .

- A patch in the seal where bonding or adhesive is missing
- A slash or slice in the package
- A leak in a corner of the package
- A swollen or dented section

> **Flexible pouches with . . .**
> - A break in the adhesive across the width of the seal
> - A slash or break in the package
> - A leak at the manufactured notch used for easy opening
> - A swollen appearance
> - A leak from any area

beaches, on ground where contact with bacteria in the soil or viscera is unavoidable. Food is placed in cool, shallow, shaded pits in the ground, lined with wood, animal skins, or leaves, and covered with mosses or leaves. The food is left to ferment for a month or two. Actually, it is not a true fermentation. There are no carbohydrates or sugars, required for true fermentation, which would produce acids and inhibit growth of the bacterium. Instead, the process is one of decomposing protein and fats. Foods prepared in this manner can lead to botulism outbreaks.

In summer, "stinkheads" (fish heads) and "stink eggs" (fish eggs) are prepared this way. Throughout the year, "stinktails" (beaver tails) and "muktuk" (whale) are prepared in a similar manner. Muktuk is the skin and a thin pinkish blubber layer immediately underneath the skin of marine mammals.

The hazard from these processings has been compounded by the introduction of plastic bags to line the pits and enclose the food. The bags promote anaerobic conditions conducive to *C. botulinum* growth and toxin production. Also, tight-lidded buckets and glass jars—also new introductions—worsen the problem. Both are used to ferment the traditional foods above ground. Like the plastic bags, they too, provide an anaerobic environment. The aboveground temperature, warmer than the pits, fosters bacterial growth, even more rapidly.

Sometimes, the glass jars are kept in houses next to stoves, at about 86°F—an almost optimal temperature for *C. botulinum* growth. Prepared in this manner, the "fermentation" time is shortened to a week, compared to months in the traditional pit burial. The newer procedure has been dubbed "fast food" production.

The traditional methods of preparation—barring the botulinal potential—might have served the people well in providing essential nutrients in their diet. The process softened fish bones and rendered them edible, and a reliable source of calcium. Also, the process released vitamin B.

In 1996, a botulism outbreak in Alaska affected a pregnant Alaskan native in her second trimester. She had eaten "fermented" whitefish. *C. botulinum* toxin types A and E were cultured from her stool. It is unknown whether the toxin diffuses passively across the placental membrane, or whether an active transport mechanism exists, or if the neuromuscular effects of the toxin on a pregnant woman could affect the well-being of the fetus. Fortunately, her offspring appeared normal.

In 2001, a botulism outbreak in Alaska affected fourteen Alaskan natives who had eaten "fermented" beaver tail and paw. To prepare this ethnic dish, the tail and paw had been wrapped in a paper rice sack, and stored three months in an entryway of a house. Additional beaver tail and paw were added to the sack as recently as a week before the food was eaten. This method of preparation was nontraditional.

The following year, another botulism outbreak occurred in Alaska. Two Alaskan Yup'iks had found a carcass of a beached beluga whale that appeared to have died several months earlier. They cut the tail fluke into pieces, and put them in sealable plastic bags. Portions were refrigerated and later distributed to fourteen family members and friends. Botulism ensued. The method of processing was nontraditional.

Alaskan foodborne botulism rates exceed those of any other state. In the period between 1950 and 2000, there were 226 cases of Alaskan natives suffering from botulism from 114 outbreaks. About 27 percent of all U.S. foodborne botulism cases occur in Alaska. Many of the cases are caused by the nontraditional methods instituted since the 1970s, with the use of sealed plastics or lidded glass containers, and storage at inappropriate temperatures aboveground or inside homes.

Hawaii, too, has been a state with botulism resulting from ethnic foods. In 1990, three adults ate a reef scavenger fish, palani. It had been purchased fresh and cleaned at a retail fish market. However, the intestines were left inside. The fish was grilled at home, and the people ate the intestines as well as the meat encasing them. Investigation showed that the fish had been kept on ice in the freezer display case of the store but the cooling equipment was malfunctioning. The internal temperature of the fish on top of the ice was as high as 52°F. For safety, such fish require proper refrigeration, and proper gutting and disposal of all internal organs.

In 2006, there were two potential cases of foodborne botulism in an elderly Asian couple in California. They had purchased commercially packaged tofu at a retail market. At home, they boiled the tofu, towel-dried it, and cut it into cubes. They placed the cubes in a bowl, covered the bowl with plastic wrap, and stored it at room temperature for about two weeks. They, they transferred the tofu to glass jars, added chili powder, salt, white cooking wine, vegetable oil, and chicken bouillon to marinate the medley at room temperature for an additional two or three days. Then, without further cooking, the couple ate the marinated tofu. The couple claimed that they had used the same procedure for more than twenty-five years. This time, their luck ran out.

Kapchunka, an ethnic fish delicacy, is enjoyed in Russian communities. It is also known as *ribeyza*, or *rostov rybez*. In the United States, it is available at specialty delicatessens, or is prepared at home. Kapchunka is made by layering whole, raw whitefish, then curing it with salt to prevent bacterial growth, and refrigerating it from two to four weeks. The excess salt is washed off, and the fish is hung to air-dry at room temperature. The fish is uneviscerated.

In 1985, an elderly Russian-American couple died in New York City from botulism after eating purchased kapchunka. Analysis by health department investigators showed that the remains of the fish in the couple's refrigerator contained botulinum toxin. The fish contained too little salt to prevent growth of the bacteria that produces the toxin. The FDA issued a nationwide Class I Recall. The agency advised the company that had processed the kapchunka that it could not resume production until it could assure the agency that the product would contain a minimum of 8 percent salt in the loin muscle of each fish.

Two years later, another botulism outbreak with kapchunka occurred in New York City. A man and his nine-year-old son were made ill from purchased kapchunka imported from Israel. Public health officials reported that there is no known method to process this type of fish and guarantee its safety. It was declared a public health hazard, and such marketed products would be subject to seizure. In 1988, the FDA banned interstate shipment of kapchunka.

Nevertheless, the file case was not closed. In 1992, botulism seized four New Jersey victims. They had eaten *moloha*, a whole, uneviscerated whitefish fermented in a container with salt and seasoning.

The Republic of Georgia is reported to have the highest nationally reported rate of botulism in the world. (Apparently, Georgia vies with Alaska.)

Between 1980 and 2002, there were 879 cases of botulism. Some 80 percent of the cases were attributed to home-preserved vegetables. The most commonly implicated are tomatoes, peppers, celery leaves, eggplant and combinations of vegetables. Other implicated foods are smoked fish and meat.

BOTULISM AFFECTS CREATURES OTHER THAN HUMANS

In 1997, 400 cows died suddenly of botulism at a dairy farm. Investigation showed that a cat accidentally had been ground up in hay, which later was spread for feed.

Large-scale farming may be involved. Larger hay bales may be riskier than formerly smaller ones. Bales have gone from about 150 pounds to as high as 1,500 pounds. Also, feed rations are mixed. Previously, cows were more likely to avoid small animals such as birds and rodents inadvertently mixed into hay spread for dairy cows.

In 1999, 140 cows died from botulism on a dairy farm. Officials withheld from market 1.5 million pounds of low-heat processed powdered milk and 700,000 pounds of butter produced by the cows at this farm. The officials were willing to release 1.8 million pounds of high-heat processed milk powder, which was deemed to have been processed at a temperature high enough to make the product safe. There was no recall of some 400,000 pounds of butter already distributed.

Wildlife, too, can succumb to botulism. *C. botulinum* can reproduce in stagnant swamps and has been linked to massive deaths of waterfowl. In 1995, botulism killed nearly 50,000 birds, including thirty different species of waterfowl in Lake Grand-Lieu in France. The type of botulism was one linked to only a few cases of human poisoning. However, people were warned not to collect or eat the dead birds. The conditions favorable to botulism production were favorable in the lake: algae blooms spread due to unusually warm weather.

During the summer of 1997, millions of waterfowl in the United States and Canada were killed by botulism, traced to the birds having eaten insect larvae and other invertebrates infected with *C. botulinum*. The birds became paralyzed, suffocated, or drowned. The type of botulism was a strain not known to harm humans.

In 2002, a rare botulism strain, type C, caused both bird and fish kills around the Great Lakes.

Indirectly, some fish kills have resulted from ballast water taken on board empty ships. As noted earlier, ballast helps ships improve stability. The water is discharged when the ship reaches the port where it is scheduled to load a cargo. Often, when ballast water is taken from shallow water it contains organisms from sediment. In 1990, researchers from Australia discovered *C. botulinum* in ballast sediment from a Norwegian vessel that docked in Queensland after visiting Singapore. The spores of *C. botulinum* types B and E were found to be able to survive in the ballast sediment stored at favorable temperatures for twenty-eight days. Other infective organisms, including cholera, have been identified in other ballast waters.

BOTULINUM TOXIN AS USEFUL THERAPY

Botulinum toxin can heal as well as harm. The neuromuscular blocking effects of the toxin can be used advantageously to alleviate muscle spasms due to excessive neural activity or to weaken a muscle for therapeutic purposes. In such applications, minute quantities of botulinum neurotoxin type A are injected directly into selected muscles.

Local injections of botulinum toxin are effective in the treatment of strabismus (cross eyes); essential blepharospasm (a spasm of the eyelid's muscles); and hemifacial spasm (a spasm of one side of the face). Injections may be helpful as well for other conditions with involuntary spasms of certain muscles, such as dystonia, (a voice disorder); achalasis (a constricted esophagus); writer's cramp and related occupational hand cramps; and problems with the urinary sphincter muscle. The toxin can help calm hyperactive muscles in disorders such as Parkinson's disease and multiple sclerosis.

Botulinum toxin has become popular for other uses. These include the temporary erasure of frown lines and wrinkles due to overactivity of certain facial muscles, stuttering, strokes, scoliosis, cerebral palsy, anal fissures, vaginismus, and excessive sweating.

It has been assumed that the action of injected botulinum toxin is localized and limited. This assumption may be wrong. Matteo Caleo and his team at the National Research Institute in Pisa, Italy, found in rat studies, that neurotoxins such as botulinum toxin can travel along nerve cells and remain active beyond the intended site of the injection.

—*Journal of Neuroscience*, April 2, 2008

CHAPTER 18

Streptococcus (Strep Infection): More Than Just a Sore Throat

Harry was recovering from a strep throat. Joe, his restaurant manager, thought it was safe for Harry to return to work, as long as he covered the lesion on his hand with a bandage.

Harry returned to work. His early morning assignment was to prepare eggs for salad. He cooked, peeled, and diced the eggs and stored them in the refrigerator. He noticed that Joe had not yet replaced the gaskets and that the appliance was not very cold. Joe said that the gaskets were hard to find, and he had more important problems. The refrigerator still functioned.

Later in the day, Harry took the eggs out of the refrigerator. He chopped some raw onions, green peppers, and parsley, and added these ingredients, along with seasonings and mayonnaise, to the eggs. As he was chopping, he had to keep adjusting the moist bandage, which kept slipping. He made a mental note to change it after he finished the egg salad. By then, the refrigerator was chock-full of other prepared foods. Harry decided it would be okay to leave the egg salad on a kitchen counter. What Harry did not know was that a few hours later, patrons eating the egg salad would become ill, and some would suffer from grave health problems.

To medical doctors, *Streptococcus* is a bacterium associated with many health disorders. To epidemiologists, it is linked to outbreaks of infectious diseases, including food- and waterborne ones. To food technologists, these bacteria have strains that assist in the fermentation of yogurt and meat products. To the general public, *Streptococcus* means "strep" throat. All these characteristics can be attributed to various streptococcal strains.

TOXINS ARE RESPONSIBLE
FOR STREP A'S VIRULENCE

A new and more virulent strain of *Group A Streptococcus* has emerged, and wreaks its damage by toxins. It secretes a protein, pyrogenic exotoxin A, which acts as a "superantigen." Common antigens, the protein fragments that stimulate the immune system into activity, activate only one in 10,000 of T cells, the key immune cells. However, superantigens stimulate as many as one in ten of the key immune cells, and trigger an uncontrolled cytokine production. (Cytokines are chemicals that transmit signals between cells.) In turn, the cytokines damage the cells that line the blood vessels so that fluid leaks out, blood flow dwindles, and tissues die from lack of oxygen.

Of the invasive *Group A Streptococcus* strains studied in the United States, most carry exotoxin A. People with severe invasive *Group A Streptococcus* infection, such as toxic shock, with or without myositis (a destruction of muscle) and necrotizing fasciitis (destruction of the sheath that covers the muscle), have fewer numbers of T cells bearing the superantigen receptors, which is characteristic of a superantigen reaction. (Formerly, necrotizing fasciitis was called malignant ulcer, putrid ulcer, or hospital gangrene. A popular current moniker is 'flesh-eating bug.')

The rapid destruction of tissue is localized. But the invasive strain of *Group A Streptococcus* may have more than one means to destroy. They may have another deadly toxin. The strains of the pathogen associated with myositis and necrotizing fasciitis secrete abnormally high amounts of a cysteine protease exotoxin B, an enzyme that destroys tissue by breaking down protein.

Humans have been exposed to *Streptococcus* through many centuries. Its role in food- and waterborne diseases may be more limited than prominent pathogens such as *Salmonella* and *E. coli,* but *Streptococcus* is an important pathogen, nevertheless, because of the range and severity of its possible health consequences that it is capable of inflicting.

Streptococci are gram-positive organisms, spherical in shape and less than two micrograms in diameter. The genus *Streptococcus* is one of only five genera in the family of Streptococcaceae with organisms that cause human disease. Some strains cause food- and waterborne infections. One group (*Streptococcus pyogenes*) produces pharyngeal infections (strep throat). Others cause the majority of streptococcal infections in newborns and in maternal post-labor delivery infections. Our discussion will be limited to *S. pyogenes* (*Group A Streptococcus*) disease.

TRANSMISSION OF INFECTION KNOWN AS STREP THROAT

Streptococci bacteria travel from person to person, by hand-to-mouth or mouth-to-mouth contact, or by droplets coughed or sneezed by an infected person, and dispersed into the air. The bacteria are highly infective. As few as ten to a hundred streptococci can be an infective dose.

Probably more than a million Americans are infected each year with group A streptococcus. Children from five to fifteen years of age are highly susceptible. About one in twenty adults become infected but have no symptoms. In some groups of children, the proportion of carriers to non-carriers can be far higher, as much as one in two children.

People can become infected from foods contaminated by infected food handlers or preparers. Or, foods can become infected by contact with contaminated water (raw oysters for example).

SIGNS AND SYMPTOMS OF STREP THROAT

The incubation period is one to four days, with an average period of twenty-four to thirty hours. Typically, it is followed by a red sore throat, swollen glands, cough, headache, fatigue, muscle soreness, and fever. The infection shows clinical signs of upper respiratory illness. Less typical are signs of gastrointestinal distress such as diarrhea or vomiting. Streptococcal infection can be confirmed by laboratory analysis of a throat sample or a sample of the suspected contaminated food.

POSSIBLE COMPLICATIONS FOLLOWING STREP THROAT INFECTION

Even weeks after the throat infection has cleared up, from 2 to 3 percent of people may develop rheumatic fever. This inflammatory illness may be marked by swollen joints, damage to the heart valves, nodules under the skin, and rashes. In turn, some cases of rheumatic fever lead to Sydenham's chorea, a severe movement disorder in which the person's arms and legs flail rapidly and uncontrollably. There also may be less severe movement disorders.

Other consequences of strep throat infection include middle ear and sinus infections, and kidney disease. A rare, but dangerous complication is streptococcal toxic-shock syndrome, marked by muscle aches, high fever, confusion, dropping blood pressure, and organ failure.

It was found that children with hyperactive behavioral disorders or learning disabilities were likely to have had a strep throat infection. Also, the blood of children with movement disorders who have had strep throat infections was found to contain four to five times more of a type of antibody that appears to affect the central nervous system than children without movement disorders. The researchers suggested that a fragment of the strep membrane resembles cells in the central nervous system. Because of the similarity, the body may continue to make antibodies, in the mistaken belief that the streptococci are continuing to cause havoc even after the infection has ceased. Earlier research had suggested that such antibodies trigger the severe movements in Sydenham's chorea. Also, severe movements possibly produced from strep infections, may trigger another disorder, Tourette's syndrome.

There are still more possible consequences from strep throat infections. Some children can develop reactive arthritis or arthralgia.

FOODBORNE CONTAMINATION BY STREPTOCOCCI

Before the advent of routine pasteurization, streptococcal-contaminated milk was relatively frequent as the cause of foodborne outbreaks from this pathogen. Now, such outbreaks are rare, but occasionally they do occur, especially with foods such as unripened cheeses. Also, before widespread and adequate refrigeration of foods, streptococcal-contaminated foods were more common. Early outbreaks resulted in scarlet fever or in rheumatic fever, two conditions controlled with the introduction of penicillin. The innovations of routine pasteurization, refrigeration, and penicillin changed the pattern of foodborne streptococcal infections.

By the end of the 1980s, it was suspected that foodborne streptococcal infections were rising in the United States, but there were no firm data. Lacking information, the Centers for Disease Control and Prevention (CDC) decided to conduct surveillance in four representative states between 1989 and 1991. It was estimated that up to 15,000 cases of invasive *Group A Streptococcus* infections were occurring annually in the United States, and were resulting in 5 to 10 percent necrotizing condition (death of cells). Since that surveillance study, there were other indications that the number of *Group A Streptococcus* infections was rising, and the infections were more virulent.

OUTBREAKS OF FOOD- AND WATERBORNE STREPTOCOCCAL INFECTIONS

In recent years, foodborne sources of streptococcal infection have been with raw oysters and other uncooked seafood from contaminated water, prawn cocktail with mayonnaise, truffles, and custard-filled cakes—an ideal medium.

Fresh, unripened cheeses have been implicated in some outbreaks. In a New Mexico outbreak, homemade queso blanco was made from raw cow's milk. Samples of both the cheese and the milk from which it was made showed *Group C Streptococcus*. The same strain was identified in the blood samples taken from the people who had eaten the cheese and developed fever and chills. Some of the affected people showed localized signs of infection, including pneumonia, endocarditis, meningitis and pericarditis. One person who had abdominal pain, underwent cholecystectomy surgery due to misdiagnosis, and another underwent a needless appendectomy. Two people died. Both had underlying medical problems. The outbreak caused public health officials to close the dairy, remove the cheese from stores, and issue a public warning.

A streptococcal outbreak occurred with egg salad. In this incident, described earlier, investigators found several risk factors that could have been responsible for the contamination. A food preparer with a strep throat had boiled, peeled, and diced the eggs. He stored the eggs in a refrigerator with a faulty seal. When the eggs were removed and made into a salad with mayonnaise, the egg salad was left at room temperature for a few hours before it was served.

Another outbreak involved a macaroni and cheese dish. The food preparer had been in a barroom brawl two weeks earlier, and had a small lesion on one hand. He covered the lesion with a gauze bandage before handling the food. The bandage itself might have been contaminated.

Many streptococcal foodborne outbreaks share several common features. Food preparers, who have strep throats and/or skin lesions from the infection, handle food. These people may cough or sneeze and the droplets may come into contact with food, or surfaces contacted by food. The contaminated foods are not cooked long enough, or they are cooked at temperatures that are too low. The foods, if refrigerated, are stored at temperatures insufficiently low due to malfunctioning of the refrigerators. When removed from the refrigerators, the foods are not served immediately, but held for some periods of time at room temperature. Any of these features are high risks for streptococcal contamination and growth in foods, and can result in foodborne outbreaks.

Streptococcal Contamination in Meatpacking Plants

Workers in meatpacking plants frequently develop *Group A Streptococcus* with skin lesions, and contaminate the meat they handle. In one outbreak within a four-month period at an Oregon meatpacking plant, there were forty-four reports involving impetigo-like lesions on the hands, wrists, and forearms of workers with strep throats. Also, six episodes of cellulites (inflammation of cellular tissue, especially purulent inflammation of loose connective tissue), and two episodes of lymphangitis (inflammation of a lymph vessel) were reported. The same epidemic strain of *Group A Streptococcus* was identified from the skin lesions of the workers as from contaminated meat in the plant.

The workers who became infected had not shared knives or gloves with other workers. The practice was that meatpackers owned and maintained their own knives and gloves. The investigators suggested that the meat was a vehicle for *Group A Streptococcus* transmission.

The workers who killed the animals and deboned them did share knives. Among those workers, the risk of infection was higher. Bones are recognized as a source of skin injury among meat workers.

In cases such as the Oregon meatpacking plant outbreak, *Group A Streptococcus* could be spread from within the plant to outside the plant. In Great Britain, for example, retail butchers and restaurant workers have been infected with epidemic *Group A Streptococcus* strains during times when outbreaks occurred in meatpacking plants. It was thought that the butchers and restaurant workers became infected by their contacts with contaminated meat delivered from the incriminated plants.

Streptococcal Contamination at Fish Farms

In the late 1990s, a newly recognized and invasive pathogen was identified in skin and bloodstream infections related to injuries inflicted in workers who prepared farmed fish. The bacterium was *Streptococcus iniae*. Two days after suffering injuries from skin cuts or punctures while preparing fresh whole fish, the workers became ill.

Fish workers who become infected with *S. iniae* may suffer bacteremic illness. Some workers have developed cellulites of the hand. Others have developed endocarditis.

S. iniae had been identified in fish in the late 1970s. However, in recent years, the bacteria appear to have mutated, and have become infectious for humans. The pathogen is found most commonly in tilapia (also known as St. Peter's fish, or Hawaiian sunfish), but it is found, too, in other farmed fish such as hybrid striped bass, rainbow trout, yellowtail, eel, and turbot. The U.S. Department of Agriculture's (USDA) Agricultural Research Service regards *S. iniae* as one of the most problematic infectious pathogens in farmed fish.

Aquaculture should be regarded as an extension of land farming, with intensively reared animals. In fish farms, the fish are in overcrowded quarters, fed an abnormal diet, and develop numerous health problems. Like land animals, the farmed fish are maintained with medications to avoid mass illnesses. In fish that have become infected with *S. iniae*, their death rate is as high as 30 to 50 percent of the group. The infected fish are not known to pose danger to fish workers with unbroken skin.

It is thought that scaling, cleaning, and removal of the fish heads and appendages at retail stores before sales might be a good practice. It could reduce the potential infection from *S. iniae* for in-home preparation of the raw fish. Also, anyone who has a hand cut or lesion should avoid handling raw fish. All raw fish should be cooked thoroughly.

CHAPTER 19

Staphylococcus (Staph Infection): A Poster Child for Antibiotic-Resistant Bacteria

Rose and Dora went over the menu together. They were planning a shower party for their good friend, Sue, and her friends. Rose and Dora would take advantage of good neighborhood shopping for the foods. Both women held full-time jobs and had no time to prepare foods.

Rose and Dora planned some appetizers, including wedges of cheese and semi-dry salami on crackers, to accompany the wine. The precooked ham and precooked turkey would be accompanied by cooked vegetables and packaged fettucini salad. All these dishes were provided conveniently by the nearby deli. Dessert would be custard-filled pastries, supplied by the bakery section of the deli. Rose and Dora ordered the items a week before the shower, and all they needed to do was to pick up the foods the day of the shower. Both the ham and turkey were presliced, and arranged artistically on plastic platters, ready to be served.

The party was enjoyed, and the women attending commented on how good the food tasted. After all of them left, Rose and Dora refrigerated the leftovers and disposed of the paper plates and the plastic cutlery. They remarked about how few dishes needed to be washed.

By the time the kitchen was tidy, both Rose and Dora began to feel queasy. Soon, both women were vomiting and had diarrhea. The next day neither of them felt well enough to go to work. One by one, the attendees at the shower contacted Rose and Dora to report their illnesses. Four of them sought medical help. Of the four, two required hospitalization. One developed endocarditis; the other, reactive arthritis. Both women had very slow recoveries.

*S*taphylococcus is a facultative bacterium, meaning that it is capable of functioning under varying environmental conditions. This is illustrated by its characteristics of being non-mobile, non-spore forming, and anaerobic, yet creating havoc. *Staphylococcus* causes foodborne illness by producing one or more enterotoxins, which are the agents totally responsible for the consequences of the infection. From 50 to 70 percent of *Staphylococcus aureus* (staph) strains are enterotoxigenic.

Seven staphylococcal enterotoxins (SE) were identified, and designated as SEA, SEB, SEC1, SEC2, SEC3, SED, and SEE. In 1996, another staphylococcal enterotoxin was discovered with contaminated cheese in Brazil, and designated as SEH. Additional SEs may exist, but to date have not been identified.

The toxins remain viable in food even if the foodborne staphylococcal bacteria are killed. SEs are heat stable, and still are viable at 212°F. Only prolonged boiling inactivates these toxins. SEs also survive in solutions of salt or sugar at levels that would kill other foodborne pathogens. The process of irradiation for preserving food is ineffective in killing SEs.

SEs play a role as superantigens. They activate T lymphocytes and cause them to proliferate. Superantigens can stimulate the production of various chemical messengers. In this respect, the SEs resemble another toxin produced by *Staphylococcus:* toxic-shock syndrome toxin-1 (TSST-1). This may explain why, experimentally, the SE strains—SEA, SEB, and SEC—can induce toxic-shock-like illnesses.

SOURCES OF FOODBORNE *S. AUREUS* INFECTION AT FARMS

Sources of *S. aureus* infection may begin in farm settings. Both dairy farms and pig farms are high-risk environments.

Mastitis, an infection of the udders of cows, is caused by staphylococcal bacteria. They destroy milk-secreting cells in the cow's mammary glands. Inside the glands, the immune cells seek out and destroy invading pathogens. However, *S. aureus* and other mastitis pathogens have capsules that make their recognition difficult for the immune cells. As a result, a dairy producer with a herd of a hundred cows can expect some fifty to eighty obvious cases of mastitis each year. Mastitis costs the American dairy industry several billions of dollars annually. According to Max J. Paape at the U.S. Department of Agriculture's (USDA) Agricultural Research Service, cows with mastitis that do not respond to antibiotic treatment are culled from the herd and sold for meat, thus increasing the amount of antibiotic residue in the human food supply.

The first transgenic cow was developed in 2001. It was cloned with a gene to resist *S. aureus*-caused mastitis. The cow was manipulated to secrete a protein, lysostaphin, to help the animal resist *S. aureus* infection. The gene for lysostaphin production was obtained from a benign species of *Staphylococcus* (*S. simulans*) that competes with its disease-causing relatives.

Pig farms serve as a setting for *S. aureus* infection and antibiotic resistance. Accounts from here and abroad have associated MRSA (methicillin-resistant *S. aureus*) with pig farms and pig farmers.

In a study conducted in France and reported in 2004, the prevalence of antibiotic drug resistance in bacteria taken from the noses, throats, and stools of pig farmers was higher than from non-pig farmers. With a few exceptions, individuals in each group had not had any antibiotic treatments during the months before the study. The prevalence of *S. aureus* in the noses of non-pig farmers was similar to that reported in the general population. The higher rate in the pig farmers suggested that it was due to their work environment.

A 2005 study in France confirmed pig farming is a risk factor for increased nasal colonization with *S. aureus*. The strains found in farmers were not found in nonfarmers, suggesting the transmission between pigs and farmers. Also, transmissions of MRSA can go from farm to farm, as breeding pigs are bought and sold.

In the Netherlands, contact with pigs is recognized as a risk factor for persons to become MRSA carriers. From 2004 to 2005, MRSA was cultured from Dutch patients who had contact with pigs. The investigators also found MRSA carriers among pig farmers.

In 2006, a Dutch farmer contacted the Pig Health Unit of the Veterinary Faculty of Ulrecht University, the Netherlands, to report an outbreak among his pigs of exudative epidermitis. This is a highly infectious disease among suckling and weaning piglets in which secretion oozes through an inflamed outermost skin layer. The farmer operated a breeding farm with 200 sows. He was experiencing a high preweaning mortality rate (20 percent) in piglets caused by this skin infection. Laboratory analysis confirmed *S. aureus* infection, which was resistant to multiple drugs, and was MRSA. The investigators thought that the piglets were infected through contact with the sows. Identification of MRSA with the piglets was unexpected. The case was the first report of culturing MRSA from clinically diseased pigs.

Seventy percent of 209 pigs and nine of fourteen workers on seven linked farms in Iowa and Illinois were found to be carrying a new strain of

MRSA (ST398). This new and fast-spreading strain has been found in 12 percent of retail pork and other meat samples tested in the Netherlands by Dutch researchers. There is concern that the strain ST398 of MRSA poses a risk to the food supply.

Lynn Knipe, associate professor of animal sciences, and her team at Iowa State University in Ames, conducted a survey to determine the frequency of five pathogenic microorganisms on pork at the time of slaughter and further processing. Among the pathogens studied was *S. aureus*. The researchers collected ham and pork loin samples three times, over a period of three months, under normal conditions in three meat plants. Each time, they took samples from fifteen carcasses at five distinct points in slaughter and processing. *S. aureus* and *Salmonella* were the two most prevalent pathogens found. A significant increase in the occurrence of *S. aureus* was identified in samples taken as the pork carcasses progressed through different operations in the plants, up to the stage where pork cuts were trimmed. In general, the frequency of contamination by all the pathogens increased significantly during the handling steps after slaughter.

TRANSMISSION OF *STAPHYLOCOCCUS*

Most animals, except cows, pigs, kittens and monkeys, are moderately insensitive to SEs. Not so with people. The amount of SEs needed to cause human illness is unknown, but as little as 1 microgram of SEs in 100 grams of food will induce gastrointestinal symptoms. SEs resist proteolysis by enzyme activity. The toxins pass, without any loss of their own activity, through the stomach, to the intestinal tract, where they stimulate emesis (the act of vomiting) and diarrhea.

Humans are common reservoirs for *S. aureus*. More people are colonized by the bacteria but are asymptomatic than people who show signs of infection. From 20 to 50 percent of healthy individuals who carry *S. aureus* colonize the bacteria in the throat or nose, on the skin, or in the stool. Colonization is especially likely to occur if the skin is broken, which allows staphylococci to form abscesses at the site, or to invade the body and travel through the bloodstream to infect the kidneys, tissues, or bones. If staphylococci invade a woman's pelvic area at the time of childbirth, the newborn may become colonized and infect others by direct contact.

A carrier is a person who looks asymptomatic but harbors the infection within his or her body, and can infect others. Young children tend to be colonized carriers of staphylococci because of their frequent contact with respiratory secretions contained in "runny noses." From 10 to 35 percent of children are staphylococcus carriers, and 35 percent of the general adult population are carriers.

People who are most likely to be staphylococcus carriers and transmitters are health-care workers, who spread the infection from one patient to another by contacts; patients with dermatologic conditions; patients with long-term in-dwelling intravascular catheters; persons with insulin-dependent diabetes; and injection-drug users.

In terms of staphylococcus foodborne contamination, any carrier who handles or prepares food can be responsible for infections.

SIGNS AND SYMPTOMS OF STAPHYLOCOCCAL INFECTION

Signs of staphylococcal infection can begin as quickly as thirty minutes after consuming staphylococcal-contaminated food, but more commonly, it is from two to four hours; on rare occasions, after eight hours. The illness begins with the classical signs of abdominal cramps, diarrhea, nausea, vomiting, low-grade fever, and muscle soreness. Occasionally, the infection is accompanied by headache, weakness, dizziness, chills, and perspiration.

The infection affects the upper gastrointestinal tract. Often, it is mistaken for streptococcal infection, which affects the lower gastrointestinal tract. *Streptococcus* is an infection of longer duration than *Staphylococcus*, which lasts for only one to three days. Although death is a rare outcome, possible health consequences are numerous.

Both the time of the onset of *Staphylococcus* and the severity of the symptoms depend on the amount of toxin(s) consumed, and the individual's susceptibility to the toxin(s). The toxins can produce illness after consumption of as little as 0.1 to 1 micrograms of enterotoxins.

Much raw meat is contaminated with *S. aureus*, but the strains are less likely to be entero producing than strains from humans. Humans are the largest reservoir for enterotoxin-producing *S. aureus* strains. The presence of these microbes in food is likely to indicate poor hygiene by an infected food handler or preparer.

SOME CONSEQUENCES FROM STAPHYLOCOCCAL INFECTION

The short-lived infection can cause skin infections, including boils, abscesses, impetigo, and pusticular acne. In turn, breaks in the skin can cause the staphylococci to travel through the bloodstream and cause abscesses in the body's internal organs.

Because the infection is so highly contagious, it has what has been termed a "ping-pong effect." It can pass back and forth, more than once, between people in contact with each other. Some settings include close living quarters in military barracks; contact sports, especially those that are apt to inflict skin cuts, as well as shared athletic equipment; and children sharing toys, soap, and towels.

Prisons have close living quarters. In 2002, more than 900 inmates in a Los Angeles, California, prison became infected with MRSA. Close contact is another factor. Many free-living homosexual men in Los Angeles also became infected. Many, but not all of them, were HIV-infected as well. The boils and abscesses were on their hands, legs, chests, buttocks, and genitalia. The infection even attacked intact skin.

Some long-range consequences of staphylococcal infection include acute septicemia, bacteremia, endocarditis, urinary tract infection, and reactive arthritis. Co-infection of *S. aureus* with other infections often develops into severe necrotizing pneumonia. *S. aureus* pneumonia has been complicated further by the emergence of MRSA as a cause of infection among individuals in a community without traditionally recognized

S. AUREUS: A FACTOR IN OBESITY?

Bifidobacteria dominate in the guts of healthy breast-fed infants, and are associated with a well-functioning immune system. This beneficial organism has been linked to a reduced likelihood of childhood obesity.

A study at the University of Turku in Finland compared the intestinal flora in infancy of twenty-five overweight seven-year-olds and twenty-four normal weight seven-year-olds. Studies of their feces samples had been recorded earlier, when the children had been six months of age, and again at twelve months of age.

It was found that *Bifidobacteria* were twice as abundant in the stools of the infants who grew up with normal weight than those who became overweight. The overweight children had more *S. aureus* in their guts as infants than the normal weight ones. Moreover, *S. aureus* has been associated with chronic low-grade inflammation, which is another factor linked to obesity.

—*American Journal of Clinical Nutrition*, March 2008

MRSA risk factors. *S. aureus* infection can complicate cases of measles. During the 1968 to 1969 influenza epidemic, co-infection with *S. aureus* led to a relatively high mortality rate of 33 percent. Fatality was rapid, within twenty-four hours of hospitalization.

FOODBORNE SOURCES OF *S. AUREUS*

Many foods support the growth of *S. aureus* and its toxin formation, except those with a pH of less than 5.0. The toxins are produced over a wide range of temperatures. Growth of *S. aureus* and its toxin production may be restricted by other competing microorganisms (for example, spoilage organisms in raw food). Foods with low-water activity, such as ham, cured meat, and sweet cream products, do not support the growth of spoilage organisms, so the staphylococci can grow unchecked unless storage temperatures prevent their growth.

Staphylococcus-contaminated milk is a common source of SEC and SED. SEs are present in raw milk from mastitic cows. Commercially packaged foods are sources of *Staphylococcus* contamination, but are less common. If previously cooked protein foods such as meat or poultry are temperature abused, they become sources of SED. Cross-contamination of cooked foods by raw foods, especially raw meat, has caused some outbreaks.

Only a third of food handlers and food preparers, from whom staphylococci have been isolated, displayed any symptoms of an active staphylococcal infection. Therefore, there are probably many asymptomatic carriers who are in contact with foods.

Contamination of Cooked, Frozen, and Cured Foods

Foodborne *S. aureus* can contaminate previously cooked foods, either not recooked or recooked improperly, or stored improperly. Common sources are meats, especially cured hams and vacuum-packaged Genoa and semi-dry salami, precooked turkey, salads with eggs, potatoes, and macaroni, and cream-filled baked goods. Other foods, less commonly contaminated, have included cooked shellfish and finfish, clam chowder, chocolate milk, whey powder and milkshakes, cheese, whipped butter, vegetables, and fruits. Food recalls due to *S. aureus* contamination have included numerous incidents with canned mushrooms imported from China, canned lobster bisque, and bean curd. Japan conducted a recall after more than 7,000 people were made ill by *S. aureus*-contaminated canned low-fat milk.

Typical cooking temperatures do not destroy staphylococcal toxins. Foods contaminated with the toxins may appear, smell, and taste normal. When leftover foods are reheated, the cooking temperature may not be sufficiently high, or the cooking time may not be long enough to kill the toxins that have survived and multiplied from *S. aureus* contamination. The heat may be high enough to kill competing pathogens, which affords the *S. aureus* toxins greater opportunities to develop and thrive. The toxins can survive at 212°F. Merely bringing food to a boil is insufficient. Prolonged boiling is necessary.

Temperature abuse is another factor. If food is contaminated with *S. aureus,* allowing cooked food to remain at room temperature permits toxin formation and proliferation. It is an all-too-common experience, after the repast of a social gathering, to see the turkey or beef roast resting on a kitchen counter for hours while the social activity continues. Or, another type of temperature abuse occurs when frozen food is thawed improperly at room temperature, instead of being allowed to thaw in a refrigerator.

Foods in which staphylococci survive, but do not grow, may be hazardous if the food is used as an ingredient, along with other foods in which the staphylococci can grow. An example is a convenience food product such as precooked pasta salad, which will be discussed shortly.

Although salt acts as a preservative with many food products, the *S. aureus* toxins are highly resistant to salt. Salt-cured ham is a common vehicle for enterotoxic staphylococci. It would seem that the high salt level added to processing the ham would be protective. Yet, the toxins can grow and thrive in salt solutions. The salt content of precooked packaged ham may be as high as 3.5 percent, yet provide an ideal growth medium for *S. aureus* and its toxins.

Drying, freezing, and heating will injure or stress *S. aureus* cell walls so that the pathogen is unable to form colonies in the presence of salt. But the injured cells have an ability to repair themselves and continue to form colonies in the presence of salt.

Contamination of Precooked Foods

S. aureus is one of the most common types of food poisoning associated with precooked pasta products. Often, such products are wrapped in modified atmosphere packaging (MAP). John R. Mount and his associates in the Department of Food Science and Technology, at the University of

Tennessee in Knoxville, studied the survival of *S. aureus* in MAP-packaged cooked fettucine noodles. They found that intentionally contaminated cooked pasta product had to be stored at near-freezing temperature in order to prevent bacterial growth in the packaged product.

A notable outbreak from a tortellini pasta product at a luncheon held at the posh Waldorf-Astoria Hotel in New York City in 1993 made 180 people ill. The investigators traced the pasta product back to its manufacturers, Nuovo Pasta Productions, located in Stratford, Connecticut. Investigators found that the plant had numerous deficiencies. Ingredients were held at room temperature for extended periods of time. One food handler had an open cut on his finger. Pasta drying and freezing racks were not sanitized between production runs. The product manufacturing dates and codes did not correspond to actual production dates. Employees used cases marked with previous lot numbers to pack a new day's production. The hoppers and rollers in the forming equipment were cleaned inadequately between uses. The pasta kneader-sheeter had dough adhering to it from previous runs even after the appliance had been cleaned. Fluorescent light fixtures lacked protective coverings. One employee wore jewelry.

Because the products of Nuovo Pasta Productions were shipped interstate, the federal Food and Drug Administration (FDA) was involved. As noted earlier, the agency can *request* but *cannot mandate* recalls for such products. (In contrast, the sister agency USDA can close down operations in meatplants if the agency deems a problem to be a threat to human health.) Nuovo refused to initiate a voluntary recall. In an act of "gentle persuasion" the FDA agents suggested that Nuovo should contact its liability insurance carrier to find out if its policy would cover a company leaving a product on the market, knowing that the product is a potential health hazard.

Finally, Nuovo recognized that a product recall was in its own best interest. The company mailed a recall letter to some twenty distributors. The original outbreak had been on November 7, 1993. The recall letters went out nearly two months later, on December 29, 1993. In January 1994, the plant was inspected. Some *S. aureus* was still identified, but not at levels requiring regulatory actions. The inspectors deemed that the levels were not likely to produce toxins.

In February 1994, Nuovo recalled and destroyed products. The recall involved sixty-five different varieties of pasta products, distributed for restaurant and institutional use.

Unsuitable Packaging and *S. aureus*-Contaminated Food

Both canned and fresh mushrooms have been vehicles for *S. aureus* contamination. The problem with canned mushrooms probably is due to insufficient heat during retorting (cooking). The problem with fresh mushrooms differs, and packaging may be involved.

Using polyvinylchloride (PVC) plastic overwrap to seal packages of fresh mushrooms creates a near-anaerobic environment that allows enterotoxigenic strains of *S. aureus* to grow. Stefan Martin and his colleagues in the Department of Food Science at Pennsylvania State University, University Park, noted that *S. aureus* normally does not compete well with other food bacteria. Experimentally, by overwrapping the packages, the unventilated mushrooms intentionally inoculated with *S. aureus*, grew the bacteria after four days. Ventilated-packaged mushrooms suppressed the growth of *S. aureus*, and after several days of storage, no enterotoxins were detected. However, temperature-abused packages led to growth of *S. aureus* in the ventilated packages that exceeded the growth in the unventilated ones. The researchers recommended that fresh mushroom packages be ventilated and stored refrigerated during distribution as well as in retail stores. The FDA entered into an agreement with the mushroom industry that all fresh mushroom packaging be ventilated. However, this practice is not required by law.

THE ANTIBIOTIC-STAPHYLOCOCCAL CONNECTION

From the beginning, staphylococci were linked to penicillin, the first manufactured antibiotic. Sir Alexander Fleming (1881–1955), a Scottish

NEW FOOD TECHNOLOGIES INCREASE STAPHYLOCOCCAL INFECTION RISKS

"Consumer demand for more 'fresh' refrigerated foods and the use of new technologies, such as modified atmosphere packaging and sous vide, which alter the natural microbial flora of foods, leave us only one tenuous safeguard—the refrigerated distribution system," noted *Food Technology* (Dec 1990). In the case of *S. aureus*, even refrigeration is an inadequate safeguard.

bacteriologist, was interested in antibiotic substances that would be non-toxic to animal tissues. In the late 1920s, Fleming was researching influenza bacteria. He noted that a mold contaminant had developed accidentally on an old staphylococcal culture. The mold had created a bacteria-free circle around itself. Experimenting with it, Fleming found that a liquid made from the mold culture prevented staphylococcal growth, even when the solution was diluted a hundredfold. Fleming named the manufactured antibiotic penicillin because it was derived from the mold, *Penicillium.*

Penicillin was hailed as a "wonder" or "miracle" drug because it could control bacteria, yet had remarkably few harmful effects. Science writer Nicolas Rasmussen, in describing penicillin, noted that it made possible for humans to escape the "ancient ecological constraints and reach for total rationalistic dominance of living nature." Rasmussen views penicillin as "the technological fix . . . [that] enables a massive scale-up in factory farming, making gigantic feedlots and chicken batteries that previously had been foiled by infectious diseases not just possible but economical." Further, the introduction of penicillin reflected "the ascendancy of technology as the vehicle to health [and] brought with it a rise in the status of drug firms, and a decline in the status of doctors whom patients came to regard less as founts of wisdom than as conduits of pills."

Increased Use of Antibiotics

After penicillin's success, pharmaceutical companies developed numerous antibiotics. These drugs were regarded as so miraculous that they were proposed as routine additives to crop sprays, in animal feed, and in food preservatives. It was suggested that blight on some fruits, and diseases of other crops might be eliminated with penicillin use. Foods such as hamburgers could be sanitized, if another group of antibiotics, tetracyclines, were applied in massive doses.

There was some reason for such optimism. Penicillin had subdued some serious diseases such as scarlet fever. But, as early as 1942, Fleming warned the medical profession about the emergence of antibiotic-resistant strains of staphylococci. By then, researchers discovered that bacteria contain an enzyme that can break off penicillin's molecular core.

Howard W. Florey, co-developer with Fleming of penicillin, also decried the overuse and misuse of penicillin. Prophetically, Florey warned that penicillin's ineffectiveness might already be developing. He cited clinical cases that required four to eight times the initial antibiotic dose in order to control infections. Florey noted that some coliform organisms actually *increased* during the course of penicillin treatment. He warned that other bacteria could emerge whose potential for infection or harm as yet was barely comprehended.

Despite these early warnings, popular scientific accounts from 1942 through 1948 heralded every newly developed antibiotic as part of the growing consortium of wonder drugs that would eliminate infectious diseases that had been scourges through the centuries.

In the 1950s, methicillin, a semi-synthetic penicillin, was introduced. It allowed for relaxation of traditional hygiene with people and with farm animals. Many dairy cows, for example, were being treated with penicillin for mastitis due to a staphylococcal-related infection. A 1955 market survey showed that nearly 12 percent of 474 milk samples selected nationwide, were contaminated with penicillin. Meat, poultry, and eggs, when tested, were showing residues of antibiotics.

Staph Infections Spread, Unchecked

At the same time, a new phenomenon emerged: staph infections in hospitals, long-care nursing homes, and other institutions where large numbers of people are confined, and in contact with each other. For decades, such infections have raged. They have not been contained, and have worsened. The staphylococcal infections in such settings became resistant to antibiotics. First, they became resistant to penicillin, the antibiotic long in use. In 1952, all staphylococcal patients had responded to penicillin treatment, but by 1980 that number dropped to 10 percent. A similar pattern followed with other antibiotics, with fewer and fewer of them effective for controlling infections. Methicillin resistance to *Staphylococcus aureus* became so common that its acronym MRSA came into widespread usage. A wild strain of *Staphylococcus* acquired a mobile genetic element containing a gene for methicillin resistance, which can cause severe skin and soft tissue infection. The infection, untreated, can lead to toxic shock syndrome, or can reach the lungs and cause pneumonia.

Vancomycin, one of the last bows in the quiver of antibiotic treatment, also has become ineffective. Hospitals and other institutions continue to struggle in combating MRSA and its consequences.

As staph infections continue in institutions, the problem has become even more widespread in community settings, involving the general pop-

STAPHYLOCOCCAL INFECTIONS IN HOSPITALS

Staphylococcal infections in hospital settings are not new. The renowned bacteriologist, Robert Koch (1843–1910) isolated and cultivated staphylococci from surgical infections. Since then, we have learned that high-risk factors for hospital patients to acquire MRSA infections include: persons who have had antibiotic treatment prior to hospitalization; being placed in an intensive-care unit; undergoing surgery; and those who are in contact with other people in the hospital who are MRSA-infected (for example, other patients, hospital staff, and visitors).

Hospital health-care workers can be transmitters of MRSA if they fail to wash their hands after physically examining one patient before examining the next. Healthy people can carry staphylococci in the nose and throat, as well as on skin and hair. One reported case described how a surgeon infected a patient during an operation from the surgeon's nasal secretions.

MRSA can be transmitted in hospital settings by fomites, such as stethoscopes and other hand-held instruments, catheters, and dialysis equipment. Even neckties and jewelry can be transmitters. The staphylococcus toxins can withstand hot water and some disinfectants commonly used in hospitals. Some institutions now use self-sterilizing bedsheets.

ulation. Presently, the issue of staphylococcal infection encompasses agricultural practices, food handling, and preparation practices, as well as institutional and community practices. All these factors are interwoven in any discussion of foodborne outbreaks of *S. aureus.*

Strangely, the CDC does not include staphylococcal cases in its list of notifiable infections. Yet, *S. aureus* is highly infectious. In earlier years, the CDC *did* include this pathogen in its Annual Summary of Notifiable Infectious Diseases. Without data of reported laboratory-confirmed cases, it is impossible to have any idea regarding the extent of current staphylococcal infections in the United States. One can assume that the numbers are large, combining foodborne sources along with institutional and community sources. Also, one can assume that the total numbers are large because everyone either has experienced staph infection personally, or has had a family member, friend, neighbor, or relative who has had the infection in recent times.

THE QUEST FOR NONRESISTANT ANTIBIOTICS

Because antibiotics become ineffective, many pharmaceutical companies have discontinued spending the effort and money required for research and development of new antibiotics. Other drugs are more attractive to develop if they are likely to have long-lasting sales, and fewer uncertainties. As a result, in recent years, few new antibiotics have been developed.

Antibiotics are derived from naturally occurring substances. It was logical to search for naturally occurring substances that might have similar effects, without the drawback of bacterial-resistance development.

Two antibiotics were discovered inadvertently in soil fungus, and in experiments, they inhibited *S. aureus* growth. Robert A. Baker, a chemist at the USDA's Agricultural Research Service at Winter Haven, Florida, and his team were examining the association of soil fungus with citrus diseases. The antibiotic compounds were unknown previously, and were found to inhibit the growth of MRSA bacteria.

Christoph Schempp and his colleagues at the University of Freiburg, Germany, found that hypericum, a chemical contained in the plant, St. John's wort, inhibited the growth of MRSA. This herbaceous plant is used medicinally to treat skin injuries, burns, and other ailments.

A fraction in cultured tissues of lettuce and cauliflower was described as "highly and consistently inhibitory" of *S. aureus* growth, by Gordon Campbell and a team at the University of New Brunswick in Canada. The researchers were looking for plant substances with antimicrobial activity. They suggested that the use of cultured plant tissues should be investigated for various bactericidal substances of medical interest.

Scientists associated with the National Agricultural Research Foundation in Greece found experimentally that high concentrations of oleuropein and phenolics, both extracted from olives, were able to inhibit the growth of *S. aureus* and its production of enterotoxin B.

Atsuyoshi Nishina and his colleagues at Nippon Oil and Fats Company in Tokyo reported that bamboo extract inhibited the growth of *Staphylococcus* species. The chemists pulverized bamboo bark and dissolved the powder in an alcoholic base. Then, they isolated four extracts from the liquid mixture. The extracts were especially effective against staphylococci.

A compound isolated from plants used traditionally in Native American medicine may be a key discovery for the development of drugs to treat MRSA, according to Kim Lewis at Tufts University's Biotechnology Center in Medford, Massachusetts, and Frank R. Stermitz at Colorado State University in Fort Collins. Jointly, they led a team of researchers who isolated a substance from the leaves of barberry plants. Coupled with antibiotics, the compound inactivated strains of *S. aureus* that are mainly responsible for MRSA. The basis for combining the two components was that one undermines the bacteria's defense mechanism, and the other kills it. Medicinal plants adopted this two-pronged strategy during their evolution.

New Zealand honey from bees working the manuka bush is considered inedible due to its bitterness. However, the honey has a potential use as a therapy for MRSA. This honey, applied to wound dressings, appeared to control staphylococcal infections. To understand its mechanism of action, Rose Cooper and her colleagues at the University of Wales Institute in Cardiff, United Kingdom, used an electron microscope to observe *S. aureus* growing on petri dishes. Many of the bacteria were immobilized after encountering manuka bush honey. The *S. aureus* cells began to divide, but then stopped. The researchers are attempting to identify the component(s) that interfere with *S. aureus* cell division. Sterile manuka bush honey has been available by prescription in the United Kingdom since 2004.

These are some of the investigations in the quest for nonresistant antibiotics to control *S. aureus.* One researcher predicted, "Plants may hold the key to ultimate antibiotics."

In discussing penicillin, Nicolas Rasmussen, mentioned earlier, suggested that instead of regarding antibiotics as miracle drugs, they should be viewed as "limited resources that require stewardship . . . In an era that increasingly assumes that science and technology bring costs with every benefit and rejects rationalist fantasies of nature forever dominated by one fix after another, the promise that chemistry will always stay ahead of bacterial evolution seems hollow . . . If our culture's flagging trust in technological institutions like the drug industry means that after forty years, we finally heed calls to limit antibiotic use in agriculture and outpatient medicine, then this may be one tragicomedy with a happy ending."

CHAPTER 20

H. pylori: A Dramatic Discovery in Gastroenterology

In the early 1980s, the internist and the pathologist took turns peering into the microscope. They were convinced that the unidentified corkscrew-like bacteria were pathogenic. But they were unable to convince the medical establishment. To prove the pathogenicity, the internist boldly ingested the bacteria and waited. Within a few days, he became ill.

An old adage previously held that stomach ulcers arose from "hurry, worry, and curry." It was thought that a lifestyle with emotional stresses and anxieties, accompanied by too much alcohol, tobacco, and caffeine, plus a diet rich in spicy foods, led to stomach ulceration. The common belief was that all these factors produced too much stomach acid. The solution was to reduce the stomach's acid level. The old dictum was "no acid, no ulcer."

CONVENTIONAL VIEW OF STOMACH ULCERS

It is true that ulceration can result from the highly acidic stomach acid and pepsin (a digestive enzyme) contacts at the submucosal or muscular layers of the stomach. But mucus production by the mucous-secreting cells of the stomach and the duodenum usually provide adequate protection. Certain drugs, such as steroids and non-steroidal anti-inflammatory drugs (NSAIDs), over time, may contribute to ulceration by inhibiting production of an enzyme (cyclooxygenase) that produces prostaglandins, which help protect against mucosal damage.

Routinely, people with peptic ulcers were advised to follow a bland diet, and to drink milk. Later, the milk recommendation was revised. Although milk does have a buffering action on gastric acid, the calcium and hydrolyzed milk proteins that it contains actually *stimulate the production of more acid.*

There was scant evidence that the caffeine in coffee induces peptic ulcer disease, or interferes with healing. Tea, cola drinks, 7-Up, and even decaffeinated coffee stimulate acid secretion just as much as regular coffee. Even the advice to avoid spicy foods did not appear to be valid. A study led by N. Kumar, of men with duodenal ulcers, demonstrated that hot chili peppers eaten daily did not show any reduction in the rate of healing, compared to a control group.

CONVENTIONAL TREATMENT AND ITS LIMITATIONS

Conventional medical treatment for stomach ulcers focuses mainly on antacids and H2-receptor antagonists such as cimetidine (trade name, Tagamet) to block the production of gastric acids. The term H2-receptor antagonists sometimes is shortened to H2 antagonists, or H2 blockers. This treatment can be effective in reducing acidity and allows time for the inflamed ulcerated area to heal. However, the treatment deprives the body of the beneficial effects of stomach acid, which protects the body against many of the intestinal pathogens such as *Salmonella*, *Shigella*, and enterotoxic *Escherichia*. Also, the stomach acid is necessary for digestive activity, and lacking adequate acid lowers the body's absorption and utilization of nutrients.

The H2-receptor antagonists, widely used to treat peptic ulcer, suppress symptoms but fail to cure the disease. People may be asymptomatic after this treatment, but endoscopic examination after a year has shown many relapses—up to 80 percent. After two years, relapses were 100 percent.

Even persons given maintenance therapy with continued use of H2-receptor antagonists had a cumulative recurrence rate of 48 percent after one year. Some individuals seemed to require permanent therapy.

The results of treatments were discouraging. What was missing from the therapy that might permit stomach ulcers to heal, and not require repeated treatment?

A DRAMATIC DISCOVERY

In the early 1980s, J. Robin Warren, a pathologist at the Royal Perth Hospital in Western Australia, kept finding strange occurrences of apparently infectious organisms in the stomachs of people who previously had gastric resections for peptic ulcer disease. He brought the finding to the attention of a colleague at the hospital, Barry J. Marshall, a resident in internal medicine. The finding piqued Marshall's curiosity as well.

Marshall applied scientific methods in an attempt to document the association of the infectious organism with gastritis and peptic ulcer disease. (Gastritis is a term used to describe a group of conditions characterized by inflammation of the mucous membrane lining the stomach.) By 1981, Marshall and Warren detected a corkscrew-like bacterium in biopsy specimens from patients with histologic gastritis. (Histologic refers to the structure, composition, and function in tissues that display the condition.) They noticed inflammation at the site of the bacterium in the gastric mucosa (a protective mucous lining of the stomach).

Out of curiosity, Marshall and Warren performed biopsies on every patient undergoing endoscopy in 1981. They found these corkscrew-like bacteria in some 600 patients. Marshall and Warren were unable to identify the bacterium with any known ones. They termed them *Campylobacter*-like organisms, with the acronym CLO.

At first, the two men focused on gastritis. They found that nearly all patients with type B antral gastritis (a region of the stomach) were infected with CLO. Then, they discovered that nearly all patients with peptic ulcer disease, and most with gastric cancer, also were infected with CLO. The bacterium was present in at least 90 percent of all duodenal ulcers, and in 60 to 80 percent of all gastric ulcers.

Mode of Action

The following year, Marshall and Warren succeeded in culturing the organism from the stomach. This led to the discovery that the bacterium had unique characteristics. It had an ability to produce the enzyme urease; a feature not shared with other *Campylobacter* species. The organism did not rightly belong to the *Campylobacter* genus. As a matter of fact, the bacterium did not seem to belong to any other known genus.

In April 1982, Warren was culturing this unusual bacterium. Then, the hospital experienced an outbreak of antibiotic-resistant *Staphylococcus aureus* (staph infection, see Chapter 19). For a few days, Warren's laboratory was overwhelmed with work on this infection, and his work with petri dishes containing the strange bacterium had to be set aside. The petri dishes remained in an incubator for five days, which was three days longer than standard procedure. However, the tardiness proved to be fortuitous. The elapsed time was sufficient for the bacterial colonies to become visible microscopically. Marshall and Warren decided to rename the newly identified bacterium, *Campylobacter pyloridis*. (By 1989, the organism would be renamed once again. It was given a new genus, and renamed *Helicobacter pylori*, which remains as its name.)

The Thunder of Silence

By 1983, Marshall and Warren had studied the bacterium thoroughly and were convinced that it was implicated in gastric ulcers and gastric cancer. They were ready to announce to the medical world that the bacterium caused peptic ulcer disease. Marshall was confident that the finding would receive immediate and universal acceptance in the medical community, as well as by pharmaceutical companies. The two men suggested that from now on, peptic ulcer therapy would consist mainly of treatment with antimicrobials, and that a brief treatment would eradicate the bacterium and heal the ulcer permanently.

Marshall and Warren's announcement was met with a thunder of silence. Doctors were skeptical that a bacterium could survive stomach acidity. Most of their colleagues at the hospital thought that the hypothesis was so preposterous that they declined even to look at the bacterium in the microscope. A few who did declared the bacterium as "aberrant" or an anomaly. Medical journals rejected articles submitted by Marshall and Warren. There was a certain degree of snobbery; a hospital in Perth was regarded as a backwater institution. The inference was that medical breakthroughs emanate from prestigious institutions.

The pharmaceutical companies were disinterested. They were content with their large profits that flowed from continuous sales of Tagamet and Zantac (its largest competitor), used over and over again in traditional treatment of gastric ulcer therapy. According to reporter Jerry E. Bishop, who wrote later in the *Wall Street Journal* in 1994, the continued use of conventional therapy with H2-receptor antagonists would cost a patient more than $11,500 for fifteen years of maintenance, and frequent relapses. Stomach surgery performed when stomach ulcers bleed repeatedly costs about $18,000. These figures were for 1994. According to Bishop, the H2-receptor antagonists comprised a huge market, estimated at $5 billion annually worldwide. Zantac had sales of $3.5 billion in the fiscal year ending in 1993. This amount represented nearly half of the company's total sales. Tagamet, the original H2-receptor antagonist, represented another billion dollars in annual sales. In contrast, Marshall's suggested antimicrobial treatment would have cost, in 1994 figures, about $925 for a one-time cure.

Draconian Action

Finding no receptive audience to investigate the connection between the infective organism and stomach ulcers, Marshall took bold action. As he recalled later, "To prove that people without gastritis could catch *H. pylori*, in 1984 I decided to infect myself. One week after drinking a culture of *H. pylori*, I developed severe gastritis and we cultured the germ from my biopsies."

Marshall was able to demonstrate that stomach ulcer is an inflammatory condition of gastric mucous-secreting epithelium, variously termed "type B gastritis," "antral gastritis," "active chronic gastritis," "superficial gastritis," or "acute gastroduodenitis." *H. pylori*, nearly universally present in these conditions, is found adhering to the gastric mucosa. The bacteria do not attach to the cells of intestinal type, so they are not found in the duodenal cap, except on islands of the gastric epithelium.

SOME UNSUNG HEROES

After Dr. Marshall was convinced that he and Dr. Warren had identified an unrecognized pathogen, he searched the literature to learn if there had been earlier investigators. He found that a century earlier there had been some investigators. Among them was a German doctor, named Boettcher. However, his work was not recognized by others, and the doctor was discouraged from further study of the bacterium.

In 1940, Dr. A. Stone Freedberg, an American researcher, identified a corkscrew-like bacterium in the stomach of ulcer patients in Boston, Massachusetts, where he practiced. But other scientists failed to confirm his findings. Dr. Herman L. Blumgart, his superior, suggested that Freedberg move on to another project, with something easier to prove. Freedberg abandoned the project with the bacterium.

H. pylori's Survival in a High-Acid Environment

One of the reasons that the medical community was so skeptical of Marshall's claim was due to the conventional wisdom that bacteria cannot survive in a highly acidic stomach. *H. pylori* turned out to be an extremely hardy bacterium, and able to resist the highly acidic environment of the stomach. To date, it is the only known bacterium with this capability. It has high urease activity. This enzyme acts on urea (a chemical waste product) present in the stomach, and produces a cloud of ammonia and bicarbonate. This action raises the local pH surrounding the bacterium. Using their flagella, *H. pylori* then migrate through the mucus layer to the mucous-secreting cells, where they attach to the cell membrane and cause damage to the microvilli and cytoskeletal web. They destroy the intercellular junctions, trigger inflammation, and severely reduce the cell's ability to manufacture mucus. In addition, *H. pylori* produces protease (a protein enzyme) and a lipase (a fat enzyme). Both enzymes digest the mucus layer. With the mucus layer compromised, gastric acid and pepsin are able to attack the gastric epithelium and produce ulceration.

If Marshall and Warren had proposed their hypothesis in more recent times, the idea that a bacterium could survive in the highly acidic environment of the stomach would not have seemed so outrageous. Since then, we have learned that other bacteria not only exist but actually *thrive* in other harsh environments of extreme cold and extreme heat. Some are found in thermal vents and in volcanoes. Others can live in extremely saline salt flats, and even in granite. In truth, no part of the planet is free of bacteria, and this is especially the case within the human body that houses rich sources of nutrients that allow both beneficial and pathogenic organisms to thrive.

NEWER FINDINGS

After Marshall and Warren's seminal work, there have been additional findings about *H. pylori.* Inoculation of different species of *Helicobacter* into the stomachs of experimental animals also led to gastric mucosal inflammation in the animals, as it had in humans. By 1997, in addition to *H. pylori* in humans, at least eighteen other *Helicobacter* species were identified. Only one appears in humans.

Marshall and Warren's investigations related *H. pylori* infection to various types of gastric ulcers. Later studies have shown that these infections, if not eradicated, can lead to stomach cancer. A 1991 study, led by Julie Parsonnet, showed that nearly 90 percent of patients who underwent gastrectomy for intestinal-type stomach cancer also had *H. pylori* infection. Parsonnet reported, "Ours is the first study to show a direct association between *H. pylori* and gastric cancer."

Chronic *H. pylori* infections may be carcinogenic because they cause chronic local inflammation and trigger inflammatory cells to release mutagens. Inflammation also stimulates cell division, which makes cells vulnerable to carcinogens.

Over time, the frequent use of heavily smoked and salted or poorly preserved foods may lead to atrophic gastritis and make the gastric mucosa more susceptible to cancer development. Foods relatively rich in nitrates, nitrites, and secondary amines (for example, bacon, frankfurters, and smoked ham) can combine to form N-nitroso compounds known as nitrosamines. These compounds have been shown to induce gastric tumors in animals. Moreover, anaerobic bacteria, which often colonize in stomachs that already are affected by atrophic gastritis and intestinal metaplasia, may convert nitrates and nitrites to potentially carcinogenic compounds. A diet with an abundance of fruits and vegetables that contain adequate quantities of vitamin C (ascorbic acid) exerts a buffering effect against nitrosamines.

In 1994, the World Health Organization (WHO) classified *Helicobacter pylori* as a carcinogen.

Recently, with growing interest in the role of genes in health and disease, some attention has been given to *H. pylori*. In a study conducted at Wayne State University in Detroit, Michigan, researchers found some strains of *H. pylori* that harbor a gene that may be implicated in a large share of stomach cancers. Individuals infected with a strain of *H. pylori* CagA (an acronym for cytotoxin-associated gene-A) are sixteen times more likely to develop premalignant stomach growths than individuals infected by a strain of *H. pylori* that lacks the gene. Ikuko Kato, a cancer epidemiologist who coauthored the study, reported that "it matters what kind of *H. pylori* a person has. It affects the risk of developing these precancerous lesions." People with these lesions, called dysplasias, are up to 100 times more likely to develop stomach cancer as are people without them.

Marshall and Warren's Legacy

Marshall's dramatic self-inflicted infection proved the connection between *H. pylori* and stomach ulcers. Gradually, the medical community begrudgingly changed its attitude and therapy. By 1994, the National

Institutes of Health (NIH) issued a Consensus Statement on *"Helicobacter pylori* in Peptic Ulcer Diseases."* The Consensus Statement was extraordinary. It did not *recommend* but *required* doctors to follow the treatment regimen originally outlined by Marshall and Warren, using antimicrobials to eradicate the bacterium. The treatment for gastric ulcers underwent a sea change.

The following year, Robert Glickman, the Herman L. Blumgart Professor of Medicine at Harvard Medical School and Chair of the Department of Internal Medicine at Beth Israel Hospital in Boston, proclaimed, "the role of *Helicobacter pylori* in gastrointestinal disease is one of the most dramatic discoveries in gastroenterology." Other kudos abounded.

In 2005, the pioneering work of Marshall and Warren was acknowledged both in worldwide recognition and monetarily. The Nobel Prize in Physiology and Medicine was awarded to Marshall and Warren for their innovative work that revolutionized the treatment of stomach ulcers. The *Journal of the American Medical Association (JAMA)* declared in its November 9, 2005 issue that the "controversial hypothesis" of the two men was "dogma-shattering" and took years to gain acceptance.

THE GENOME OF *H. PYLORI* IS SEQUENCED

In the late 1990s, researchers at the Institute for Genomic Research (presently, the J. Craig Venter Institute) announced that they had completed the genome of *H. pylori.* The 1.7 million-pair sequence was obtained and analyzed by Jean-Francois Tomb and J. Craig Venter of the Institute and forty coworkers. The group believes that the sequence data will be useful for developing antibacterial and antiulcer drugs. Russell F. Doolittle of the Center for Molecular Genetics at the University of San Diego, California, called the study a tremendous accomplishment involving "breathtaking" speed of data generation and "insightful and thorough" genetic analysis.
—*Nature,* 1997

Marshall and Warren's legacy extends far beyond their work with *H. pylori.* Their findings encouraged many other researchers searching for causes of many chronic diseases to consider, for the first time, the possibility of infectious agents as factors. The researchers began to seek out possible infectious agents as factors in many chronic diseases of unknown etiology.

HOW IS *H. PYLORI* TRANSMITTED?

Writing in the June 2000 issue of the *Journal of Bacteriology*, an international group of scientists suggested that *H. pylori* did not evolve in prehuman ancestors over millions of years. Rather, the bacterium is a more recent phenomenon, and was transmitted from animals to humans when agricultural practices and population densities increased some 10,000 years ago. The scientists analyzed DNA from samples of more than 500 strains of *H. pylori* from five continents. The analyses showed five different genetic types. Each was associated with a different area of the world, with a link between proteins produced by the *H. pylori* CagA gene and proteins found in various animal hosts, including both domesticated animals and rodents. The ancestors of European strains of *H. pylori* might have come from mice or sheep, and ancestors of Asian strains, from cats, pigs, or Mongolian gerbils. All these animals can be infected with certain *H. pylori* strains recovered from human patients.

David Y. Graham, at Baylor College of Medicine in Houston, Texas, believes that humans might not have had a long history with *H. pylori*, but acquired the infection only after they began to domesticate sheep. Shepherds in modern Italy are about eighty times as likely to be infected with *H. pylori* as are their non-shepherding siblings or the general population. In the July 10, 1999 issue of the *Lancet*, Graham recorded that 60 percent of raw milk samples from sheep on Italian farms contain traces of DNA from *H. pylori*. This suggests that the bacterium could have been transmitted to people centuries ago from sheep, via its original host: raw milk. Graham's findings reinforce those of the international group of scientists noted above.

H. pylori and Transmission Person to Person

H. pylori can be transmitted from person to person. In a clinical research unit in a hospital in Northern California, asymptomatic *H. pylori* infected and non-infected adults were studied. All of the infected individuals were given a cathartic and an emetic. The lead researcher, Julie Parsonnet, reported in 1999 that fecal and oral shedding of *H. pylori* from otherwise healthy but infected adults was confirmed from stools, air, or saliva, before and after a cathartic and emetic, and from vomitus during emesis. All the samples of vomit from infected individuals grew *H. pylori,* often in large amounts. Air samples taken during the vomiting of some individuals grew *H. pylori.* Saliva taken before and after emesis grew low amounts of *H. pylori.* The study showed that *H. pylori* can be cultivated from vomit, and occasionally from saliva and cathartic-induced stools. The organism is potentially transmissible during episodes of gastrointestinal tract illness, especially when the individual vomits.

In view of this study, it is not surprising that gastroenterologists are exposed frequently to *H. pylori*-infected patients. As a group, gastroenterologists have twice the expected rate of *H. pylori* infection of the general population. For these doctors, the infection is an occupational risk.

H. pylori and Environmental Settings

H. pylori can be transmitted orally-orally, or orally-fecally. A study was conducted to assess the rate of intrafamily transmission in a general population, and the role of a family's social background. Campogalliano, a town of about 5,000 people in Northern Italy, was chosen for the study. The overall prevalence of *H. pylori* infection was found in more than half of the population of the town. Children in families with both parents infected had a significantly higher prevalence of *H. pylori* infection than children in families with only one parent, or neither parent infected. The socioeconomic status was related independently to the infection rate in children. Those from blue-collar or farm-worker families had a greater risk of infecting their children than did white-collar worker families. The researchers concluded that *H. pylori* infections cluster within families belonging to the same population. The socioeconomic status may be another risk factor, with large families and crowded living conditions.

In a study of a rural community in the Colombian Andes in South America, multiple routes of *H. pylori* infection were found. Nearly 700 children, two to nine years of age, were examined. Their overall prevalence of *H. pylori* infection was 69 percent. The prevalence increased with age, with 53 percent of children two years of age infected up to 87 percent of children nine years of age. More boys than girls were infected. The strongest predictor of the infection rate was the number of people within a household, and especially the number of children. The larger the household, and the greater the number of children, the greater was the risk for *H. pylori* infection. Multiple routes of transmission were person to person; swimming in polluted rivers, pools, and streams; eating raw vegetables frequently; and having contact with sheep.

Gastroenterologist Peter Grübel, while working in Africa, wondered if the high infective rate of *H. pylori* in developing countries might be related to the constant presence of many houseflies on everything. Later, while working at St. Elizabeth's Medical Center in Boston, Massachusetts, Grübel suggested that the common housefly might be an unrecognized factor in *H. pylori* infection transmission. In a study published in the June 1997 issue of the *Journal of Clinical Microbiology*, Grübel and his colleagues reported on their work. They exposed one group of adult houseflies to a culture of *H. pylori* on petri dishes, and another group to a sterile dish. Bacteria clung to the skin of the exposed flies for up to twelve hours. The bacteria were detected in those insect guts and found in their excrements for up to thirty hours after the original exposure. No bacteria were detected in the control flies. The researchers suggested that *H. pylori* can be transmitted from human excrement by the common housefly, which then, by crawling on food, can contaminate it. However, the housefly is only a potential carrier, not a proven reservoir.

PREVENTING HOUSEFLIES FROM CONTAMINATING FOOD

Prepare food in a screened area. Keep raw flesh foods refrigerated until you prepare them. If you serve food outdoors at barbecues or picnics, keep the foods on platters covered so that flies cannot alight on them.

H. pylori and Oral Transmission

Australian public-health researchers investigated the risk factors in *H. pylori* infection. The bacterium was known to be cultured from samples of dental plaque taken from patients. When teeth are scaled during dental cleaning, some of the loose plaque may be ingested. This can lead to the stomach becoming infected with *H. pylori*. The researchers suggest that less frequent teeth scaling may reduce the risk for *H. pylori* infection.

Other oral transmissions may result from certain cultural traditions. In some societies, people eat communally and share bowls and cutlery. Also, in areas such as West Africa, it is common for mothers to chew food before offering it to infants. There is a high rate of *H. pylori* infection among children in West Africa.

H. pylori and Transmission Via Food

Raw poultry has been identified as a vector for *H. pylori* infection. A study of the bacteria in broth, in a saline solution, and in raw chicken found that the bacterium remained viable in all three media when they were held at room temperature. The *H. pylori* survived for twenty-four hours in the raw chicken, and could be kept alive for several days longer even after the raw chicken was refrigerated. The results demonstrated that improperly stored raw food, especially of animal origin, may be a vector for *H. pylori*.

CAN CHOPSTICKS TRANSPORT *H. PYLORI*?

Sharing chopsticks can transmit *H. pylori* bacteria. Because the bacterium is found in saliva and in dental plaque an oral-oral transmission is possible. An epidemiological study conducted by a group of Hong Kong researchers led by W. K. Leung, reported in 1998 that Chinese people who use chopsticks had the highest *H. pylori* seroprevalence (present in serum). The researchers cultured saliva and chopstick washings from twenty-seven patients with *H. pylori* infection, to learn whether chopsticks could transmit the bacteria to other family members. The researchers detected *H. pylori*-specific DNA in the saliva of ten of the patients. However, *H. pylori*-specific DNA was detected in only one individual, both in the saliva and in the chopstick washings. The researchers concluded that transmission of *H. pylori* by chopsticks may be a rare event but it can occur.

H. pylori and Transmission Via Water

Water, like food, can transmit *H. pylori*. The bacterium can enter well water from human and animal waste through sewage that enters poorly constructed or damaged wells, or wells that are poorly located. In a 1994 to 1995 survey conducted by Kansas State University researchers of wells examined in the Midwest, on average, 60 percent of all private wells, and 80 percent of all dug wells failed to meet safe drinking water standards. Other studies found that 65 percent of private well-water samples contained *H. pylori*.

The bacterium is found in untreated sewage, which supports the finding that *H. pylori* is transmitted through fecally contaminated water. This finding explains why the infection incidence is so high in developing countries where proper sanitation and clean water are lacking.

In a study in Colombia, researchers from the Massachusetts Institute of Technology in Cambridge, found *H. pylori* in contaminated drinking water in Narino, an area with one of the world's highest prevalence of ulcers and gastric cancer. More than 90 percent of the population was infected with *H. pylori*. This was the first attempt to examine environmental water samples for *H. pylori*.

H. pylori as a Multifactor Public Health Issue

Obviously, *H. pylori* infection is a multifactorial problem. To sum up, among the risk factors is low socioeconomic status. In turn, this is related to other factors, such as overcrowded living conditions with large families and many children. Young children can excrete *H. pylori* bacteria and cause fecal contamination of the living environment. A lack of a fixed hot-water supply or access to clean water also is related to the low socioeconomic status. Dirty drinking water, contaminated food, and poor sanitation are all aspects of the problem. Eradication of *H. pylori* needs to encompass a number of factors.

AVAILABLE TESTS TO CONFIRM *H. PYLORI* INFECTION

In order to detect infection with *H. pylori*, a doctor may recommend one or more of the following tests:

- Biopsy specimen
- C-urea antibody test
- Endoscopy diagnosis
- Enzyme-linked immunosorbent assay (ELISA)
- Serologic test
- Serum antibody test
- Stool antigen test
- Urease test

TREATMENTS TO ERADICATE *H. PYLORI*

Treatments to eradicate *H. pylori* in a person consist of several antibiotics and bismuth subsalicylate (a product such as Procter & Gamble's Pepto-Bismol). Unfortunately, antibiotics often cause gastrointestinal side effects such as abdominal pain and diarrhea. Some of the antibiotic treatment is ineffective, which leaves the patient vulnerable to even nastier and less manageable strains of *H. pylori* infection.

In cases of antibiotic ineffectiveness, an endoscopic biopsy may be performed. This procedure can be done in an outpatient medical office. After the patient is given a mild sedative, a flexible scope is slid down the throat into the stomach, from where a tissue sample is extracted. It is studied to identify *H. pylori.* Another test, noninvasive, is the breath test, which sniffs out byproducts generated by *H. pylori.* Also, there is an antibody blood test. However, none of these tests identify the *H. pylori* strain, so they do not reveal which antibiotics might be the most effective.

Because of the limitations of antibiotic therapy, there has been a search for some alternative therapies. To date, none have been shown to be as effective as the conventional treatment, but some may be helpful as adjuncts.

An Alternative Treatment: Probiotics

In a 2001 pilot study led by A. Armuzzi, *Lactobacillus GG,* a probiotic, was given along with conventional treatment to patients with *H. pylori* infection. The probiotic substantially reduced the intestinal side effects and improved the patients' tolerance for the treatment.

In 2005, probiotics were studied with mice, in an attempt to learn if probiotics might reduce the risk for *H. pylori* colonization in the animals' digestive tracts. K. C. Johnson-Henry led a team of researchers to test the validity of a claim for a branded product consisting of a blend of two probiotics (*L. rhamnosus* strain 0011 and *L. acidophilus* strain R0052). The claim for the product was that this blend would suppress colonization of *H. pylori* strain SS.

Thirty female mice were divided into four groups. All groups were intentionally infected with *H. pylori.* They were given, respectively, sterile water (the controls); probiotics in sterile water; a challenge orogastrically with *H. pylori;* and pretreatment with probiotics in drinking water prior to, and following, the challenge with *H. pylori.* The researchers examined tissue samples from the stomachs of the animals to determine *H. pylori* colonization, mucosal inflammation, and epithelial cell apoptosis (cell death). The sterile water did not affect the overall wellbeing of the mice. The other groups, given *H. pylori* and probiotics, showed *Lactobacillus* species to be excreted in the stools over the duration of the treatment. Pretreatment with probiotics reduced *H. pylori* growth up to 100 percent. Moderate to severe *H. pylori*-induced inflammation in the gastric antrum (stomach cavity) of the mice was reduced up to 71 percent by probiotic pretreatment. However, the pretreatment did not prevent *H. pylori*-induced apoptosis in the gastric mucosa. The results suggested that the branded product containing two strains of *Lactobacillus* could be a safe and effective treatment to prevent infection, and to improve the eradication of *H. pylori*. However, it would not replace conventional therapy. Rather, it would be a useful adjunct.

An Alternative Treatment: Lactoferrin

Lactoferrin is a protein found in human and cow's milk. It has bacteriostatic and bacteriocidal activity against many organisms. It has the ability to bind to iron and prevent iron from being utilized by bacteria for their growth. Also, lactoferrin appears to cause adverse changes in bacterial membrane permeability. Lactoferrin seemed like a promising candidate as an adjunct to conventional therapy for *H. pylori* eradication.

In 2004, in a study led by F. DiMario, fifty patients with dyspepsia and gastritis, who were infected with *H. pylori*, were assigned randomly to receive treatment for one week with standard antibiotic treatment, or the treatment combined with lactoferrin (200 milligrams twice a day). After eight weeks of treatment, the patients' *H. pylori* status was assessed by the breath test or an *H. pylori* stool antigen test. The eradication rate was 100 percent in the group receiving the addition of lactoferrin to the conventional therapy, compared with only 76.9 percent in the group receiving the conventional therapy. The results of the study suggested that *H. pylori* can be eradicated efficiently by adding lactoferrin to the antibiotic treatment.

An Alternative Treatment: Plant Compounds

Numerous active principles in plants, especially herbs, have been suggested to combat *H. pylori*. To date, findings indicate that they would be useful adjuncts rather than replacers of conventional treatment. Among these substances are: garlic, thyme, ginger, turmeric, jalapeño pepper, cranberry, rhubarb root, cinnamon, licorice, goldenseal, bloodroot, green tea, mastic gum, bee propolis, and essential oils of verbena and lemon grass. Of all these substances, *Allium sativum*, an active principle in garlic, has received much attention. This constituent shows antimicrobial activity against *H. pylori* both in vitro and in vivo. Using garlic in the diet may help prevent *H. pylori* from colonizing in the stomach and may provide a low-cost intervention strategy that is harmless but effective in populations at high risk for stomach cancer, especially if antibiotic resistance and the risk of reinfection are high.

Gail B. Mahady led an in vitro screening program at the College of Pharmacy of the University of Illinois, Chicago, of crude plant extracts and natural compounds known to inhibit *H. pylori* growth. Of the initial thirty plant extracts and isolated chemical compounds tested, seventeen were found to inhibit the growth of fifteen different strains of *H. pylori*. The active chemical constituents in these plants were identified as berberine, sanguinarine, chelerythrine, protapine, and allicin. The most active components were isoquinoline alkaloids. The strongest inhibitory action against *H. pylori* was from goldenseal (*Hydrastis canadensis*), bloodroot (*Sanguinaria canadensis*), turmeric (*Curcuma longa*), and garlic (*Allium sativum*).

In 2000, Israeli scientists at Tel Aviv University investigated the ability of medicinal plant extracts to inhibit in vitro growth of *H. pylori*. The highest activities were found in water extracts of thyme (*Thymus vulgaris*). Alcoholic extracts of the herb also were quite strong in activity. An alcoholic extract of cinnamon (*Cinnamomum zeylanicum*) showed strong activity. A dried thyme water extract inhibited *H. pylori* growth completely in vitro, either in an agar or liquid medium.

Herbal treatment for *H. pylori* infection might be used most appropriately when conventional treatments have failed, or they are considered inadvisable or inappropriate. Conventional treatments usually are given for a brief period of one to two weeks. Herbal treatments may need to be given for longer periods of four to six weeks or more, to have some degree of effectiveness. Some herbal therapies can be incorporated into the diet, and used as an ongoing practice to prevent reinfection, after the bacterium is eradicated. Extended herbal therapy might be appropriate if ongoing exposure to persistent *H. pylori* infection is a potential risk factor for cardiovascular disease in many people.

Gowsala P. Sivam and colleagues at the Cancer Prevention Program of the Fred Hutchinson Cancer Center in Seattle, Washington, noted that the incidence of gastric cancer is lower in individuals and in populations with a high intake of vegetables containing thiosulfates such as allium. These substances in vegetables, especially garlic, can act as antibiotics. In 1997, the group reported that a garlic extract, with a known thiosulfate concentration, was effective in inhibiting *H. pylori.* Even a low thiosulfate concentration was effective.

In clinical trials, M. Yang reported in the *Journal of Traditional Chinese Medicine* that rhubarb root eradicated 89 percent of *H. pylori* infection in fifty-three patients.

It is recognized that cranberry has anti-adhesive ability in the urinary tract and prevents bacterial infections. Can it be useful as well in therapy to eradicate *H. pylori* infection? In a randomized, double-blind, placebo-controlled trial with 189 patients, cranberry showed some helpful activity in 14.4 percent of patients, compared to only 5.4 percent in the control group. Positive results were found after thirty-five days of treatment, and after ninety days as well. The results showed a low rate of success, but nevertheless did show some activity. The researchers suggested that cranberry juice might be a useful adjunct to other treatments for *H. pylori* eradication.

Sulforaphane, a powerful compound found in cruciferous vegetables such as broccoli, cabbage, and kale, shows some promise as a potential treatment for *H. pylori* infection, according to a study conducted by researchers from Johns Hopkins University in Baltimore, Maryland, and at the National Center for Scientific Research in Paris, France. The lead author, Jed W. Fahey, reported that infection rates of *H. pylori* run as high as 80 percent of the population in parts of Central and South America, Africa, and China. In those areas, stomach cancer is the leading cause of all cancer deaths. Yet, antibiotics may be prohibitively expensive or difficult to deliver. The amount of sulforaphane used in the study was comparable to what one might expect to be consumed by a person eating a diet rich in cruciferous vegetables. Broccoli contains far more sulforaphane than other cruciferous vegetables, and broccoli sprouts have the most. Although the study was conducted in a laboratory setting, encouraging people to grow and consume these vegetables might achieve results easier than depending on antibiotic treatment.

Mastic gum is a resinous exudate gathered from the stem and main leaves of a plant, *Pistacia lentiscus.* It grows in the Mediterranean region, especially on the Greek island of Chios. The ancient Greeks used mastic gum for stomach distress. Currently, the leaves are eaten in the Mediterranean area. Low doses of mastic gum have been found useful in eradicating *H. pylori* infection. In a letter to the *New England Journal of Medicine* (Dec 24, 1998), Farhad Hewez at the Barnet General Hospital in the United Kingdom, and several researchers from University Hospital at Nottingham, also in the United Kingdom, reported that one milligram of mastic gum taken per day for two weeks "can cure peptic ulcers very rapidly." Clinically, mastic gum has been reported to be effective in the treatment of benign gastric ulcers and duodenal ulcers. In rat studies, mastic gum showed cytoprotective and mild antisecretory properties. Studies showed mastic gum effective against at least seven different strains of *H. pylori*. The mechanism is thought to be due to structural change induced within the *H. pylori* cell by the mastic gum, which causes the bacterium to weaken and die.

EDIBLE OILS AND *H. PYLORI*

Linoleic acid, a major component of many edible oils, inhibits the growth of *H. pylori*. Linoleic acid is found in some commonly used oils, such as olive oil and sunflower seed oil. Also, it is abundant in fish oil. Duane Smoot at Howard University Hospital in Washington, D.C., has been investigating oils high in linoleic acid for their potential use in *H. pylori* treatment.

An Alternative Treatment: Nutritional Supplements

Certain nutrients, such as vitamin C and beta-carotene, have been suggested for treatment of *H. pylori* infection. Some of the evidence is derived from in vitro tests. As with the herbal treatments based on in vitro tests, the studies with nutrients do not necessarily translate to in vivo outcomes.

There is evidence that low vitamin C concentrations in gastric juice in the presence of *H. pylori* infection play a role in the pathogenesis of gastric cancer. *H. pylori*, as a carcinogen, also reduce the concentration of vitamin A, an anticarcinogen, in gastric juice by inhibiting intragastric (within the stomach) secretion of this vitamin. Thus, by increasing the concentration of vitamin C in gastric juice, there might be beneficial results against *H. pylori* infection.

To test the value of vitamin C supplementation with people infected with *H. pylori*, M. Jarosz led a team of researchers to study sixty persons with dyspeptic symptoms, and with proven chronic gastritis and *H. pylori* infection. The people were divided into two groups. They were assigned randomly to receive either antacids (the control) or vitamin C for four weeks. The vitamin C was administered in four divided doses daily: 2 grams one time, and then 1 gram three times. Only fifty-one people completed the study. The *H. pylori* infection was unchanged in the control group. The average total vitamin C concentration in their gastric juices also remained unchanged. In the vitamin C-treated group, *H. pylori* infection was eradicated in eight of twenty-seven people (30 percent) who completed the treatment. Four weeks after the treatment ended, vitamin C concentrations in gastric juice had more than doubled in patients with successfully eradicated *H. pylori* infection, but remained unchanged in those patients whose infections persisted. These results suggest that supplementation with vitamin C can increase gastric juice vitamin C concentrations and may eradicate *H. pylori* in some people with chronic gastritis.

Although vitamin C supplementation with 5 grams daily eradicated *H. pylori* in only 30 percent of the patients, it is possible that larger dosages of vitamin C supplementation might be effective for a larger percentage of patients. Many individuals can tolerate 10, or even 20 grams of vitamin C daily, if the vitamin is taken in divided doses and swallowed along with food.

Hui-Min Zhang led a team at the Toyko-based Research Institute of the International Medical Center of Japan to study the role of vitamin C with *H. pylori*, using both in vitro tests and in vivo tests with laboratory animals. The group found that high vitamin C concentrations were able to inhibit up to 90 percent of *H. pylori* cultured in petri dishes. Then, in 1997, the group reported that administered high vitamin C concentrations significantly slowed the growth of *H. pylori* in the stomachs of Mongolian gerbils.

Pelayo Correa, at Louisiana State University in New Orleans, administered 30 milligrams of beta-carotene, or 2 grams of vitamin C, daily for six years to one group of volunteers with precancerous changes in their stomach cells. A second group underwent the standard fourteen-day antibiotic treatment. A third group was given various combinations, or a placebo. After three years, and again, after six years, the guts were examined by endoscopy or biopsy. All three treatments (beta-carotene, vitamin C, and antibiotics) resulted in an increased rate of cell regression or return to normal. In treatment of nonmetaplastic atrophy (a type of precancerous cell change), people who received the beta-carotene were 5.1 times more likely to improve than those taking placebos. Those taking vitamin C or antibiotics were 5.0 times and 4.8 times, respectively, more likely to improve. Similarly, people with intestinal metaplasia (another type of precancerous change) were 3.4 times more likely to improve with beta-carotene; 3.3 times more with vitamin C; and 3.2 times more with antibiotics. The study suggested a benefit from vitamin supplementation for retarding the progression of premalignant gastric lesions.

These antioxidant vitamins play an important role. Chronic infection with *H. pylori* depletes the gut of antioxidant vitamins, probably because the antioxidants attempt to quench the large number of free radicals generated by localized inflammation. The free radicals, if not quenched, can mutate stomach wall cells, which increase the risk for stomach cancer development.

Angelo Zullo at Sapienza University in Rome, Italy, led a team of researchers to evaluate fifty-eight patients with precancerous intestinal metaplasia after they had received antibiotic treatment for *H. pylori* infection. Half of the patients were given either 500 milligrams of vitamin C daily for six months, or no further treatment. At the end of the six months, the researchers found a reversal of intestinal metaplasia in about one-third of the patients taking vitamin C. In contrast, only one patient (3.4 percent) from the other group showed improvement. Zullo noted that ascorbic acid (vitamin C) is the main antioxidant in gastric juice in the stomach, where its concentration normally is four times more than in the plasma.

An Alternative Treatment: Combining Elements

In 2004, scientists at the Shinshu University in Japan, led by Masatomo Kawakubo, announced their discovery of a built-in defense mechanism in the body that protects it from *H. pylori* damage. They found that a component of gastric mucous secretions—designated as a mucin-type O-glycan—is present within the deeper regions of the gastric mucus. It can inhibit the growth and motility of *H. pylori* in culture by interfering with cell-wall biosynthesis. Thus, cells of the gastric mucus appear to protect themselves from *H. pylori* infection by secreting O-glycans that possess strong antibiotic activity.

Using these various fragments of information concerning the activity of nutrients in eradicating *H. pylori* infection, C. Kockar and colleagues tried various combinations to learn which ones might be the most effective. They reported their experiment and results in 2001. Working with 210 patients with *H. pylori* infection, confirmed by gastric biopsies, they assigned them randomly to one of seven treatment groups. The treatment was for fourteen days, and consisted of one of the following:

1. Standard eradication treatment with antibiotics and acid-secretion inhibitors

2. Standard treatment plus 1 gram of vitamin C daily

3. 1 gram of vitamin C daily

4. Standard treatment plus 120 milligrams of beta-carotene daily

5. 120 milligrams of beta-carotene daily

6. Standard treatment plus allicin daily

7. 1,200 micrograms or 4,200 micrograms of allicin daily (the dose of allicin was unclear)

Four weeks after the treatment period, gastric biopsies were repeated. The eradication rates were as follows:

1. Standard treatment: 66.7 percent

2. Standard treatment plus vitamin C: 50 percent

3. Vitamin C: 10 percent

4. Standard treatment plus beta-carotene: 50 percent

5. Beta-carotene: 0 percent

6. Standard treatment plus allicin: 90 percent

7. Allicin: 23.3 percent

In the Jarosz study discussed earlier, supplementation with vitamin C had been 5 grams a day—five times the amount in the study led by Kockar. That study achieved eradication success in 30 percent of the patients, which was three times higher than in the Kockar study. This would suggest that the success rate with vitamin C in the Kockar study might have been higher if a larger amount of vitamin C had been used. However, the earlier study was faulty in interpreting the results. Assessment of the patients was made when the treatment ended, rather than a more appropriate period a month after the treatment. Consequently, it was not possible to distinguish between a transient suppression of *H. pylori* from true eradication.

In the Kockar study, both vitamin C and allicin eradicated *H. pylori* infection in a small proportion of patients. These treatments are safe, and without the high incidence of side effects from the conventional treatment. The vitamin C and allicin treatments if combined, and with vitamin C used at a higher level, might be helpful for some patients. A follow-up can determine whether the treatment was successful. If not, additional treatment with conventional therapy might be necessary.

UNANTICIPATED CONNECTIONS

The development of stomach cancer in people with *H. pylori* infection that is untreated or unsuccessfully treated was discussed earlier. However, there are a number of other unanticipated connections with the bacterium, which are linked to an assortment of health problems and diseases.

H. pylori and Malabsorption

Much of the reduction in gastric acid output linked to aging is not a natural decline, but caused by *H. pylori*-induced atrophic gastritis. Ultimately, this condition can lead to nutrient malabsorption, especially of folic acid, vitamin B_{12}, vitamin C, iron, and other nutrients, and lead to malnutrition. How does this develop?

Folic acid: H. V. Markle at Centenary Health Centre in Scarborough, Ontario, Canada, suggested a link between the increased risk of coronary heart disease and reduced folate levels induced by *H. pylori* infection. Markle proposed that there was a relationship between the changes caused in gastric juice by *H. pylori*-induced gastritis, and the reduced bioavailability of folates. Gradually, chronic subclinical atrophic gastritis can destroy the capacity of the gastric mucosa to produce acid. Eventually, the gastric pH rises. Elevated gastric pH and damage to the gastric surface in the epithelium are associated with lower levels of ascorbic acid concentration in gastric juice. The reduced gastric juice ascorbate may affect the bioavailability of dietary folates. Decreased folates cause an increased blood concentration of homocysteine, an independent risk factor for atherosclerosis. Both *H. pylori* infection and coronary artery disease occur more frequently in individuals with poor socioeconomic status, who are less likely to have sufficient folate intake in the diet or to supplement with folic acid to maintain an adequate folic acid level. Poor folate status, in itself, also may be a factor in the promotion of carcinogenesis.

Vitamin B_{12}: Vitamin B_{12} is another nutrient that may be linked to *H. pylori* infection-induced malabsorption. Among other effects, *H. pylori* infection causes acute gastritis, as well as hypochlorhydria (a low level of hydrochloric acid) or achlorhydria (a lack of hydrochloric acid). Ultimately, this deficiency can lead to vitamin B_{12} malabsorption in some people. Other factors may be involved to induce this malabsorption.

In vitro studies show that acid and pepsin are critical in splitting cobalamin (vitamin B_{12}) from food binders in the stomach. In vivo studies of the gastric secretion in fifteen patients showed lower acid secretion in three of them with severe food-cobalamin malabsorption compared with only mild malabsorption or normal absorption in the others. This suggests that gastritis, with diminished acid secretion, is related to a failure to absorb food-derived cobalamin.

Iron: Iron malabsorption is associated with *H. pylori* infection. Alaskan Inuits have a higher intake of dietary iron than similar general populations elsewhere in the United States. It was puzzling to investigators in the Centers for Disease Control and Prevention's Arctic Investigations Program (AIP) in Anchorage. The Inuits' diet consists of many iron-rich foods such as meat and cold-water fish. Yet, when examined, iron-deficiency anemia was prevalent. This health problem has long been recognized in Alaskan Inuits of all ages and of both sexes. The AIP examined the possible relationship between the anemia and *H. pylori* infection. A study of stool-blood content in healthy Inuit adults from Southwestern Alaska revealed that abnormal stool-blood loss was common in the population. Endoscopy of those with the highest stool-blood loss showed chronic active gastritis caused by *H. pylori* infection in all but one person.

Another team of researchers led by Ray Yip studied the Yupik Eskimos living along the coast of the Bering Sea. The survey showed that iron deficiency was nearly eleven times higher in Yupik men, and four times higher in Yupik women, than in the general U.S. population. The Yupik diet was not deficient in iron. Endoscopic evaluation showed grossly abnormal-appearing gastric mucosa in 97 percent of the individuals examined. Factors such as alcohol use or recent NSAID treatment were not associated with the endoscopic findings, but *H. pylori* was. Previously, *H. pylori* infection had not been recognized as a cause of chronic blood loss or iron deficiency. Infection with this pathogen was judged to be a reasonable cause of occult blood and anemia in this group of people.

Ascorbic acid: *H. pylori* infection causes low ascorbic acid levels in gastric juice caused by a combination of decreased secretion and increased oxidation of ascorbic acid (rendering its antioxidant activity ineffective). As discussed earlier, *H. pylori* infection is associated with increased risk for gastric cancer. An important causation of gastric cancer is the conversion of food-derived nitrates, nitrites, and amines into carcinogenic nitrosamines. This reaction is inhibited by ascorbic acid. Therefore, the association of *H. pylori* infection with gastric cancer may be related to ascorbic acid depletion. As noted, *H. pylori* infection also may cause hypochlorhydria, and this could lead to multiple nutritional deficiencies, and overgrowth with bacteria and fungi in the small bowel. Thus, eradication of *H. pylori* might be more important than previously recognized in order to maintain good nutrient absorption and prevent malabsorption.

H. pylori and Failure to Thrive

The geriatric failure to thrive (GFTT) syndrome is reflected in failing mobility, a tendency to fall, and a general loss of interest. GFTT patients lose their ability to perform basic activities of daily living, and mental functioning declines. It had been considered that GFTT was part of a normal aging process. However, some cases have been ascribed to *H. pylori* by Valery A. Portnoi at Genesis Physician Services, in Washington, D.C. She found cases in which GFTT, as well as anorexia (loss of appetite, which may result from disease), were associated with *H. pylori* infection. These conditions were reversed after the patients were given treatment for *H. pylori*. They regained weight, and were restored to physical and intellectual functioning, which continued over a six-month period of follow-up observations.

H. pylori and Skin Diseases

Infection with *H. pylori* has been implicated in the development of chronic skin disorders. One is rosacea, a chronic skin disease resulting from an upset in the normal functioning of the immune system. Rosacea is characterized by redness over the nose and cheeks, especially during and after periods of physical exertion. Other symptoms include skin bumps or pimples, a swollen nose, and small, dilated blood vessels in the skin. It was noted that individuals treated for *H. pylori* infection with antibiotics resulted in the relief of symptoms of rosacea. In many cases, the eradication of *H. pylori* resulted in complete clearance of rosacea, which is a skin disorder that is difficult to eradicate.

Allergenic skin conditions may have strong links with *H. pylori* infection. Eradication of the bacterium resulted in 73 percent of patients with chronic urticaria (hives), reported Akiko Shiotani and colleagues.

According to Mikihisa Sakurane and colleagues, "in chronic skin diseases, persistent infection with *H. pylori* may be an eruption trigger and may cause deterioration of the disease into an intractable and chronic form."

Other chronic skin diseases may be connected with *H. pylori*. Anyone suffering from a chronic skin condition should be tested for *H. pylori* infection during the treatment of the skin condition.

H. pylori and Coronary Heart Disease

Is *H. pylori* infection a risk factor for coronary heart disease? A team led by Nizal Sarrafzadegan from the Isfahan Cardiovascular Research Center in Iran attempted to answer this question. They examined patients with confirmed cases of acute and chronic coronary syndromes to learn if there was any association with *H. pylori*. Also, they examined the possible influence of *H. pylori* infection on the fibrinogen (coagulation) levels in the patients. Indeed, they found a significant relationship between *H. pylori* infection and acute myocardial infarction (heart attack). Also, fibrinogen levels were significantly higher among patients with *H. pylori* infections than among those without the infection. The results supported the hypothesis that *H. pylori* may influence acute myocardial infarction by enhancing thrombosis (blood clot formation within a blood vessel), and possibly is mediated by raised fibrinogen levels.

Only about half of all coronary artery disease can be explained by the usual risk factors. Some researchers suggest that *H. pylori* infection may be an important link in atherosclerosis development. The strongest evidence for an association between infectious agents and cardiovascular disease is for *Chlamydia pneumoniae*. However, a role for *H. pylori*, too, is beginning to emerge.

A virulent strain of *H. pylori* associated with coronary heart disease was reported in Scotland by R. K. Singh and colleagues.

Another study suggested that inflammation induced by *H. pylori* infection contributes to the early state of atherosclerotic development in young men, reported by Y. Saijo and colleagues.

The presence of *H. pylori* infection nearly doubles the risk of developing heart disease. This conclusion was reached in two different studies. One study was conducted by a team led by M. A. Mendall; the other, by M. Gunn and colleagues.

Hugh S. Markus led a study that demonstrated chronic *H. pylori* infection to be associated with ischemic heart disease, and also to be an independent risk factor for ischemic cerebrovascular disease. The bacterium may be a factor in furthering the development of atherosclerosis.

The mechanism of hardening of the arteries may be related to chronic inflammation of blood vessel walls caused by infectious microbes. As noted earlier, *H. pylori* and *C. pneumoniae* are prime candidates. Also, there may be overactivity of the immune system affecting vessel walls, with infectious microbes playing an indirect role.

The virulence of the *H. pylori* species appears to be a key factor in its association with heart disease. In a study led by Vincenzo Pasceri of Catholic University of the Sacred Heart in Rome, Italian researchers described eighty-eight people with ischemic heart disease, and a control group of eighty-eight healthy people, matched by socioeconomic status and body mass index (a widely used diagnostic tool to identify weight problems). Some 62 percent of the people with heart disease also were found to be infected with *H. pylori.* The infection rate in the control group was 40 percent. A particularly virulent *H. pylori* strain that contained the CagA gene affected 43 percent of the study participants. In comparison, only 17 percent of those infected with a strain lacking the gene were affected. The finding strongly suggested that the association between *H. pylori* and heart disease is related to the strength of the bacterial strain. Additional infectious agents also are associated with heart disease. As already indicated, *C. pneumoniae* is one. Another agent is the cytomegalovirus.

H. pylori and Strokes

The CagA gene of *H. pylori* has been implicated as a trigger of strokes. In a study led by Antonio Pietroiusti of Tor Vergata University in Rome, low-grade inflammation, such as the body's response to a chronic infection, may precede stroke as well as heart disease. Linking an inflammation to any specific infection is difficult. However, Pietroiusti and his team showed that the particularly virulent gene of *H. pylori*, CagA, is associated with large-vessel strokes. The attack is triggered when blood vessels to the brain are blocked by fatty plaque. The CagA gene of *H. pylori* produces potent toxins that are thought to attack plaque-lined blood vessels, and result in inflammation. The CagA gene of *H. pylori* was identified in 43 percent of 131 people who had suffered from large-vessel stroke, and in 20 percent of sixty-one people who had suffered from a stroke triggered by a blood clot from another part of the body.

H. pylori and Organ Disorders

Problems with organs of the body, including the gallbladder, liver, and eyes, appear to have surprising linkages to *H. pylori* infections. In time, additional ones may be discovered.

Cancer of the gallbladder is the greatest cause of cancer mortality in Chilean women. The incidence rate for this tumor varies widely worldwide, being about ten times higher in high-risk than in low-risk populations. This suggests that environmental aspects such as infectious microorganisms, carcinogens, and nutrition are probable factors in the pathogenesis of cholecystitis (inflammation of the gallbladder). Because several *Helicobacter* species can colonize in the liver of animals and induce hepatitis, a study was conducted to determine whether *Helicobacter* infection in humans is associated with cholecystitis. The study was led by James G. Fox from the Division of Comparative Medicine at the Massachusetts Institute of Technology in Cambridge. The researchers studied bile or gallbladder tissue taken from forty-six Chileans with chronic cholecystitis who were undergoing surgery. The researchers cultured the specimens and tested for *Helicobacter* species. Recovery of the *Helicobacter* species from frozen specimens was unsuccessful, but thirteen of twenty-three bile samples and nine of twenty-one gallbladder tissues were positive for *Helicobacter*. The findings suggest an association of bile-resistant *Helicobacter* species with gallbladder disease.

The liver is another organ that may be affected by *H. pylori* infections. Within the genus of *Helicobacter* is one species, *H. hepaticus*, which is associated with chronic hepatitis and hepatocellular neoplasia in laboratory mice. Most *Helicobacter* species identified to date are associated characteristically with (and named after) specific mammalian host species in which they generally inhabit the gastrointestinal tract, with or without causing gastritis or other chronic inflammatory disease. There is a broad potential host range for some species of the bacterium. *H. pylori*, originally isolated from humans, more recently has been isolated from the domestic cat. This suggests that *H. pylori* may be a zoonotic pathogen, one that is transmissible from a companion animal to humans.

Whether or not *H. hepaticus,* in itself, is capable of infecting humans, it does demonstrate that liver tissue can be infected persistently by at least one member of the genus *Helicobacter.* Liver cancer can be a long-term consequence of such infections. It raises the question: can liver cancer in humans be induced by presently unrecognized bacterial infection?

Acute peptic ulcer and upper gastrointestinal bleeding reportedly occurs in more than a third of all cirrhotic patients in Italy. In a case-controlled study, led by Antonio Ponzetta from the Department of Gastroenterology at the Giovanni Battista Hospital in Turin, ulcers were examined in 45 male patients with hepatitis B virus-associated cirrhosis of the liver, and 310 age-matched blood donors who lived in the same area. Antibodies against *H. pylori* were present in 89 percent of patients, and in 59 percent of blood donors. This very high incidence of *H. pylori* may explain the frequent occurrence of gastroduodenal ulcers in cirrhotic patients.

H. pylori may be associated with another organ, the eye. Jannis Kountouras led a study in Thessalonica, Greece, and documented a high incidence of *H. pylori* infections in patients with glaucoma. The infection was detected in 88 percent of all glaucoma patients studied. Eradication of the *H. pylori* infection was judged to be beneficial for the glaucoma parameters, which suggests a possible causal link between the infectious organism and the eye disease.

H. pylori and Other Health Conditions

There is some suggestive evidence that connects *H. pylori* to numerous other health conditions. The following are brief descriptions.

- A study of 275 atopic patients with symptoms of peptic ulcers showed that sinusitis and exercise-induced anaphylaxis can be induced by *H. pylori.* Of the patients, 19 percent were found to have either IgE or IgG antibodies against *H. pylori.* The researchers suggested that appropriate antibiotic therapy for the *H. pylori*-induced ulcers would resolve the allergy symptoms in these patients. Because *H. pylori* also is a suspected cause of hypochlorhydria, which impairs the digestion of protein, individuals with food allergies should be checked for *H. pylori* infection.

- M. Pocecco and colleagues in Italy found that the prevalence of asymptomatic infection with *H. pylori* was significantly higher in young diabetics than in controls. Some of the diabetic children had abdominal complaints. Gastroduodenoscopy revealed gastric inflammation and the presence of *H. pylori*. A significant association appeared between cow's milk protein antibodies and *H. pylori* antibodies in the diabetic group, but not in the control group. Often, the association between *H. pylori* infection and the response to cow's milk protein was present in the onset of diabetes.

• Does *H. pylori* infection play a role in the causation of Sjögren's syndrome? N. Giordano led a team of researchers who studied this syndrome, a slow, progressive autoimmune disease that typically manifests as arthritis. The researchers tried to learn whether *H. pylori* plays any role in this syndrome. Gastric biopsies from four patients with Sjögren's syndrome showed that three of them were infected with *H. pylori*. They were given medications to eradicate the infection. After the bacterium was eliminated, some of the clinical symptoms of the syndrome, such as dry eyes and dry mouth, were reported to improve dramatically. The researchers concluded that *H. pylori*, along with other infections, may play a role in the causation of Sjögren's syndrome.

• *H. pylori* may play a role in another autoimmune disease, idiopathic thrombocytopenic purpura (ITP). This condition is characterized by a low platelet count. As a result, there is a tendency for blood to leak out of tiny blood vessels. Nobuyuki Shigeto and his colleagues examined sixteen patients with ITP and found that *H. pylori* was present in 87 percent of them. The investigators were able to eradicate *H. pylori* successfully in 64 percent of the infected patients, which led to a complete remission of ITP in more than half of these patients.

• Can *H. pylori* be linked to severe morning sickness in pregnant women? About one in 1,000 pregnant women experience a severe form of morning sickness, with nausea and vomiting. It is known as *hyperemesis gravidarum*. Women with this condition may vomit three or more times daily. They experience weight loss and have an imbalance of electrolytes. Both conditions may lead to malnourishment. These unpleasant events can continue throughout the pregnancy. Researchers at the University of Vienna, Austria, led by P. Frigo, found that more than 90 percent of pregnant women who suffer from *hyperemesis gravidarum* were infected with *H. pylori*. The researchers suggested that in the early phase of pregnancy the changes in a woman's body fluid concentration affect the acidity of the stomach. In turn, this may activate latent *H. pylori* residing in the stomach.

- Could there be a link between *H. pylori* infection and sudden infant death syndrome (SIDS)? This possible connection was proposed by C. Phillip Pattison and Barry J. Marshall, who first identified the bacterium. Jointly, the two doctors proposed this idea in 1997 in *Medical Hypothesis*, a journal that provides a forum for speculative theories.

  Although the prone sleeping position is one of the major risk factors for SIDS, Pattison and Marshall were impressed by a number of epidemiologic similarities between SIDS and *H. pylori* infection. Both are more common in males; in poor and nonwhite populations; and in large families and crowded living conditions. Both conditions can produce growth retardation in children, and have been shown to cluster in families. C-urea breath tests have shown that children may be infected with *H. pylori* before they are three months old.

  As for the mechanism that might link the infection with SIDS, the two doctors proposed a hypothesis. Although *H. pylori* infection in children usually is asymptomatic, its presence could lead to the synthesis of the inflammatory cytokine interleukin-1, which can produce fever, activate immune response, and increase deep sleep. Under these conditions, terminal hypoxia (a reduction of oxygen in body tissues below physiologic levels) could result from the combination of a relatively minor respiratory or enteric infection, and a prone sleep position. In an alternative scenario, the large amount of urease produced by *H. pylori* could be aspirated in gastric juice, reach the alveolae in the lungs, react with plasma urea, produce ammonia toxicity, and lead to respiratory arrest.

- Does *H. pylori* play a role in cholera epidemics? D. R. Nalin at the Merck Research Laboratories in West Point, Pennsylvania, suggests that it does. Cholera epidemics frequently occur in tropical countries where hypochlorhydria (described earlier) is common. Hypochlorhydria increases the susceptibility to cholera, a serious infection from *Vibrio cholerae*. Hypochlorhydria can be caused by childhood malnutrition, and *H. pylori* is thought to be related to this condition. *V. cholerae* exist in copepods (marine crustaceans) with chitin (hard, protective coverings). The *V. cholerae* can adhere to the chitin and provide a passage through the gastric acid barrier in the human stomach. Further studies are needed to determine the role of *H. pylori* in cholera epidemics.

STEPS YOU CAN TAKE TO PREVENT
STOMACH ULCERS AND *H. PYLORI*

- Eat ample amounts of green leafy vegetables. They are rich in folic acid. Also, eat ample amounts of cruciferous vegetables such as broccoli and kale.

- Eat ample amounts of vegetables containing lycopene, a phytochemical. Tomatoes are a good source. Eat produce with high levels of beta-carotene. These are foods that range in color from yellow to orange, such as squashes, sweet potatoes, and cantaloupes.

- Eat foods that contain vitamins A, C, and B_{12}, and selenium.

- If you are a mother, breastfeed your infant. There are protective effects of specific human milk IgA against *H. pylori*, according to the findings of J. E. Thomas and co-researchers. For example, *H. pylori* are ubiquitous in West Africa. However, when mothers breastfeed their infants through the first two years of life, IgA in breast milk can protect infants against early acquisition of infections, including *H. pylori*. The breastfeeding may be crucial in delaying the onset of *H. pylori* infection and in maintaining the integrity of the gastric acid barrier throughout the vulnerable weaning period.

- Consume plain whole-milk yogurt that contains live active cultures. The probiotic bacteria in the yogurt helps maintain the beneficial microflora in the stomach, and wards off colonization of pathogens such as *H. pylori*, among others.

- Limit or avoid eating nitrated foods such as frankfurters, luncheon meats, bacon, and smoked hams.

PART FOUR

Reducing Your Risk of Foodborne Illness

CHAPTER 21

The Semmelweis Solution

In the 1840s, up to 30 percent of women who gave birth in European hospital maternity wards died of puerperal fever. This bacterial infection (septicemia) can be in the female genital tract after childbirth.

A Hungarian-born obstetrician, Ignaz Philipp Semmelweis (1818–1865), practicing in the Vienna General Hospital, noted that frequently interns and physicians came from the autopsy department where they had performed dissections, and then examined birthing mothers. Also, it was common practice for surgeons to wear bloody leather aprons, similar to those used in butchering operations. The interns and the surgeons would wash their hands *after* they assisted in childbirth or performed surgery, but *not before*.

While puerperal fever raged in hospital settings, Semmelweis knew that women who were assisted by midwives and gave birth at home remained relatively unaffected by this scourge.

Semmelweis concluded that puerperal fever was septic and contagious, and it was preventable by good hygiene. As assistant professor in the maternity ward of the hospital, in 1847 Semmelweis ordered the interns to wash their hands with soap and water, and sanitize their hands with chlorinated lime *before* contacting patients. As a result of this regulation, the maternal death rate in the ward dropped from 12.24 percent to 3.04 percent by the end of 1847, and to 1.27 percent by the end of 1848.

THE LOW-TECH, LIFE-SAVING ACT OF HANDWASHING

Despite this dramatic achievement, Semmelweis encountered strong and, at times, vicious opposition from hospital officials. In 1850, disillusioned, Semmelweis left Vienna, and became professor of obstetrics at the University of Pest Hospital in Hungary. While there, Semmelweis enforced handwashing procedures, and reduced the death rate for women from puerperal fever to 0.85 percent. However, Semmelweis's findings and publications on the subject were resisted by hospital and medical authorities in Hungary and elsewhere. Depressed by ridicule, Semmelweis suffered a nervous breakdown, and was placed in a mental hospital in Vienna. Ironically, the pioneer in handwashing died of an infection from a

PERSONAL HYGIENE: AN OLD TRADITION

Many cultures have viewed personal hygiene, including handwashing, in a socio-religious context of purity. Early hygiene practices were recorded in ancient Mesopotamia, Assyria, Babylon, and Phoenicia. The Phoenicians are credited with the invention of soap in 600 B.C. Hygienic tradition developed in Asia, Greece, and Rome. Illness prevention was embodied in the Greek, and later, Roman goddess of health, personified as Hygeia.

The Bible provided instructions on handwashing and hand-drying practices for those attending the ill, dying, or dead. In short: wash hands vigorously in running water and dry them in sunlight. These recommendations sound familiar in modern times, with our principles of handwashing: friction, dilution, disinfection, and drying.

Early rabbinical literature mandated washing hands and feet daily. Additional handwashing was prescribed during specific occasions to maintain good health: after arising from a night's sleep, after urinating and defecating, and before eating.

In the twelfth century, Moses Maimonides, a Jewish scholar and philosopher, was appointed as physician to an Egyptian sultan. Maimonides talked and wrote about the importance of handwashing and hand drying, as well as of environmental hygiene. The sultan was never ill during Maimonides' presence in his court, and the sultan attributed his good health to Maimonides' encouragement to practice good personal hygiene.

By the Middle Ages, people crowded into European cities with little or no personal or environmental hygiene. Western civilization slid into a stagnant period. For about a thousand years, personal hygiene was neglected, and practiced mainly by monks and religious orders. Centuries passed until Semmelweis, Holmes, and others demonstrated the importance of handwashing.

serious scalpel wound on his right hand. He was a victim of the scourge against which he had fought so valiantly.

On the American side of the Atlantic Ocean, as early as 1843, Dr. Oliver Wendell Holmes preached handwashing to his medical colleagues. As with Semmelweis, Holmes's recommendations had little impact at the time on obstetric practices.

Louis Pasteur's germ theory of disease gradually brought recognition to the importance of handwashing to the medical profession, as well as to food handlers and preparers. The intertwining of practices in medical facilities and food preparation facilities with handwashing were similar to the intertwining with staph infection more recently.

HANDWASHING HABITS TODAY

Fast forward to the end of the twentieth century. In 1995, the American Medical Association (AMA) felt it necessary to remind health professionals to wash their hands. In a resolution titled "Ten Dirty Digits," the AMA reported that only 14 to 59 percent of doctors routinely washed their hands between patient encounters; nurses, 24 to 45 percent; and other health-care workers, 23 to 73 percent. Despite in-service education, lectures, automated water-and-soap dispensers, and other measures, handwashing rates remained dismally low. Duncan W. Clark, a specialist in preventive medicine, who wrote the AMA resolution, noted that 1997 would be the 150th anniversary of the efforts of Semmelweis to emphasize the importance of handwashing.

At the same time, what was the record of food handlers and preparers? For foodservice settings, the Food and Drug Administration (FDA), in its 1997 Food Code, called for food handlers and preparers to clean their hands and exposed portions of their arms with a cleaning compound immediately before engaging in food preparation, including work with exposed food, clean equipment, utensils, and unwrapped single-service and single-use articles, as well as the customary handwashing after food handling. Also, foodservice workers were cautioned not to wash their hands in sinks used for food preparation, or in service sinks used to dispose of mop water and similar liquid waste.

Despite the Food Code, an FDA report, compiled in 2000, found that workers in the food retail industry had a poor record of handwashing. Grocery store employees had 78 percent compliance, and fast-food service employees averaged only 55 percent compliance. In an additional report, the FDA found that 30 to 45 percent of employees at restaurants and supermarkets were out of compliance. Improper handwashing was the main reason.

In 2005, the FDA revised the Food Code. The agency defined proper handwashing techniques as using a good hand soap, rubbing hands vigorously for at least 15 seconds, followed by a thorough rinse under clean running water. The revised Food Code also recommended that handwashing sinks be located conveniently, within easy and unobstructed access to employees, and that the sinks have an adequate flow of heated water.

During the same period, what were the handwashing practices of the general public? In a survey, conducted by the American Society for Microbiology, in partnership with Bayer Corporation Pharmaceutical Division, more than 2,000 people were observed in public toilets in five large American cities. The researchers hid themselves in bathroom stalls, or pretended to comb their hair while observing the practices of the public-toilet users. Only 60 percent of people using the public toilets in Penn Station in New York City washed their hands; 78 percent, at Navy Pier in Chicago; 71 percent, in a casino in New Orleans; 69 percent, at Golden Gate Park in San Francisco; and 64 percent, at a major baseball field in Atlanta. Also, perception did not match reality. The survey noted that 94 percent of adults reported that they always washed their hands after using public toilets, yet on average, only 68 percent were observed doing so. Women washed their hands more frequently than men—74 percent and 61 percent, respectively.

Lifestyle Trends Discourage Handwashing Habits

The terms "dashboard dining" and "deskfast" have come into usage as time-pressed Americans eat wherever and whenever they can. The American Dietetic Association, in cooperation with ConAgra's Food Foundation Home Safety program, surveyed more than 1,500 working men and women. About 62 percent reported that sometimes, or often, they are too busy to sit down and eat meals. Furthermore, 90 percent admitted to doing other things while preparing meals, without washing their hands between operations and food handling. Some 35 percent admitted to multitasking at their desks: using computers, reading, making and receiving phone calls, writing, doing calculations, or cleaning the work area—all done while eating. Of this group, 31 percent reported that they did not wash their hands consistently as they switched from tasks to foods.

THE ART OF HANDWASHING

Handwashing would seem like a straightforward procedure. It is not. The practice may be too infrequent, too brief, not thorough, or ineffective. According to sanitarians, up to a third of the general public do not wash their hands after using toilets (corroborating the findings cited above) and those who do, often fail to wash their hands thoroughly. The importance of this finding is noteworthy. It is estimated that some 10 to 30 percent of all foodborne illnesses result from poor personal hygiene of food handlers and preparers. Also, it is estimated that the implications of poor personal hygiene habits by food workers possibly could be responsible for up to 80 million cases of illnesses and 10,000 deaths a year in the United States.

These are collated recommendations for *everyone before handling food.*

Wash Hands *After* You . . .

- Use the toilet
- Handle uncooked foods, especially raw meats, poultry, eggs, and fish
- Touch anything that might contaminate hands, such as contact with doorknobs or unsanitized work surfaces
- Touch hair, face, body, clothing, apron, towel, etc.
- Insert or remove contact lenses
- Shake hands
- Sneeze, cough, or blow the nose
- Smoke, eat, drink, or chew gum or tobacco
- Use any cleaning, polishing, or sanitizing agent
- Clear tables
- Take out garbage
- Pet or touch cats, dogs, reptiles, or exotic animals
- Treat a wound, or touch a sick or injured person
- Change a diaper

Food handlers and preparers who work continuously should wash hands at least every hour, and change to new gloves frequently.

Washing Hands *Properly* and *Effectively* Involves Several Steps . . .

1. Wet hands with hot running water

2. Apply soap to hands, including wrists, palms, back of hands, fingers, around and under nails

3. Rub hands together vigorously for at least 10 to 15 seconds, scrubbing all surfaces

4. Use a nailbrush

5. Rinse hands thoroughly under running water

6. Dry hands with an air dryer, or a clean disposable towel

A SANITARIAN'S WISH

"If food-safety professionals were given one wish, we would unanimously ask that the human species be given a re-evolution, with the dominant gene encoded for the characteristic of habitual and thorough handwashing."
—Robert W. Powitz, Ph.D., M.P.H., forensic sanitarian

What does the act of thorough handwashing with soap achieve? The main effect is to loosen the oil and dirt that hold germs, and allow the rinsing water to carry them away. One study showed that regular soap-and-water handwashing carried away 96 percent of staph bacteria. The detergent action of all soaps breaks down the fatty coatings on many viruses. A 1993 study showed that handwashing disposed of the viruses that cause both hepatitis A and polio.

Pay Special Attention to Fingernails

In handwashing, special care needs to be given to the area around and under the fingernails. More than 95 percent of hand flora reside in the nail region. These places are difficult to clean.

Sanitarian Robert W. Powitz suggests a do-it-yourself demonstration that provides a learning experience about fingernails and handwashing. Although the demonstration is intended as an educational tool to teach food handlers and preparers the importance of hand cleanliness, the exercise would work equally well with children.

HANDWASHING: SCIENCE VS. PRACTICE

"There is a treasure trove of handwashing science lying dormant, awaiting implementation. Year after year, the bank of scientific knowledge grows, yet foodborne illness risks associated with poor handwashing in the food industry persist. Science and technology are on an obvious path of continuous improvement, but handwashing frequently—and therefore adequately as a food safety measure—is not. Unfortunately, the assets that handwashing science offers us remain frozen, yielding an unnecessary high level of risk to the food industry and to its customers."
    —Jim Mann, Founder and Executive Director, Handwashing for Life
    Institute, and Handwashing Leadership Forum

Put equal amounts of ground cinnamon or paprika in a small bottle. Add some vegetable oil. Cap the bottle and shake well to obtain a colored emulsion. Apply the mixture liberally to the hands, making certain that the colored emulsion shows around and under the fingernails. Wash your hands. On the first try, most of the mixture can be washed off, but some will remain around and under the nails. For this area, scrub vigorously with a nailbrush, to dislodge the emulsion.

Powitz claims that if everyone would start their shift with a good handwashing, including the use of a brush, and wash frequently thereafter, problems with food cross-contamination would no longer be a problem. Nails should be kept short and clean. The wearing of artificial nails is linked to poor handwashing practices. Some food plants, restaurants, and other institutions where food is handled or prepared, prohibit the use of artificial nails. It is even more difficult to keep the area around and under the nails clean with artificial nails than with natural ones.

HAND CLEANSERS

Plain Soap

We still apply the term "soap" to bars and liquids that are no longer soaps as we knew them in the past. Most present soaps are detergents.

A study led by Elaine L. Larson from Columbia University's School of Nursing in New York City, demonstrated that plain soap used for handwashing was just as effective as antimicrobial soaps. There was no difference in the number of symptoms of infection, types of infection, or rates of infection. Larson concluded that "it doesn't matter what you clean with. What matters more is that you clean."

The findings of Larson's team were reinforced by guidelines issued by the Association for Professionals in Infection Control and Epidemiology (APIC). For general patient care, APIC recommended the use of plain soap, rather than antimicrobial soap (to be discussed shortly).

Alcohol-Based Antiseptic Hand Cleansers

Alcohol-based gels as antiseptic hand cleansers are regarded as a supplement to, but not as a replacer of, plain soap and water washing. The alcohol-based cleansers are useful as hand antiseptics when clean running water is unavailable. They are quick, convenient, and portable. However, these products are not recommended for hands that are heavily soiled with dirt or body fluids.

Both the Centers for Disease Control and Prevention (CDC) and the APIC guidelines recommend that when an alcohol-based gel is used, an adequate amount of the gel should be applied so that all areas of the hands are completely covered. The hands should be rubbed together vigorously until they are dry. If the hands are dry in less than 10 to 15 seconds, an insufficient amount of the gel has been applied.

The FDA recommends that the alcohol concentration in such products be from 60 to 95 percent for the greatest germicidal efficiency. If you purchase such products, read the label information. The alcohol may be termed ethanol, ethyl alcohol, or isopropanol.

Some of these products are ineffective in reducing bacterial counts on hands. One commercial substandard product, seized by the FDA, contained only 49 percent ethanol as the active ingredient. The label claimed that the product reduced germs and harmful bacteria by 99.9 percent. Yet, in testing, after the cleanser was applied to the hands and handprints impressed on agar plates, the product resulted in an *increased* concentration of bacteria. None of the other hand cleansers, with high-alcohol contents, showed this effect. The substandard product was sold at stores of a deep-discount chain, suggesting that low-economic groups in the population may be at greater risk of purchasing an ineffective product.

Several Internet sites provide directions for making a bubble-gum-scented child hand cleanser with 33 percent isopropanol as the sole active ingredient. Such a product is likely to be ineffective, and to give parents or caregivers a false sense of safety.

Antimicrobial Products

In 1972, antimicrobial soaps were introduced in health-care settings for surgical scrubs. With growing public awareness of foodborne disease outbreaks and well-publicized food recalls, the marketplace was receptive to products that would kill pathogenic microbes.

HYPE, MISLEADING INFORMATION, AND SCAMS

Many companies producing disinfectants for years, decided to replace the word with antibacterial after focus groups determined that 'antibacterial' would sell more products than 'disinfectants.'

The front label of a dishwashing liquid declared that the product was "antibacterial." On the back label, the product was designated only to be antibacterial if used as a hand soap, not as a dishwashing soap. The company was able to use the conflicting claims on the front and back panels, because the company had sought approval from the FDA, which regulates such products, but had not sought approval from the Environmental Protection Agency (EPA), which regulates antimicrobial claims for cleansers and detergents.

Antibacterial window-cleaning liquids have been promoted to give a "germ-free shine." What the consumer may not realize is that the solution must remain on the glass for at least ten minutes before it can kill germs.

In 1997, the EPA charged Microban Products Company, located in Huntersville, North Carolina, with making "unsubstantiated public health claims" for its pesticide Microban Plastic Additive "B." In a civil complaint, the EPA charged that Microban claimed that products treated with its pesticide protect children from infectious diseases caused by E. coli and other bacteria. In fact, the treatment was approved *solely to protect the plastics in products from deteriorating.* The EPA warned, "If parents and child-care providers believe that toys are sanitary or self-sanitizing, they may not practice standard hygiene to prevent transmission of harmful germs, or be as careful as they should be."

Antibacterial toothbrushes have been promoted to prohibit growth of bacteria. The fine print reveals that the antibacterial agent prohibits "the growth of bacteria that may affect the plastic in the handle."

In the late 1980s, Dial was the first antimicrobial soap introduced to the general public. By the mid-1990s, not only were antimicrobials added to many liquid and bar soaps, but also their use extended to many personal care and household items. Nothing was overlooked. From 1992 to 1998, some 673 antimicrobial products were introduced. The development was regarded as a major marketing feat of the 1990s. The phenomenon was highly profitable. Often, the products sold at a higher price than their untreated counterparts. Their annual sales to consumers have become a billion dollar business in the United States.

Among the germ-proofed kitchen products are detergents and dishwashing liquids, kitchen sponges, cutting boards, countertops, faucets, kitchen utensils, trash bags, and even dog or cat feeding bowls. Germ-proofed products extended to the bathroom with toothpastes, denture cleaners, toothbrushes, and mouthwashes; liquid and bar soaps; deodorants; cosmetics; skin cleansers, lotions, and creams; acne medications, diapers, baby wipes, and cotton swabs; shower curtains and shower stalls; and even cat litter.

Other areas in the house were not overlooked. Antimicrobial-treated paints and wallpapers, carpeting, curtains, blankets, clothing, underwear, sweat socks, hunting clothing, children's toys and highchairs, ballpoint pens, plastics, keyboards, stair railings, and window-cleaning solutions were some of the products.

As might be expected, the antimicrobials permeated every aspect of health-care facilities. Hospital instruments, appliances, sheeting, and hospital clothing were among many of the treated objects.

By 2009, 75 percent of all liquid detergents and 30 percent of all bar soaps contained antimicrobial compounds.

A BRIEF HISTORY OF TRICLOSAN

The antimicrobial agent that accounted for the marketing phenomenon is a chlorinated aromatic compound with antibacterial, antifungal, and antiviral properties. The trade name is Triclosan when used in detergents; Microban, in plastics and clothing; and Biofresh, in acrylic fibers.

Triclosan, now generic, originally was registered as a pesticide with the EPA. As a chlorophenol, this chemical is in a group of substances suspected as human carcinogens. Triclosan is categorized as a persistant organic pollutant (POP). It is known to cause skin irritation and photoallergic contact dermatitis if one is exposed to this chemical along with sunlight.

Triclosan as a Toxic Agent

Triclosan is a hormone disruptor and has been shown to interfere with thyroid metabolism in frogs. In mouse studies, triclosan lowered the body temperature and had a depressant effect on the central nervous system. In toxicological studies with rats and rabbits, triclosan was linked both to decreased birthweight and decreased survival.

If triclosan is swallowed accidentally, even a very small amount can lead to a cold sweat, followed by circulatory collapse, convulsions, coma, and death.

Triclosan is lipophilic (meaning that is has an affinity to bind with fat). It attaches to fatty tissue, and can accumulate in the liver, kidneys, and lungs.

Triclosan in dishwashing detergent causes additional exposures through inhalation and dermal absorption. Residues of triclosan can remain on dishes and cutlery if the items are not rinsed thoroughly.

Due to the numerous applications of triclosan in consumer products, inevitably, increasing amounts of it are being found as residues accumulating in humans. It has been identified in the umbilical cord blood of newborn infants, and in breast milk.

Discovery of Triclosan's Many Damaging Effects

The triclosan-treated detergents and soaps, drained from sinks, ultimately reach wastewater treatment plants. These facilities are not equipped to remove triclosan from the water. Chlorine, used commonly as a water disinfectant, dissipates quickly, but triclosan often survives sewage treatment. It was found that only about 21 percent of the triclosan entering water treatment plants breaks down. (When it does break down, triclosan degrades to methyl-triclosan, which is even more lipophilic and bioavailable than its parent compound.)

At the water treatment plant, if the wastewater contains triclosan, and chlorine as well, the two chemicals can combine and form chloroform, a suspected carcinogen.

The chemical structure of triclosan is similar to the chemical structure of dioxin—one of the most toxic of all known chemicals. If both triclosan and chlorine are in the water, and the water is exposed to sunlight, dioxin can form. Dioxin is an acknowledged carcinogen.

Most of the triclosan that enters the water plant does not break down. It accumulates in solid sludge. A small amount remains in the liquid stream. The solid sludge may be hauled to farms where it is applied to soils as fertilizer. Presently, it is not known if the triclosan present in the sludge (along with the heavy metals) accumulates in the soils and is taken up by crops that enter the food supply. The triclosan remaining in the liquid stream flows into water bodies. Triclosan has been detected in water discharged from treatment plants, and found to be absorbed and bioaccumulated in aquatic organisms such as algae. Going up the food chain, the triclosan can reach fish, and ultimately the food eaten by humans and other creatures.

Worldwide Concerns Mount

By the early 2000s, scientists from several European governments issued warnings about the hazards of triclosan. Scientists in Denmark cautioned against the routine uses of antimicrobials in household and personal care products. Similar warnings were given by scientists in Finland and Germany. In the United Kingdom, four major grocery chains announced that they would not sell triclosan-containing products. The soap and detergent manufacturers in Europe agreed to hold production levels of antimicrobials to 1998 levels.

In the United States, health professionals voiced concerns. A study funded by the National Institute of Nursing Research, found no evidence to suggest that the use of antibacterial soap with triclosan provided any benefit over plain soap in reducing bacterial counts, or rate of infections in healthy persons in household settings. There was concern that the extensive use of the antibacterial products in community settings might provide a suitable environment for the emergence of drug-resistant bacteria.

In 2002, the Council on Scientific Affairs of the American Medical Association voiced similar concerns. The Council opposed the routine use of antimicrobially treated products.

The APIC (mentioned earlier), comprised of some 12,000 doctors, nurses, and other health-care workers who oversee infection control in medical facilities, reported that there is "no proven infection-prevention benefit in the use of these products."

No studies had been conducted to demonstrate that use of antimicrobials in kitchens actually decreased the incidence of foodborne diseases. In 2003, researchers for the *Journal of Community Health* conducted a survey. They followed adults in 238 households in New York City for nearly a year. They found that there was no difference in the numbers of microbes on hands whether people used ordinary soap or antimicrobial soap. At least four other large studies showed similar findings. The results of these studies led to a question: Do these antimicrobials cause more harm than good, by creating antibiotic-resistant bacteria? One study concluded, "The use of common antimicrobials for which acquired bacterial resistance has been demonstrated should be discontinued in consumer products unless data emerge to conclusively show that such resistance has no effect on public health and that such products are effective in preventing infection. Ultimately, antibiotic resistance must be controlled through judicious use of antibiotics by health-care professionals and the public."

Long Overdue FDA Regulation

The FDA, which regulates triclosan, had been passive in allowing the antimicrobial products to flood the marketplace. The agency was shaken by the voiced concerns of the medical community. Long overdue, the FDA finally focused on the issue. In 2005, an advisory panel appointed by the agency on non-prescription drugs, gave testimony on "several decades worth of clinical data," indicating that antimicrobial detergents and soaps "are no more effective than soap and water in reducing infections." The panel concluded that home use of antimicrobial detergents and soaps "poses unacceptable risks of environment contamination and contribute to the evolution of antibiotic resistance."

In the same year that the report from the advisory panel was issued, analysts at Datamonitor, an independent research-based analysis firm, released some pertinent figures. About 1,500 new antimicrobial products had been introduced in the United States since 2000. By 2006, up to a million pounds of triclosan were added yearly, solely to personal care products. This amount did not include the numerous other products containing triclosan.

The widespread use of triclosan encourages complacency. It is a poor substitute for good hygiene.

Overuse of triclosan reduces the time when it becomes ineffective. Already, several bacterial strains grow readily on triclosan; one even may use triclosan as an energy source. Considering the fact that bacteria frequently acquire new traits from one another by exchanging genes, triclosan's effectiveness may be doomed.

Due to the extensive use of triclosan, by 2009 this antimicrobial and its breakdown products were identified as widespread environmental contaminants in waterways, fish, foods, and in human milk, serum, and

THE ACTION OF TRICLOSAN

When triclosan was first introduced in consumer products, it was thought that the chemical killed microbes in multiple ways, rather than like most antibiotics that kill a single protein. Later, it was learned that triclosan's main method of killing is very specific. It inhibits an enzyme involved in fatty acid synthesis. Some bacteria with mutations in the enzyme's gene can resist triclosan. Also, an antibiotic commonly used to treat the tuberculosis bacteria targets the same enzyme, raising the possibility that triclosan will lead to new drug-resistant strains of the microbe.

Another way that bacteria fend off triclosan is that nearly all strains of *Pseudomonas aeruginosa* (a deadly bacteria that often infects people with weak immune systems) thwart triclosan due to the action of efflux pumps that inactivate the antiseptic action of the antibacterial agent. When the gene for one key pump mutates, the bacteria quickly regain their defense against triclosan by increasing the production of other efflux pumps. Triclosan's prevalence may promote the development of multiple drug-resistant microbes.

urine. Triclosan was identified in a large number of water samples, according to chemist Weilin Shelver at the U.S. Department of Agriculture's (USDA) Agricultural Research Service (ARS) in Fargo, North Dakota. There is growing concern about triclosan's impact on antimicrobial resistance, as well as on the environment, wildlife, and human health.

SAFETY MEASURES TO REDUCE FOOD CONTAMINATION

Gloved or Barehanded Food Preparers?

At first glance, it would appear that the wearing of gloves by food preparers offers a good barrier against food contamination, especially with ready-to-eat foods, and would be safer than food preparation with bare hands. The answer is not simple, nor clear-cut. Gloves *can* act as a safety barrier, but with certain qualifiers.

The gloves must be intact. They must not have any breaks, tears, leaks, abrasions, or punctures. Unfortunately, it has been found that half the time, glove wearers fail to notice punctures. When tested, the leakage rate was 2.5 percent among randomly selected gloves. As a precautionary measure against defective gloves, the *British Journal of Surgery* advised surgeons to use a double set of gloves. This recommendation might not be acceptable to food handlers and preparers.

Bacteria on gloved hands can double every forty minutes when the hands are dry, and every fifty minutes, when wet, according to Mary Lou Fleissner, an epidemiologist at the Indiana State Board of Health. Tasks such as peeling shrimp or shucking oysters make it difficult to maintain the integrity of gloves. Also, a glove can tear from long fingernails and artificial fingernails. A glove traps heat and moisture, which can liquefy any nail contamination and release it if the glove is not intact.

A deteriorated glove can transfer fragments of the glove into food. Some gloves are manufactured in bright colors so that such fragments can be identified in food products. Another approach is to make 'detectable' gloves. A substance incorporated into the glove intentionally as an adulterant sets off a metal detector in a food-processing line.

Gloves must not be used repeatedly, for an unduly long period. Discarding such gloves is cost effective. One food corporation reported that the outlay of fifty cents for a new pair of gloves is far less costly than to pay for hepatitis claims.

There are important rules for glove use:

- Gloves must be kept clean. Food preparers do not always recognize that the gloves are dirty. When this happens, noted Charles Otto, an FDA staffer, "gloves make the problem worse."

- The worker must have clean hands before donning the gloves. A survey conducted by the U.S. Food Standards Agency found that less than half of food workers wash their hands when they should, and a third of caterers fail to wash their hands after using toilets. The current Food Code requires workers to spend at least 20 seconds in handwashing. However, in a study published in the *Annals of Internal Medicine* (Jan 1998), there was only marginal benefit in the 20 second handwashing over a 10 second handwashing.

- Gloves must be suitable for the specific food processing or preparation task. For example, some gloves are made from materials that do not resist heat, fat, alcohol, oxygen, ozone, or ultraviolet light, or other things that can affect the integrity of the gloves. Gloves differ in their densities, tensile strength, durability, and puncture-resistance. Some are loose fitting; others snug. Some become stiff and brittle.

- Gloves must be tolerated. Formerly, it was common to use latex gloves from natural rubber. Then, it was discovered that latex can be allergenic for food workers who are sensitive to latex. Also, the foods, in contact with the latex gloves, could be contaminated with latex, and subsequently induce reactions in consumers who are sensitive to latex. The American Academy of Allergy, Asthma, and Immunology recommended that latex gloves *not* be used by food handlers and preparers. Some states banned use of latex gloves, while others required restaurants to post warnings.

   Latex gloves were replaced by synthetic rubber substitutes, notably by polyethylene, polyvinyl chloride, polyurethane, nitrile, and neoprene. Each one has certain advantages and drawbacks. For example, some of these synthetic rubber substitutes contain chemicals that induce reactions, such as irritant dermatitis and chemical sensitivity dermatitis; others contain bisphenol A, a hormone disruptor.

- Gloves should be comfortable to wear. Workers have complained that some gloves fit poorly, or create excessive hand sweating. Some gloves now have disposable absorbent inserts to absorb sweat produced inside the gloves.

   Is food that is prepared by gloved workers much safer than food that is prepared barehandedly? One study reported in the *Journal of Food Protection* (Apr 2005) did not find a great difference between the two. Researchers purchased about 400 plain flour tortillas from fast-food restaurants and analyzed the tortillas for *S. aureus, E. coli,* and other foodborne pathogens. About 46 percent of the samples handled by gloved workers were contaminated, and about 52 percent, handled by barehanded workers. The apparent failure of gloved workers to prevent, or at least reduce contamination, is thought to be due to the tendency of workers to wear the same pair of gloves for extended periods, and to wash their hands less frequently when they use gloves.

Monitoring Handwashing

If employees use the same restrooms in restaurants and food supermarkets as customers, the obligatory sign "workers must wash their hands before returning to work" may be reassuring to customers. Unfortunately, the practice is not always followed by employees.

In large institutions where food handlers have their own bathroom facilities, attempts have been made to educate workers about the importance of handwashing. For example, an industry-sponsored "Handwashing Olympics" was organized to encourage innovative techniques that encourage proper handwashing. One entry was the use of a special solution applied to the hands before washing. The person then washes his or her hands, using the person's customary procedure. If the handwashing is not thorough, the solution still left on the hands is visible under ultraviolet light.

Another handwashing training kit is a portable viewing box. The employee applies soap to his or her hands, washes, and then thrusts the hands into a viewing box. Viewed under a black light, all the missed spots show up. For cross-contamination training, an invisible powder is placed on the person's hands or other surfaces with which the employee would come in contact. After washing hands and surface, the black light reveals where the powder is still present, demonstrating how infectious pathogens can be spread from hands to surfaces, and can cross-contaminate.

At many large plants where food is handled or prepared, automatic washing facilities make handwashing easy for employees. The person stands at a station and plunges his or her bare or gloved hands into two cylinders. Photo-optical sensors activate the unit, which cleanses the hands using a timed jet spray of a water-containing sanitizing agent. Cycle counters on the units keep track of the number of handwashes per day. Field studies showed an initial high acceptance, although over time use tended to taper off. However, surveys showed that the automatic washing units were used three times as frequently as traditional manual washing methods. In addition, touchless handwashing stations have similar devices as those familiar to the general public: infrared sensors that detect the presence of hands and dispense a pre-measured amount of water and soap; automatically flushed toilets; and motion-activated rollers that dispense paper toweling.

Despite these attempts to make voluntary handwashing by food handlers and preparers a routine habit, surveys show dismal results. One large company survey tracked 1.3 million employee work hours, in several food service locations within food plants. There was regular observation of handwashing performances, and interviews with employees and supervisors, as well as with soap suppliers. The survey found that, on average, food service employees used the handwashing facilities less than once daily.

After electronic handwashing control and verification systems were installed at test locations and employees were given individual codes for activating water flow, the number of handwashings per day increased dramatically at each location. But after the handwashing systems were removed, handwashing performances returned to the former poor record, averaging less than one handwashing per employee per day.

Because voluntary compliance was so poor, plant supervisors realized that more draconian methods were needed, beyond education and coaxing. Personal hygiene of food handlers and preparers was essential for public protection. Keeping a watchful eye on an employee's personal hygiene strengthens food safety. To ensure handwashing, another step was taken: automatic surveillance.

A high-tech approach, Hygiene Guard can track whether kitchen staff in restaurants, including the chef, food preparers, dishwashers, and waiters, actually use soap dispensers and wash their hands after using toilets. Under the system, each employee is required to wear a battery-powered "smart badge." Unless an employee uses the soap dispenser and stands for a required period of time in front of a sink with running water, an infraction is recorded by the badge, which communicates with sensors in the bathroom. The sensors are connected to a computer in the manager's office. In some instances, the badge will flash. Also, the badges beep periodically to remind employees to wash their hands frequently.

Privacy advocates complain that such devices represent an unprecedented intrusion. The device has been dubbed "Big Brother in the Bathroom." It is part of a growing trend to monitor employees electronically. Despite the protest, such devices are attractive to restaurants, hotels, hospitals, and other institutions, where food safety is an issue that looms large.

The CDC rates poor personal hygiene of food handlers and preparers along with improper temperature control as the two most significant factors leading to foodborne illness. According to the CDC, handwashing is one of the "most important means of preventing the spread of infection." The importance of low-tech, thorough, and frequent handwashing to prevent foodborne diseases cannot be overstated. Washing hands does not require much thought or effort, but it does require awareness.

CHAPTER 22

Food Safety in Your Kitchen

The safety of our food supply depends on many components from farm to fork, including growers, processors, shippers, distributors, and retailers. The safety also depends on protective regulations, and enforcements by vigilant inspectors at the federal, state, and local levels. As individuals, we exert little control over food safety before purchase. However, we, too, bear responsibility in our own kitchens, to make certain that safe food is kept safe.

PRACTICE FOOD SAFETY AT HOME

Several studies and surveys have found that food-handling practices within American home kitchens contribute to foodborne illness. For example, in 1998, in a multistate survey, the Centers for Disease Control and Prevention (CDC) found that 20 percent of food preparers did not wash their cutting boards with soap or bleach after using the boards to cut raw flesh foods. Some people continued to take unnecessary risks, such as eating undercooked meat or eggs, and consuming raw milk and raw shellfish.

The CDC's findings were confirmed by another survey conducted during the same year. Audits International, in Highland Park, Illinois, studied consumer home food-handling practices in 121 households in 82 cities in the United States and Canada. The company found that 74 percent of consumers failed to meet *minimum* food safety standards. There was at least one *major* food safety violation in 60 percent of the homes. Poor practices included cross-contamination of foods, improper dishwashing practices, incorrect food preparation, and improper cooking of leftover foods. The people who had faulty practices either did not know the proper procedure, or they failed to pay close attention to what they were doing (*Food Technology*, Feb 1998).

In 2004, Janet B. Anderson, a dietitian at Utah State University in Logan, and her colleagues found ninety-two women and seven men who were willing to prepare foods in their own kitchens in their usual manner, while having their actions videotaped. The volunteers were assigned to prepare one of three entrées (meatloaf, chicken breasts, or marinated fish) along with a fresh vegetable salad.

In reviewing the videotaping, the researchers noted numerous food-handling practices that would increase the risk of foodborne illness. Handwashing was inadequate. One-third of the volunteers failed to clean surfaces during food preparation. With unwashed or inadequately washed hands, nearly all the volunteers cross-contaminated raw flesh foods with unwashed vegetables and ready-to-eat foods numerous times during food preparation. Many of the volunteers undercooked the meat and poultry entrées. Perhaps what is needed is a home-kitchen Hazard Analysis and Critical Control Point Program (HACCP, see inset on page 209). Except for the record keeping and its verification, the other principles could be applied as helpful tools to ensure food safety in the home kitchen.

Store Shelf-Stable Foods Properly

Many foods can be stored at room temperature for lengths of time. The area should be dry. Some foods, notably potatoes, need to be stored in darkness. For many foods, an open shelf or a closed cupboard provide good storage conditions, as long as the foods are kept out of bright sunlight. They should be away from the stove and refrigerator exhausts. Extreme heat (over 100°F) or extreme cold (below 32°F) can harm canned goods. Otherwise, they are safe to use, even when they are stored for lengthy time periods. Dry foods, such as beans, can be stored safely in tightly closed glass jars, and kept for long periods at room temperature.

Low-acid canned foods, such as meat and poultry, stews, soups (except tomato), pasta products, potatoes, corn, carrots, spinach, beans, beets, peas, and pumpkins can be stored from two to five years. High-acid canned foods, such as tomato products, fruits, sauerkraut, and foods in vinegar-based sauces or dressings, can be stored for twelve to eighteen months. Some canned hams are shelf-stable, but make certain that they are. Any canned hams labeled "keep refrigerated" must be treated as perishable.

UNDERSTANDING FOOD DATING TERMS

- **"Use by"** dates are determined by the product's manufacturer. There is some flexibility. The product may still be satisfactory and safe for a short time after expiration of the "use by" date. Some grocery stores pull the products off the shelves and cover "the use by" date with a sticker that may read "manager's special" with a discounted price.

   As long as a product is wholesome, it is legal for a retailer to sell fresh and processed meat and poultry products beyond the expiration dates on the packages.

   Federal regulations required a "use by" date on baby foods and infant feeding formulas. Make certain that the dates on these products have not expired.

   Dating on other products is not required by federal regulation. However, many states require dating for some perishable foods.

- **"Sell by"** dates guide the store manager to determine how long to offer the product for sale. If you find that a product is still being sold with an expired date, bring it to the attention of the section or store manager.

- **"Best if used by"** or **"Best if used before"** is not a safety date, but a recommendation for a time of peak flavor or quality in a product.

   When buying dry or canned foods make certain that the date (if given) on the package or can has not expired. At times, this information is coded, for use by the processor or grocery store, in the event of a recall. Don't buy any packages that are broken or appear to have experienced tampering. As noted previously in the discussion of botulism (see pages 256–257), don't purchase any cans that are bulging, rusty, or swollen. Dented cans may, or may not be safe. Keep unopened dry foods in their original containers. Once opened, transfer dry food products to airtight glass containers. Label them. Stock canned goods so that you can use the older stored ones first.

Store Refrigerated Foods Safely

The cool temperature of the refrigerator helps to maintain the freshness of perishable foods and keeps them safe by inhibiting or retarding the growth of most bacteria. Remember, however, that some microorganisms can continue to grow and multiply in refrigerated foods. (See the discussion on the psychrophilic characteristic in Chapter 8 on *Listeria*.)

Maintaining freshness in refrigerated produce varies with different foods. You can observe declining food quality when broccoli florets yellow, celery goes limp, and apple skins shrivel. Plan to use produce at its prime. Use perishable foods before they show telltale signs of decline. For example, use watercress promptly, and reserve cabbage for later use. Discard any food that becomes moldy, slimy, or foul smelling. Follow the wise adage: "If in doubt, throw it out."

Keep a thermometer in the refrigerator where you can read it easily. Maintain a temperature of 40°F or lower in the appliance. Check the temperature periodically. Although 40°F may be suitable for summertime, you may need to adjust the cold control for wintertime to prevent milk, lettuce, green peppers, and other sensitive foods from freezing.

Do not overload the refrigerator. Air must circulate to cool all foods. On the other hand, the freezer works efficiently when it is well stocked, with a minimum of air.

Transfer any unused portions of foods from open cans to inert (glass, not plastic) containers with covers, and refrigerate them. Metals and other substances in cans, once opened and in the presence of oxygen, can interact unfavorably with food.

Store meats, poultry, and fish in the coldest part of the refrigerator— usually at the back. Keep eggs in their original cartons, not in built-egg slots provided in some refrigerator doors.

Store Perishable Foods Safely

Many supermarket wrappings are permeable to air. Such wrappings may be adequate for storing foods briefly in the refrigerator, but inadequate for longer freezer storage. If you plan to freeze foods, overwrap the original packaging with tight, heavy-duty foil, plastic wrap, freezer paper, or a ziplock bag. Try to exclude as much air space as possible. Adequate packaging helps to prevent "freezer burn," a condition that denotes deterioration of quality. However, food that shows freezer burn is still safe to eat.

In freezing foods at home for future use, label the contents and date of freezing. Plan to rotate, by using the longest stored items first.

Raw foods from animal sources require prompt refrigeration. Their refrigerator and freezer shelf life varies. Be guided by the following chart.

FOOD	REFRIGERATOR SHELF LIFE	FREEZER SHELF LIFE
EGGS		
Egg whites or yolks	2–4 days	12 months
Whole eggs	3 weeks	Not applicable
FISH	1–2 days	Not applicable
CHEESES		
Cottage cheese	5 days	Not applicable
Soft cheeses	2 weeks	4 months
Hard cheeses	3–4 months	6 months
ICE CREAM	Not applicable	1–3 months
BUTTER	1 month	3–6 months
MEATS		
Raw meats	1–2 days (ground meat or stew meat, fresh pork sausages); 3–5 days (lamb or pork chops, steaks, roasts of beef, veal, lamb, or pork)	1–2 months (pork sausage); 3–4 months (ground or stew meats); 4–6 months (lamb or pork chops, roasts of lamb, pork, or veal); 6–12 months (roast of beef or steak)
Cooked meats and meat dishes	3–4 days	2–3 months
Processed meats (bacon, frankfurters, half-cooked or fully cooked ham, luncheon meats, smoked sausages)	3–5 days (luncheon meats, half-cooked and fully cooked ham); 7 days (unopened vacuum-sealed package) or until the "use by" or "sell by" date expires; 7 days (opened package bacon, frankfurters, smoked sausage)	1–2 months
POULTRY		
Raw poultry (chicken, duck, goose, turkey)	1–2 days	9 months (parts of chicken or turkey); 1 year (whole chicken, turkey, duck, or goose)
Cooked poultry	1–2 days (with broth or gravy); 3–4 days (without broth or gravy, or cooked casseroles)	3–4 months (cooked casseroles); 4 months (without broth or gravy); 6 months (with broth or gravy)

Thaw Foods Safely

Thaw frozen foods properly to keep them safe. *Thaw in the refrigerator, not on the kitchen counter at room temperature.* Although freezing foods at 0°F inactivates most pathogens such as bacteria, yeasts, and molds, it does not destroy them. After food is thawed, any pathogens already present can become activated, and under favorable conditions can multiply to high levels. Adequate cooking of properly thawed foods will prevent foodborne illness.

Frozen food can be thawed simply by transferring the frozen container from the freezer to the refrigerator. This procedure takes time for thawing, and it is best to plan ahead. To hasten the thawing, place the container in a pan of water in the refrigerator. To hasten the thawing even more, transfer the frozen food to a suitable container and use the microwave oven.

Clean the freezer regularly with a sanitizing solution. If the freezer and the refrigerator units are cleaned at the same time, it is helpful to transfer any items from the freezer and refrigerator to a portable ice chest or cooler, kept at a low temperature with gel packs or ice cubes.

PRACTICE SAFETY IN PREPARING FOODS

Safe practices in preparing foods have been mentioned throughout this book. They are important enough to bear repetition.

Bacteria multiply between 40°F and 140°F, termed the "danger zone." Harmful bacteria that cause many cases of food poisoning cannot be seen, smelled, or tasted. It is important to keep cold foods cold (40°F or lower) and hot foods hot (above 140°F). Do not allow perishable foods to remain at room temperature for more than two hours; in very hot weather, allow even less time. In practical terms, this means that you may have to excuse yourself from the dinner table with guests, and refrigerate the remains of a roast and other foods.

To hasten the cooling of a large volume of leftover food, such as a soup or a stew, divide it in shallow pans and refrigerate them. When the food has cooled, transfer it into suitable containers for the refrigerator or freezer.

Marinate raw flesh foods in the refrigerator. Unless you plan to cook the marinade along with the food, discard it. The mixture contains raw juices from the flesh foods.

Stuffing placed in the cavity of whole poultry can interfere with thorough cooking of the bird. Cook the stuffing separately from the poultry.

Use a traditional oven to cook roasts and whole poultry. Microwave oven cooking may not penetrate the interior of the food sufficiently, or it may cook the food unevenly. If viable pathogenic organisms are present, they may not be killed.

Wash your hands, cutting knives, and surfaces frequently. This mantra warrants endless repetition.

Sanitize Kitchen Surfaces and Sinks

A sanitizing agent such as the common household bleach is useful to clean kitchen surfaces and the kitchen sink. A tablespoon of bleach to a gallon of water is a common recommendation. However, some groups recommend different proportions of bleach to water—all the way up to three-quarters of a cup of bleach to a gallon of water. This proportion may be overkill. Usually, the large amount is recommended by the sellers of bleach. Strong solutions may be appropriate for cleaning floors or diaper pails, or for unusual circumstances such as after an area has been flooded, especially to get rid of mold, or if vomit has contaminated an area.

For normal cleaning of kitchen surfaces and sink, a more dilute formula is effective, and less likely to discolor countertops. Various governmental agencies and extension service personnel offer additional suggestions:

- Allow the bleach solution to remain on the surface for a few minutes to do its work.

- Use paper towels (not dishcloths or sponges) to wipe it off.

- Make a new sanitizing solution every time you clean the surfaces and sink. Once mixed with water, the bleach can dissipate and the solution loses its effectiveness.

- Clean the kitchen sink drain and drain disposal periodically with a mild solution of bleach in water. Pour the solution down the drain and allow it to remain for a few minutes before flushing it down with running water.

- Avoid scented bleaches. Usually, they are not as strong as regular unscented bleach, which make them less effective for sanitizing purposes. (Scented products should be avoided for other reasons, too. They are sensitizing agents that can provoke adverse reactions, and they add to environmental pollution.)

Cutting Boards: Some Surprising Findings

With the introduction of plastic cutting boards, it was assumed that they were more hygienic than wooden ones. It was thought that the plastic cutting boards were impervious, could be cleaned thoroughly, and were safer than porous wooden ones in which microorganisms could lodge. These untested assumptions led the USDA, as well as many extension-service educators, to urge food preparers to choose plastic over wood, and for sanitarians to endorse plastic cutting boards for commercial settings.

In 1993, unexpected findings were reported by microbiologists at the Food Research Institute of the University of Wisconsin in Madison. Dean O. Cliver and Nese O. Ak attempted to find ways to decontaminate wooden cutting boards and make them as safe as plastic ones. To their surprise, they found that pathogens disappeared on wood, but thrived on plastic.

Cliver and Ak intentionally contaminated both plastic and wooden cutting boards with two nonpathogenic strains of *Escherichia coli*, the virulent *E. coli* O157:H7, *Listeria innocus*, *L. monocytogenes*, or *Salmonella* Typhimurium. The researchers reported that "bacteria inoculated onto plastic blocks were readily recovered in minutes to hours, and would multiply if held overnight." However, "recoveries from wooden blocks, regardless of new or used status, differences increased with holding time." Clean wood blocks usually absorbed the inoculum completely within three to ten minutes. If the fluids contained the amount of bacteria likely to come from raw meat or poultry, the bacteria generally could not be recovered after entering the wood. At much higher levels, the bacteria might be recovered after twelve hours at room temperature and with high humidity, but their numbers were reduced by at least 98 percent, and more often by more than 99.9 percent. The small remainder was removed readily with hot water and detergent. Cliver and Ak concluded that "cross-contamination seems unlikely if the bacteria cannot be recovered by the procedures used in these experiments."

Surprised by the results, the researchers repeated their experiments several times. Each time, after exposure of only three minutes, in each type of wood tested, more than 99.9 percent of the bacteria disappeared. Yet all the bacteria on plastic surfaces survived. Old knife-scarred wood performed as well as new wood in its antibacterial effect. Yet, similarly, scarred plastic seemed to *encourage bacterial growth*. Bacteria survived even after scrubbing the plastic with soap and hot water.

In 1994, Cliver and Ak, joined by C. W. Kaspar, conducted additional studies with blocks of plastic, hard rubber, and nine different hardwoods. Bacteria were applied in a nutrient broth or chicken juice. Then, the bacteria were recovered by pressing the blocks onto agar as a nutrient. Bacteria inoculated onto plastic blocks were recovered readily after minutes to hours. They multiplied when held overnight. Recovery from the wooden blocks generally was less than from the plastics.

Although new plastic cutting-board surfaces were relatively easy to clean and were microbiologically clear, plastic boards with extensive knife scars were difficult to clean manually, especially if they had chicken fat deposits on them. Cleaning of the wooden boards with hot water and detergent generally removed remaining bacteria, regardless of the bacterial species, wood type, or whether the wood was new or old.

Additional follow-up studies were performed by microbiologists at the University of Michigan. Viable bacteria were detected on wooden cutting boards scanned by an electron microscope. But the researchers concluded that as long as the surfaces were maintained hygienically, and sanitized frequently, there would be no danger of cross-contamination either from a wooden or a plastic cutting board.

In early 1997, Cliver, joined by P. K. Park, updated the test findings at the University of Michigan. Cliver and Park used an electron microscope and scanned three types of plastic cutting boards. There were new surprises. The scanning revealed that plastic cutting boards, rather than being smooth and impervious, had holes, grooves, punctures, and cavities. All could harbor bacteria that would resist being dislodged during manual cleaning. Polyethylene and foamed polypropylene were found to contain holes and perforations, even when the plastics were new. During normal use, these surfaces acquired a number of deep knife-mark grooves, punctures, and cavities. Although acrylic cutting boards acquired fewer knife marks, with use, they became far more splintered and fractured. All three surfaces were inoculated with a nutrient broth containing *L. monocytogenes, S. aureus,* and *E. coli.* Vigorous washing with detergent and hot water failed to remove the bacteria from the cavities in the boards. Dried bacteria deposits formed a biofilm-like attachment to the surface of the acrylic boards. These results help to explain the earlier findings that the surfaces of used plastic were more difficult to clean manually than old wooden surfaces.

Cliver further updated his findings. In 2000, he reported that cutting boards made of close-grained hardwoods, such as maple, resist bacteria better than plastics. The cuts into hardwoods can actually trap bacteria in the grain and prevent them from resurfacing.

The final word on cutting boards probably has not been made. An additional material that has been introduced in the field is hard rubber. The Sani-Tuff rubber cutting board is used in many restaurant kitchens, and it is available for home use, too. It is claimed that the surface is non-porous and will not trap water or juices, and it resists bacterial growth. Because the board is made of rubber, it is claimed that most knife marks reseal themselves. However, if there are cuts in the board, it is claimed that the board can be sandpapered until it is smooth again. To clean the

THE MYTH OF THE UNWASHED WOODEN SALAD BOWL

From the 1930s through the 1960s, many Americans thought that in order to make a proper green leaf salad, a wooden salad bowl should merely be wiped between uses, but never washed. The idea was that the unwashed bowl would soak in the oil and vinegar dressing and, over time, would "cure" the wood. In turn, the cured wood would improve the salad it held. In truth, the oil turned rancid, the bowls became smelly, and the bowls became havens for pathogens.

The myth of the unwashed wooden salad bowl was perpetrated by food writer George Rector, to embellish a story that was printed in the popular the *Saturday Evening Post* magazine (Sept 5, 1936). Rector exploited the feeling of intimidation that many Americans experienced by snobbish French gourmets. Rector described green leaf salad as the most finicky of dishes to perfect. Rector claimed that the secret of making the perfect green leaf salad was to rub a clove of garlic into the wooden salad bowl, and never wash the bowl after preparing salads. Of course, the advice was a hoax. Rector knew that the practice had never been a French custom. He not only had worked in Parisian restaurants, but also in his cookbook (*A La Rector: Unveiling the Culinary Mysteries of the World Famous,* 1933) had included French salad recipes that were free of garlic. For a generation, many Americans tossed salads in rancid bowls, laden with microorganisms, and felt virtuous that they were approaching salad-making perfection.

board, it is advised to use soap and water. Being made of rubber, the board is not dishwasher safe. The board has been certified by the National Sanitation Foundation, an organization that tests products for their ability to resist bacterial growth, as well as their durability.

Whatever type of cutting board you choose, keep it clean. Wash it with hot soapy water, especially after you have used it for handling raw flesh foods. Allow the board to air-dry or use clean paper towels. Sanitize it frequently with household bleach. Rinse the board well in clear running water.

If possible, invest in two cutting boards, whatever your choice of material(s). Reserve one board for cutting raw flesh foods, and the other for cutting all other foods, such as bread, raw vegetables, and raw fruits. By having two separate cutting boards, you prevent cross-contamination, and reduce your risk of foodborne illness.

Clean Fruits and Vegetables Thoroughly

In the mid-1990s, numerous commercial products were marketed, allegedly to remove pesticide residues, waxes, and dirt from produce. These costly items—dubbed "boutique products"—exploited public fears. Such products promised more than they could deliver. By the 2000s, the awareness of foodborne illnesses provided another incentive to market these cleansers. Such products then were touted for their ability to rid produce of pathogens, with more hype than effectiveness. Are these products needed to clean produce?

Both the Food and Drug Administration (FDA) and the Environmental Protection Agency (EPA) recommend that consumers simply wash produce thoroughly under clean running water. Vigorous scrubbing of foods such as apples or potatoes can be done easily. For crinkly greens, such as kale or curly parsley, more time and care are needed. Although packages of mixed greens or baby spinach may state that the products have been triple washed, still it is a good practice to wash them at home under running water before using them in salads.

A study was done about how consumers commonly wash apples, and how effective the practices were to eliminate *Salmonella* on apples. The researchers applied *Salmonella* to the skins of intact apples. Then, the apples were washed under running water, or washed in water with vinegar added, or in water with a dilute solution of household bleach. The apples were scrubbed from five to thirty seconds, rinsed, and dried with clean paper towels. The simple combination of water, scrubbing, rinsing, and drying reduced somewhat the *Salmonella* on the surfaces of the apples. The use of the vinegar or bleach solutions resulted in a significant reduction of the pathogen. The researchers concluded that consumers can be educated to follow simple washing procedures with produce as with apples. The researchers suggested that consumers should not eat the hard-to-clean portions of the blossom and stem areas of the fruit.

THE MYTH OF THE FIVE-SECOND RULE

The so-called five-second rule claims that if you accidentally drop food on the floor but retrieve it within five seconds, the food is safe to eat. An experiment, conducted in 2003, challenged the five-second rule. Jillian Clarke, a high-school intern at the University of Illinois led a team of students who inoculated clean floor tiles with *Escherichia coli.* Then, they placed gummy candies and cookies on the tiles. Within five seconds, the foods became contaminated. Clarke's team found that the smoother the floor, the more readily the *E. coli* transferred to the food. They also studied human reactions. Cookies and candies were more likely to be picked up and eaten unwashed than raw cauliflower or broccoli. Yet, all these foods can be contaminated in less than five seconds.

In 2007 Paul L. Dawson and his colleagues at Clemson University in South Carolina also tested the rule. Bacteria on a contaminated surface such as a floor reside in the dirt (known to sanitarians as a biofilm). The amount of the dirt, and hence the number of bacteria that will adhere to—say a dropped slice of bologna—on a tile, wood, or carpeted floor depends on the area of contact and the mutual stickiness between the dirt and the bologna. These are not time-dependent qualities.

The findings of Dawson's team confirmed the findings of Clarke's team. Dawson reported that "food contact time had no effect on the percentage of [bacteria] transferred. Over 99 percent of bacterial cells were transferred from the tile to the bologna after five seconds of bologna exposure to tile." Furthermore, "transfer from carpet to bologna was very low (less than 5 percent) when compared with the transfer from wood or tile." The researchers suggested that the difference most likely is because the area of contact increases with surface smoothness, from carpet to wood to tile.

SAFE PRACTICES: A KITCHEN CHECKLIST

- Pay special attention to the cleanliness of hard-to-clean kitchen equipment, such as the can opener, meat grinder, meat slicer, food processor, etc.

- If you use a dishwasher, make certain that it functions properly. The water should be hot enough to sterilize the soiled items. The rinsing cycle should clear items of adhered debris and detergent. One early study found that 45 percent of all dishwashers functioned poorly or operated imperfectly. Dishes retained an average bacterial load of 410 colonies per washed dish. Some 15 percent of the washed utensils even exceeded that level (*Journal of Environmental Health*, Sept 1990).

- If you wash dishes by hand, use hot water and soap or detergent. Make certain to rinse washed dishes and implements *under running water* to rid them of residual soap or detergent. Air dry in a rack, or use a clean towel. Change towels frequently.

- Keep the kitchen (as well as the rest of the home) free of insects and rodents.

- Do not allow companion animals to be on kitchen work surfaces.

- Do not allow these animals to lick the leftovers on plates used by humans.

- Teach young children basic principles of safe food preparation, including safe cooking in the microwave oven. With lifestyle changes, many young children now share responsibilities in the kitchen. The emphasis on convenience diverts attention from safe methods of cooking, as well as other kitchen practices.

The suggestions in this chapter should help you to keep foods safe in your kitchen. In addition, lifestyle and food choices, discussed earlier, will help you avoid foodborne illnesses and the chronic health problems that can follow.

Safe and enjoyable eating. Good health.

Main Sources

Chapter 2

Acheson, D, "Long-term consequences of foodborne disease." *Fd Qual*, Sept–Oct 2000; 29: 31–33

Appelbaum, JS et al, "*Yersinia enterocolitica* endocarditis." *Arch Intern Med*, 1983; 143: 2150–2151

Archer, DL, "Enteric microorganisms in rheumatoid disease: causative agents & possible mechanisms." *J Fd Prot*, 1985; 48: 538–545

—— & FE Young, "Contemporary issues: diseases with a food vector?" *Clin Microbiol Rev*, Oct 1988; 1(4): 377–398

Ascherio, A et al, "Epstein-Barr virus antibodies & risk of multiple sclerosis." A Prospective Study. Original Contribution. *JAMA*, Dec 26, 2001; 286(24): 3083–3088

Bachmaier, K et al, "*Chlamydia* infections & heart disease linked through antigenic mimicry." *Sci* Feb 26, 1999; 283: 1335–1339

Bech, K et al, "*Yersinia enterocolitica* infections & thyroid disease." *Acta Endocrinol*, 1977; 84: 87–92

Bunning, VK et al, "Chronic health effects of foodborne microbial diseases." *World Health Stat Quart*, 1997; 50: 51–56

Calder, J, "*Listeria* meningitis in adults." *Lancet*, Aug 1977; 350(9074): 3–7

Chen, PL et al, "Extraintestinal focal infections in adults with nontyphoid *Salmonella bacteraemia:* predisposing factors & clinical outcome." *J Intern Med*, 2007; 261: 91–100

Chiodini, RJ, "Crohn's disease & the mycobacteriosis: a review & comparison of the two disease entities." *Clin Microbiol Rev*, 1989; 2: 90–117

Connor, BA, "Sequelae of traveler's diarrhea: focus on postinfectious irritable bowel syndrome." *Clin Infect Dis*, 2004; 41(Suppl 8): S577–586

Cook, I, & EH Derrick, "The incidence of *Toxoplasma* antibodies in mental hospital patients." *Austral Ann Med*, 1961; 10: 137–141

Danesh, C et al, "Chronic infections & coronary heart disease: is there a link?" *Lancet*, 1997; 350: 430–436

De Bont, B et al, "Guillain-Barré syndrome associated with *Campylobacter enteritis* in a child." *J. Pediat*, 1986; 109, 660–662

Deitch, EA et al, "Endotoxin promotes the translocation of bacteria from the gut." *Arch Surg*, 1987; 122: 185–190

Dworkin, MS et al, "Reactive arthritis & Reiter's syndrome following an outbreak of gastroenteritis caused by *Salmonella enteritidis*." *Clin Infect Dis*, 2001; 33: 1010–1014

Ebringer, A, "The cross-tolerance hypothesis, HLA-B27 & ankylosing spondylitis." *Br J Rheumatol*, 1983; 22(Suppl 2): 53–66

Ebringer, RW et al, "Sequential studies in ankylosing spondylitis; association of *Klebsiella pneumoniae* with active disease." *Ann Rheum Dis*, 1978; 37: 146–151

Gaston, JH, "How does HLA-B27 confer susceptibility to inflammatory arthritis?" *Clin Exp Immunol*, 1990; 82: 1–2

Ganem, D, "Infectious avenues to cancer." Books. Medicine. *Sci*, May 21, 1999; 284: 1279

Goldenberg, DL et al, "Bacterial arthritis?" *N Engl J Med*, 1985; 312: 764–771

Goodacre, JA et al, "Bacterial superantigens in autoimmune arthritis." *Br J Rheum*, 1994; 33: 413–419

Grant, RJ et al, "Isolated septic arthritis due to *Streptococcus bovis*." Brief Rept, *Clin Infect Dis*, May 1997

Grayston, JT et al, "A new *Chlamydia* strain, TWAR isolated in acute respiratory tract infection." *N Engl J Med*, 1986; 315: 161–168

Greub, G et al, "*Chlamydia*-like organisms & atherosclerosis." Lett. Ed., *Emerg Infect Dis*, Apr 2006; 12(4): 705–706

Gu, H et al, "Evidence of *Toxoplasma gondii* infection in recent onset schizophrenia." Abstract. *Schizophr Res*, 2001; 49: 53

Gura, T, "*Chlamydia* protein linked to heart disease." News of WK. Immunol. *Sci*, Feb 26, 1999; 283: 1238–1239

Heyma, P et al, "Thyrotropin (TSH) binding sites on *Yersinia enterocolitica* recognized by immunoglobulins from humans with Graves' disease." *Clin Exp Immunol*, 1986; 64: 249–254

Hooper, J, "A new germ theory." *Atlantic Monthly*, Feb 1999: 41–53

"Is insanity due to a microbe?" Editorial. *Sci Am*, 1896; 75: 303

Kalder, J & BR Speed, "Guillain-Barré syndrome & *Campylobacter jejuni*: a seriological study." *Br J Med*, 1984; 288: 1867–1870

Kandoff, R et al, "In situ detection of enteroviral genomes in myocardial cells by nucleic acid hybridization: an approach in the diagnosis of viral heart disease." *Proc. NAS*, 1987; 84: 6272–6276

Karmali, MA et al, "The association between idiopathic hemolytic-uremic syndrome & infection by verotoxin-producing *Escherichia coli*." *J Infect Dis*, 1985; 151: 775–782

Keat, A, "Reiter's syndrome & reactive arthritis in perspective." *N Engl J Med*, 1983; 309: 1606–1612

—— "Is spondylitis caused by *Klebsiella*?" *Immunol Today*, 1986; 7: 144–148

Kuo, C et al, "Demonstration of *Chlamydia pneumoniae* in atherosclerotic lesions of coronary arteries." *J Infect Dis*, 1993; 167: 841–849

—— & LA Campbell, "Is infection with *Chlamydia pneumoniae* a causative agent in atherosclerosis?" *Mod Med Today*, 1998; 4: 426–430

Lange, WR, "Travel and ciguatera fish poisoning." Original Investigation. *Arch Intern Med*, Oct 1992; 152: 2049–2053

Lappé, M, *Evolutionary Medicine: Rethinking the Origins of Disease*. San Francisco, CA: Sierra Club Books, 1994

Leirisalo-Repo M et al, "Microbial factors in spondyloarthropathies: insights from population studies." *Curr Opin Rheumatol*, 2003; 15: 408–412

Lindsay, JA, "Chronic sequelae of foodborne disease." Special Issue. *Emerg Infect Dis*, Oct–Dec 1997; 3(44): 443–452

Liu, Y et al, "Immunocytochemical evidence of *Listeria, Escherichi coli & Streptococcus* antigens in Crohn's disease." *Gastroenterol*, 1995; 108: 1396–1401

Mäki-Ikoa, O & K Gransfor, "*Salmonella*-triggered reactive arthritis." *Lancet*, May 2, 1992; 339 (1801): 1096–1098

Mead, PS et al, "Food-related illness & death in the United States." Synopses. *Emerg Infect Dis*, Sept–Oct 1999; 5(5): 607–624

Miller, RG, "Guillain-Barré syndrome." *Postgrad Med*, 1985; 77: 57–59, 62–64

Miller-Hjelle, MA et al, "Polycystic kidney disease: an unrecognized emerging infectious disease?" *Emerg Infect Dis*, Apr–June 1997; 3(2): 113–127

Minto, A & FJ Roberts, "The psychiatric complication of toxoplasmosis. *Lancet*, 1959 (I), 1180–1182

Mlot, C, "Chlamydia linked to atherosclerosis." Heart Disease. *Sci*, June 7, 1996; 272: 1422

Morrison, DM et al, "Colonic biopsy in verotoxin-induced hemorrhagic colitis & thrombotic thrombocytopenic purpura (TTP)." *Am J Clin Path*, 1986; 86: 108–112

"*M. paratuberculosis*: a cause for concern to the food industry?" Lab Analysis. *Fd Qual*, Aug–Sept 1999; 40: 42–43, 45–46

Neill, MA et al, "Hemorrhagic colitis with *Escherichia coli* O157:H7 preceding adult hemolytic uremic syndrome." *Arch Intern Med*, 1985; 145: 2215–2217

—— "*Escherichia coli* O157:H7 as the predominant pathogen associated with the hemolytic uremic syndrome: a prospective study in the Pacific Northwest." *Pediat*, 1987; 80: 37–40

Nelson, KB et al, "Neonatal cytokines and coagulation factors in children with cerebral palsy." *Annals of Neurology*, Oct 1998; 44(4): 665–675

Norden, CW & LM Kuller, "Identifying infectious etiologies of chronic diseases." *Rev Infect Dis*, 1984; 6: 200–213

O'Connor, S et al, "Potential infectious etiologies of atherosclerosis: a multifactorial perspective." Synopses. *Emerg Infect Dis*, Sept–Oct 2001; 7(5): 780–788

—— "Institute of Medicine Forum on Emerging Infections: linking infectious agents & chronic diseases." Conference Summ. News & Notes. *Emerg Infect Dis*, Dec 2002; 8(12): 1529–1530

—— "Emerging infectious determinants of chronic diseases." *Emerg Infect Dis,* July 2006; 12(7): 1051–1057

Oldstone, MBA, "Molecular mimicry & autoimmune disease." *Cell,* 1987; 50: 819–820

Parsonnet, Julie, *Microbes & Malignancy: Infections as a Cause of Human Cancers.* NY: Oxford U Press, 1999

Pignata, C et al, "Chronic diarrhea & failure to thrive in an infant with *Campylobacter jejuni.*" *J Pediat Gastroenterol Nutr,* 1984; 3: 812–814

Rees, JR et al, "Persistent diarrhea, arthritis, and other complications of enteric infections: a pilot survey based on California's FoodNet surveillance, 1998–1999." *Clin Infect Dis,* 2004; 38: (Suppl) 8311–8317

Report of the Task Force on Microbiology & Infectious Diseases. Natl Inst Allerg Infect Dis, NIH Publ No 923320. Bethesda, MD: NIH, Apr 1992

Rodriguez, LA & A Ruisgomez, "Increased risk of irritable bowel syndrome after bacterial gastroenteritis: cohort study." *Br Med J.* 1999; 318: 565–566

Rodriguez, LA et al, "Acute gastroenteritis is followed by an increased risk of inflammatory bowel disease." *Gastroenterol,* 2006; 130: 1588–1594

Rosenberg, IH et al, "Malabsorption associated with diarrhea & intestinal infections." *Am J Clin Nutr,* 1977; 30:1248–1253

Seppa, N, "Infections may underlie cerebral palsy." *Sci News,* Oct 17, 1998: 244

Shor, A & JI Phillips, "*Chlamydia pneumoniae* & atherosclerosis." Contemp 1999. Updates linking evidence & experience. *JAMA,* Dec 1, 1999; 282(21): 2071–2073

Stanforth, DR, "IgA dysfunction in rheumatoid arthritis." *Immunol Today,* 1985; 6: 43–45

Stanley, D, "Arthritis from foodborne bacteria?" *Agric Res,* Oct 1996: 16

Torrey, EF & RH Holken, "*Toxoplasma gondii* & schizophrenia." *Emerg Infect Dis,* Nov 2003; 9(11): 1375–1380

"Tracking molecular mimics." *Sci,* Dec 18, 1998; 282: 2161

Travis, J, "Microbe linked to Alzheimer's disease." *Sci News,* Nov 21, 1998: 325

Viitanen, AM et al, "*Yersinia enterocolitica* plasmid in fecal flora of patients with reactive arthritis." *J Infect Dis,* 1986; 154: 376

Weiss, R, "The germ of a theory: microbes may be at the core of ailments from heart disease to Alzheimer's." *Wash Post Natl Wkly Ed,* Mar 8, 1999: 8

Williams, RC, "Rheumatic fever & the *Streptococcus:* another look at molecular mimicry." *Am J Med,* 1983; 75: 727–730

Wolf, NW et al, "Immunoglobulins of patients recovering from *Yersinia enterocolitica* infections exhibit Graves' disease-like activity in human thyroid membranes." *Thyroid,* 1991; 1: 315–320

Yolken, RH et al, "Antibodies to *Toxoplasma gondii* in individuals with first episode schizophrenia." *Clin Infect Dis,* 2001; 32: 842–844

Yu, DT & GT Thompson, "Clinical, epidemiological & pathogenic aspects of reactive arthritis." *Fd Microbiol,* 1994; 11: 97–108

Chapter 3

Salmonella

Aarestrup, FM et al, "International spread of multidrug-resistant *S.* Schwarzengrund in food products." Research. *Emerg Infect Dis*, May 2007; 13(5): 726–730

"About half of feed meals, 16 percent of complete feeds found positive for *Salmonella* in CVM [Center for Veterinary Medicine] survey." *Fd Chem News*, Nov 20, 1995: 8–9

Adams, D et al, "Salmonellosis from inadequately pasteurized milk—Kentucky." Epidemiol Notes Repts. *MMWR*, Sept 14, 1984; 33(36): 505–506

Anderson, SM et al, "Multistate outbreaks of *S.* serotype Poona infections associated with eating cantaloupes from Mexico—United States & Canada, 2000–2002." *MMWR*, Nov 22, 2002; 51(46): 1044–1047

Baird-Parker, AC, "Foodborne salmonellosis." Foodborne Illness. *Lancet*, Nov 17, 1990; 336: 1231–1235

Bakalar, N, "*Salmonella,* outbreak traced to pet rodent." *NY Times*, May 10, 2005: F7

Barrett, B, "Iguana-associated salmonellosis—Indiana, 1990." *MMWR*, Jan 24, 1992; 41(3): 38–39

Beers, A, "One dead, hundreds sick from *Salmonella* outbreak in Maryland." *Fd Chem News*, Nov 10, 1997: 27

—— "*Salmonella* outbreak linked to cereal." *Fd Chem News*, June 8, 1998: 17

Bennett, G, "Cockroaches as carriers of bacteria." *Lancet*, Mar 20, 1993; 341(8847): 732

Bidol, S et al, "Salmonellosis associated with chicks & ducklings—Michigan & Missouri, Spring 1999." *MMWR*, Apr 14, 2000; 49(14): 297–299

—— "Three outbreaks of salmonellosis associated with baby poultry from three hatcheries—United States, 2006." *MMWR*, Mar 30, 2007; 56(12): 273–276

—— "Multistate outbreak of *Salmonella* infections associated with raw tomatoes eaten in restaurants—United States, 2005–2006." *MMWR*, Sept 7, 2007; 56(35): 909–911

Blythe, D et al, "*Salmonella* serotype *montevideo* infections associated with chicks—Idaho, Washinton & Oregon, Spring 1995 & 1996." *MMWR*, Mar 21, 1997; 46(11): 237–239

Boase, J et al, "Outbreak of *Salmonella*—serotype *Muenchen* infections associated with unpasteurized orange juice—United States & Canada, June 1999." *MMWR*, July 16, 1999; 48(27): 582–585

Bonland, J et al, "Multiple outbreaks of salmonellosis associated with precooked roast beef—Pennsylvania, New York, & Vermont." Epidemiol Notes Repts. *MMWR*, Nov 27, 1981; 46: 569–570

"Breaking the *Salmonella*/chicken connection, irradiation is approved for poultry processing." *Agric Res*, Oct 1981: 12

Brenner, RJ, "Curbing cockroaches & their allergens." *Agric* Res, June 1998: 4–6

Bryan, FL, "Current trends in foodborne salmonellosis in the United States & Canada." *J Fd Prot*, May 1981; 44: 394

Buchmeier, NA & F Heffron, "Induction of *Salmonella* stress proteins upon infection of macrophages." Repts. *Sci*, May 11, 1990; 248: 730–732

Burlingame, D et al, "Salmonellosis—Wisconsin." Epidemiol Notes Repts. *MMWR*, Feb 8, 1980; 29(5): 49–50

Carr, R, "Salmonellosis in a school system—Oklahoma." Epidemiol Notes Repts. *MMWR*, Feb 13, 1987; 36(5): 74–75

"Cats may pose salmonellosis risk." *Research Resources Reporter*, NIH, Sept 1979; 3(9): 7–8

Centers for Disease Control Salmonella Surveillance Report. 1984. Atlanta, GA: CDC, undated

Chatfield, D et al, "Turtle-associated salmonellosis in humans—United States, 2006–2007." *MMWR*, July 6, 2007; 56(26): 649–652

"Cockroaches can catch, spread *Salmonella* to food, water." *Fd Chem News*, Apr 11, 1994: 8–9

"ConAgra traces *Salmonella* to leaky roof sprinkler." Fd Safety. *Fd Proc*, May 2007: 14

Cook, KA et al, "Outbreak of *Salmonella* serotype Hartford infections associated with unpasteurized orange juice." *JAMA*, Nov 4, 1998; 280(17): 1504–1509

Cooke, Linda, "*Salmonella* carriers worry scientists." *Agric Res*, Jan 1993: 20

—— "Keeping 'em off the farm." *Agric Res*, Feb 1996: 4–7

Crowe, L, "Human salmonellosis associated with animal-derived pet treats—United States & Canada, 2005." *MMWR*, June 20 2006; 55(25): 702–705

Dansby, W et al, "Human *Salmonella* isolates—United States 1982." Current Trends. *MMWR*, Nov 18, 1983; 32(45): 598–600

de Jong, B et al, "Effect of regulation & education on reptile-associated salmonellosis." Research. *Emerg Infect Dis*, Mar 2005; 11(3): 398–403

de Jong, R et al, "Severe mycobacteria & *Salmonella* infections on interleukin-12 receptor-deficient patients." Repts. *Sci*, May 29, 1998; 280: 1435–1438

Dunne, EF, "Emergence of domestically acquired cefriaxone-resistant *Salmonella*-infections associated with AmpC beta-lactamose." Original Contrib. *JAMA*, Dec 27, 2000; 284(24): 3151–3156

Durham, S et al, "Subduing *Salmonella*, several strategies seem promising." *Agric Res*, Oct 2006: 14–16

Evans, M & HC Wegener, "Antimicrobial growth promoters and *Salmonella* ssp, *Campylobacter* ssp in poultry & swine—Denmark." *Emerg Infect Dis*, Apr 2003; 9(4): 489–492

Fields, PL et al, "A *Salmonella* locus that controls resistance to microbiocidal proteins from phagocytic cells." Repts. *Sci*, Feb 24, 1989; 243: 1059–1062

Finkel, E, "Australia's peanut butter crisis reaches crunch." *Lancet*, July 13, 1996; 348 (9020): 117

Finlay, BB et al, "Epithelial cell surfaces induce *Salmonella* problems required for bacterial adherence and invasion." Repts. *Sci*, Feb 17, 1989; 243: 940–943

Francis, BJ et al, "Multistate outbreak of *Salmonella poona* infections—United States & Canada, 1991." Epidemiol Notes Repts. *MMWR*, Aug 16, 1991; 40(32): 549–552

Franklin, D, "Nemo beware: fish tank can be a haven for *Salmonella*." Hlth Fitness. The Consumer. *NY Times*, Apr 18, 2006: F6

Galanis, E et al, "Web-based surveillance & global *Salmonella* distribution, 2000–2002." Synopses. *Emerg Infect Dis*, Mar 2006; 12(3): 381–388

Gensheimer, KF, "Poultry giblet-associated salmonellosis—Maine." Epidemiol Notes Repts. *MMWR*, Nov 9, 1984; 33(44): 630–631

Giljahn, LK et al, "Turtle-associated salmonellosis—Ohio." *MMWR*, Nov 28, 1986; 25(47): 733–734, 739

Harris, G et al, "Nut Recall Is Signalling Tough Stance on Safety." *NY Times*, Apr 7, 2009:

Hays, SM, "Natural microbes curb *Salmonella*, on-farm treatment could reduce cross-contamination during poultry processing. *Agric Res*, Nov 1994: 22–26

Hecht, A et al, "Contaminated pepper." Investigators' Repts. *FDA Consumer*, May 1986: 36

Hedberg, Craig W et al, "A multistate outbreak of *Salmonella javians* & *Salmonella oranienburg* infections due to consumption of contaminated cheese." Original Contrib. *JAMA*, Dec 9, 1992; 268(22): 3203–3207

Horwitz, MA, "A large outbreak of foodborne salmonellosis on the Navajo Nation Indian reservation, epidemiology & secondary transmission." *Am J PH*, Nov 1977; 67(11): 1071–1076

"Human *Salmonella* isolates—United States, 1979." Surveillance Summary. *MMWR*, Apr 25, 1980: 189–191

"Human *Salmonella* isolates—United States, 1981." Curr Trends. *MMWR*, Nov 19, 1982; 31(45): 613–615

"Human *Salmonella* isolates—United States, 1983." *MMWR*, Dec 14, 1984; 33(49): 693–695

Ingersoll, B, "U.S. to mandate testing of poultry for *Salmonella*." *Wall St J*, Feb 20, 1990: B5

"Is sunny-side up a salmonellosis haven?" Biomed. *Sci News*, Apr 16, 1988: 251

Kilness, AW, "Selenium & *Salmonella*." Clin Perspet. *Med Trib*, Jan 7, 1987: 41

Koch, Judith et al, "*Salmonella* Agona outbreak from contaminated aniseed, Germany." Dispatches. *Emerg Infect Dis*, July 2005; 11(7): 1124–1127

Landry, L et al, "*Salmonella* Oranienburg infections associated with fruit salad served in health-care facilities—Northeastern United States & Canada, 2006." *MMWR*, Oct 5, 2007: 1025–1028

Lanser, S et al, "Lizard-associated salmonellosis—Utah." *MMWR*, Aug 21, 1992; 41(33): 610–611

Larson, A et al, "*Salmonella oranienberg* gastroenteritis associated with consumption of pre-cut watermelon—Illinois." *MMWR*, Nov 9, 1979: 522–523

Lehmacher, A et al, "Nationwide outbreak of human salmonellosis in Germany due to contaminated paprika & paprika-powdered potato chips." *Epidemiol Infect*, Dec 1995; 115(3): 501–511

Levy, BS & W McIntire, "The economic impact of a food-borne salmonellosis outbreak." Original Contrib. *JAMA*, Dec 2, 1974; 230(91): 1281–1282

Levy, C et al, "Reptile-associated salmonellosis—selected states, 1996–1998." *MMWR*, Nov 12, 1999; 48(44): 1009–1013

Lipsky, S et al, "African pygmy hedgehog-associated salmonellosis—Washington, 1994." *MMWR,* June 23, 1995; 44(24): 462–463

Louie, KK et al, "*Salmonella* serotype Tennessee in powdered milk products & infant formula —Canada & United States, 1993." *MMWR;* 42: 516–517. Reprinted in *JAMA,* July 25, 1993; 270(4): 432

Lyman, DO et al, "*Salmonellae* in precooked roasts of beef—New York." *MMWR,* Aug 25, 1978: 315

Mahon, BE, "An international outbreak of *Salmonella* infections caused by alfalfa sprouts grown from contaminated seeds." *J Infect Dis,* Apr 1997; 175(4): 876–882

Memorandum: 1981 Salmonella Surveillance Data. Atlanta, GA: CDC, Mar 5, 1985

Mitchell, PP, "Eggs & *Salmonella,* FDA issues advice on avoiding contamination." *Wash Post,* Sept 21, 1988: E1

Mohle-Boetani, J et al, "Outbreak of *Salmonella* serotype Kottbus infections associated with eating alfalfa sprouts—Arizona, California, Colorado & New Mexico, February–April 2001." *MMWR,* Jan 11, 2002; 51(1): 7–9

"More than 400 cases of cantaloupe-salmonellosis reported." *Fd Chem News,* Aug 19, 1991: 45

"Multistate outbreaks of *Salmonella* serotype Agona infections linked to toasted oats cereal—United States, April–May, 1998." *MMWR,* June 12, 1998; 47(22): 462–464

"Multistate outbreak of *Salmonella* serotype Tennessee infections associated with peanut butter —United States, 2006–2007." *MMWR,* June 1, 2007; 56(21): 521–524

Murphy, J, "Studies underway to explore *Salmonella* prevalence in cattle, chickens." *Fd Chem News,* Sept 7, 1998: 25–26

Nims, LJ et al, "Salmonellosis associated with Carne Seca [beef jerky]—New Mexico." Epidemiol Notes Repts. *MMWR,* Oct 25, 1985; 34(42): 645–646

Paton, JH, "A young man who liked lizards and lost his job." Corresp. *Lancet,* May 18, 1996; 347(9012): 1376

Piagentini, AM et al, "Survival & growth of *Salmonella hadar* on minimally processed cabbage as influenced by storage abuse conditions." *J Fd Sci,* May–June, 1997; 62(3): 616–618, 631

Piergentili, P et al, "*Salmonella dublin* associated with raw milk—Washington State." *MMWR,* Aug 7, 1981; 30(30): 373–374

Pinks, DR et al, "*Salmonella heidelberg* gastroenteritis aboard a cruise ship." Epidemiol Notes Repts. *MMWR,* Apr 6, 1979; 28(13): 145–147

Pönkä, A et al, "*Salmonella* in alfalfa sprouts." *Lancet,* Feb 18, 1995; 354(8947): 462–463

"Rattlesnake meat in pills linked to salmonellosis deaths." *Fd Chem News,* Jan 9, 1995, 25

Reporter, R et al, "Reptile-associated salmonellosis—selected states, 1998–2002." *MMWR,* Dec 12, 2003; 52(49): 1206–1209

"Resistance to *Salmonella* increases, causes worry." *Am Med News,* Sept 11, 1987: 24

"Resistant *Salmonella* strains found in retail meats—CVM." [Center for Veterinary Medicine, FDA] *Fd Chem News,* Oct 22, 2001: 18

Rigau-Perez, JG, "Pet-turtle associated salmonellosis—Puerto Rico." Epidemiol Notes Repts. *MMWR,* Mar 16, 1984; 33(10): 141–142

Roberts, T & E van Ravenswaay, "The economics of food safety." *Natl Fd Rev,* Eco Res Serv, USDA, July–Sept 1989; 12(3): 1–8

Sabetta, JP et al, "Foodborne nosocomial outbreak of *Salmonella reading*—Connecticut." Epidemiol Notes Repts. *MMWR,* Nov 22, 1991; 40(46): 804–806

"Salmonella & food safety." *FSIS Background,* Wash, DC: Fd Safety & Inspection Service, USDA, Jan 1988

"*Salmonella dublin* & raw milk consumption—California." *MMWR,* Apr 13, 1994; 33(14): 196–198

"*Salmonella* found in almost all foods." In Our View. *Poultry Internatl,* Oct 1987: 6

"*Salmonella oranienburg* gastroenteritis associated with consumption of precut watermelon—Illinois, *MMWR,* Nov 9, 1979: 522–523

"*Salmonella* taints ConAgra peanut butter." *Fd Proc,* Mar 2007: 11

"*Salmonella,* the ubiquitous bug." *FDA Papers,* Feb 1967: 13–19

"Salmonellosis associated with cheese consumption—Canada." Internatl Notes. *MMWR,* July 13, 1984; 33(27): 387

Salna, B et al, "Salmonellosis associated with pet turtles—Wisconsin & Wyoming, 2004." *MMWR,* Mar 11, 2005; 54(9): 223–226

Schrader, J et al, "Salmonellosis traced to marijuana—Ohio, Michigan." Epidemiol Notes Repts. *MMWR,* Feb 27, 1981; 30(7): 77–79

Sharrar, R et al, "Multistate outbreak of salmonellosis caused by precooked roast beef." *MMWR,* Aug 21, 1981; 30(32): 391–392

Shin, Dongwoo et al, "A positive feedback loop promotes transcription surge that jumpstarts *Salmonella* virulence circuit." Repts. *Sci,* Dec 8, 2006; 314: 1607–1609

Skov, Marianne N et al, "Antimicrobial drug resistance of *Salmonella* isolates from meat & humans, Denmark." Dispatches, *Emerg Infect Dis,* Apr 2–7; 13(4): 638–641

Smith, JD et al, "Salmonellosis from homemade ice cream—Georgia." *MMWR,* Sept 25, 1981; 30(37): 467–468, 473

Strauss, E, "Anti-immune trick unveiled in *Salmonella.*" Microbiol. *Sci,* July 16, 1999; 285: 306–307

Stroh, M, "Exposing *Salmonella*'s gutsy moves." Sci News Wk. *Sci News,* Jan 27, 1992: 420

Svitlik, C et al, "*Salmonella hadar* associated with pet ducklings—Connecticut, Maryland, Pennsylvania, 1991." Epidemiol Notes Repts. *MMWR,* Mar 20, 1992; 41(11): 185–187

"Taste, bacterial-infection receptors determined." *Chem Engineer News,* June 22, 1992: 21

Ternhag, A, "*Salmonella*-associated deaths, Sweden, 1997–2003." Dispatches. *Emerg Infect Dis,* Feb 2006; 12(2): 337–339

"Tomatoes the culprit in outbreak." *Fd Qual,* Apr–May 2005: 14

Toth, B et al, "Outbreak of *Salmonella* serotype Javiana infections—Orlando, Florida, June 2002." *MMWR,* Aug 9, 2002; 51(31): 683–684

Twaddell, JC, "*Salmonella* contamination outbreaks in poultry plants across the U.S." *Fd Qual*, Aug–Sept 2006: 26–28, 30, 32, 34–35

Umland, E et al, "Outbreak of salmonellosis associated with beef jerky—New Mexico, 1995." *MMWR*, Oct 27, 1995; 44(42): 785–788

Valdezate, S et al, "*Salmonella* Derby clonal spread from pork." Dispatches. *Emerg Infect Dis*, May 2005; 11(5): 694–698

Van Beneden, CA et al, "Multinational outbreak of *Salmonella enterica* serotype Newport infections due to contaminated alfalfa sprouts." Original Contrib. *JAMA*, Jan 13, 1999; 281(2): 158–162

Waldholz, M, "Rise in *Salmonella* cases is tied to eggs formerly believed free of the bacteria." *Wall St J*, Apr 8, 1988: 13

Wegener, HC et al, "*Salmonella* control programs in Denmark." Synopses. *Emerg Infect Dis*, July 2003; 9(7): 774–780

Weinstein, JW et al, "Reptile-associated salmonellosis—selected states, 1994–1995." *MMWR*, May 5, 1995; 44(17): 347–350 [errata noted in *MMWR*, Nov 19, 1998; 48(45): 1051]

Weisse, P et al, "*Salmonella heidelberg* outbreak at a convention—New Mexico." Epidemiol Notes Repts. *MMWR*, Feb 14, 1986; 35(6): 91–92

Wheat, LJ et al, "Systemic salmonellosis in patients with disseminated toxoplasmosis." *Arch Intern Med*, Mar 1987; 147: 561–564

Zadjura, EM et al, *Food Safety & Quality, Salmonella Control Efforts Show Need for More Coordination*. Wash, DC: US General Accounting Office, GAO/RCED-92-69, Apr 1992

Salmonella Enteritidis

Altekruse, SF et al, "*Salmonella* Enteritidis in broiler chickens, United States, 2000–2005." Research. *Emerg Infect Dis*, Dec 2006; 12(12): 1848–1852

Binkin, N et al, "Egg-related *Salmonella enteritidis*, Italy, 1991." *Epidemiol Infect*, Apr 1993; 110(2): 227–237

Blumenthal, D, "*Salmonella enteritidis*, from chicken to the egg." *FDA Consumer*, Apr 1990: 6–10

Bovee-Oudenhoven, I et al, "Calcium in milk and fermentation by yoghurt bacteria increase the resistance of rats to *Salmonella* infection." *Gut*, Jan 1996; 38(1): 59–65

Buckner, P et al, "Outbreak of *Salmonella enteritidis* associated with homemade ice cream—Florida, 1993." Epidemiol Notes Repts. *MMWR*, Sept 16, 1994; 43(36): 669–671

Durham, S, "Effect of *Salmonella* on eggshell quality." *Agric Res*, Oct 2004: 19

—— "Tracking Salmonella's evolution from innocuous to virulent." *Agric Res*, Apr 2009: 8–9

Emshwiller, John R, "Shell-breaking machine runs afoul of egg producers." Enterprise. *Wall St J*, Oct 9, 1989: B2

Evans, MR et al, "*Salmonella* Enteritidis PT6: another egg-associated salmonellosis?" Dispatches. *Emerg Infect Dis*, Oct–Dec 1998, Vol 4(4): 667–669

Ewert, D et al, "Outbreaks of *Salmonella enteritidis* gastroenteritis—California, 1993." Epidemiol Notes Repts. *MMWR*, Oct 22, 1993, Vol 42(41): 793–797

Food Safety & Quality. Salmonella Control Efforts Show Need for More Coordination. GAO/RCED-92–69. Wash, DC: US GAO, Apr 1992

Grady, GF, "Salmonellosis outbreaks associated with commercial frozen pasta—Massachusetts, New Jersey, New York." Epidemiol Notes Repts. *MMWR*, June 13, 1986; 35(23): 387

Hadler, JL et al, "Salmonellosis at a resort hotel—Puerto Rico." Epidemiol Notes Repts. *MMWR*, Dec 12, 1986; 35(49): 766–767

King, N, "*Salmonella* reported in the Northeast." *FDA Veterinarian*, July–Aug 1988: 8

—— "Update on *Salmonella enteritidis* in eggs." *FDA Veterinarian*, Nov–Dec 1988: 12–13

Levine, WC et al, "Foodborne disease outbreaks in nursing homes, 1975 through 1987." *JAMA* Oct 16, 1991; 266(15): 2105–2109

Levy, M et al, "Outbreaks of *Salmonella* serotype Enteritidis infections associated with consumption of raw shell eggs—United States, 1994–1995." *MMWR*, Aug 30, 1996; 45(34): 737–742

McChesney, DG, "*Salmonella* in animal feeds." *FDA Veterinarian*, Jan–Feb 1991: 3–4

—— "Update on *Salmonella* in animal feed & feed ingredients." *FDA Veterinarian*, Sept–Oct 1994: 4–5

Mishu, B et al, "*Salmonella enteritidis* gastroenteritis transmitted by intact chicken eggs." *Ann Intern Med*, Aug 1, 1991; 115(3): 190–194

Mumma, G A et al, "Egg quality assurance programs & egg-associated *Salmonella* Enteritidis infections, United States." Research. *Emerg Infect Dis*, Oct 2004; 10(10): 1782–1787

Murphy, S et al, "Pancreatitis associated with *Salmonella enteritis*." Lettr. *Lancet*, Aug 31, 1991; 338; 571

"Outbreak of *Salmonella enteritidis* infection associated with consumption of raw shell eggs, 1991." Epidemiol Notes Reports. *MMWR*, May 29, 1992; 41(21): 369–372

Parmer, D et al, "Update: *Salmonella enteritidis* infections & shell eggs—United States, 1990." Epidemiol Notes Repts. *MMWR*, Dec 21, 1990; 39(50): 909–912

Patrick, ME et al, "*Salmonella* Enteritidis infections United States, 1985–1999." Perspect. *Emerg Infect Dis*, Jan 2004; 10(1): 1–7

Roberts, D, "*Salmonella* in chilled and frozen chickens." Lettr. *Lancet*, Apr 20, 1991 Vol 337(8747): 984–985

"Salmonellosis control in agriculture." *Bull WHO*, 1991; 69(2): 241–251

Schroeder, CM, "Estimate of illness from *Salmonella* Enteritidis in eggs, United States, 2000." Dispatches. *Emerg Infect Dis*, Jan 2005; 11(1): 113–115

Schutze, GE et al, "Epidemiology of salmonellosis in Arkansas." *Southern Med J*, Feb 1995; 88(2): 195–199

Smith, M, "Turkey-associated salmonellosis at an elementary school—Georgia." *MMWR*, Nov 22, 1985; 34(46): 707–708

Srikantiah, P et al, "Web-based investigation of multistate salmonellosis outbreak." Dispatches. *Emerg Infect Dis*, Apr 2005; 11(2): 610–612

Steinert, L, "Update: *Salmonella enteritidis* infections & Grade A shell eggs—United States, 1989." Epidemiol Notes Repts. *MMWR*, Jan 5, 1990; 38(51 & 52): 877–880

Taylor, GC et al, "Update: *Salmonella enteritidis* infections & Grade A shell eggs—United States." *MMWR*, Aug 19, 1988; 37(32): 490, 495–496

Telzak, EE et al, "A nosocomial outbreak of *Salmonella enteritidis* infection due to the consumption of raw eggs." Brief Rept. *N Engl J Med*, Aug 9, 1990; 323(6): 394–397

Salmonella Saintpaul

Jungk J et al, "Outbreak of *Salmonella* serotype saintpaul infections associated with multiple raw produce items—United States, 2008." *MMWR*, Aug 29, 2008; 57(34): 929–934

Salmonella Typhimurium

Ayala, C et al, "Multistate outbreak of *Salmonella* Typhimurium infections associated with eating ground beef—United States, 2004." *MMWR*, Feb 24, 2006; 55(7): 180–182

Brooks, JT et al, "*Salmonella typhimurium* infections transmitted by chlorine-pretreated clover sprout seeds." *Am J Epidemiol*, Dec 1, 2001; 154: 1020–1028

Cherry, B et al, "*Salmonella* Typhimurium associated with veterinary clinic." Dispatches. *Emerg Infect Dis*, Oct 2004; 10(10): 2249–2251

Cody, SH et al, "Two outbreaks of multidrug-resistant *Salmonella* serotype Typhimurium DT104 infections linked to raw-milk cheese in Northern California." Original Contrib. *JAMA*, May 19, 1999; 281(19): 1805–1810

Davis, MA et al, "Multi-drug resistant *Salmonella* Typhimurium. Pacific Northwest, United States." Dispatches. *Emerg Infect Dis*, Oct 2007; 13(10): 1583–1592

Dominguez, LB et al, "*Salmonella* gastroenteritis associated with milk—Arizona." *MMWR*, Mar 16, 1979: 117–120

Durham, S et al, "Subduing *Salmonella:* several strategies seem promising." *Agric Res*, Oct 2006; 54(10): 14–16

Ezell, H et al, "Outbreaks of multidrug-resistant *Salmonella* Typhimurium associated with veterinary facilities—Idaho, Minnesota, & Washington, 1999." *MMWR*, Aug 24, 2001; 50(33): 701–704

Frazak, PA et al, "Outbreak of *Salmonella* serotype Typhimurium infection associated with eating raw ground beef—Wisconsin, 1994, *MMWR*, Dec 15, 1995; 44(49): 905–909

Furlong, JD et al, "Salmonellosis associated with consumption of nonfat powdered milk—Oregon." *MMWR*, Mar 23, 1979: 129–130

Glynn, MK et al, "Emergence of multidrug-resistant *S. enterica* serotype Enteritidis DT104 infections in the United States." *N Engl J Med*, May 7, 1998; 338(19): 1333–1338

Helms, M et al, "International *Salmonella* Typhimurium DT104 infections, 1991–2001." Research. *Emerg Infect Dis*, June 2005; 11(6): 859–867

Hendriksen, SWM et al, "Animal-to-human transmission of *Salmonella* Typhimurium DT104A variant." Dispatches. *Emerg Infect Dis.* Dec 2004; 10(12): 2225–2227

Hosek, G et al, "Multidrug-resistant *Salmonella* serotype Typhimurium—United States, 1996." *MMWR,* Apr 11, 1997; 46(14): 308–310

Keene, WE et al, "*Salmonella* serotype Typhimurium outbreak associated with commercially processed egg salad—Oregon, 2003." *MMWR,* Dec 10, 2004; 53(48): 1132–1134

Lecos, C, "Of microbes & milk: probing America's worse *Salmonella* outbreak." *FDA Consumer,* Feb 1986: 18–21

Medus, C et al, "Multistate outbreak of *Salmonella:* infections associated with peanut butter and peanut butter-containing products—United States, 2008–2009." *MMWR,* Feb 6, 2009; 58(4): 85–90

Meunier, D et al, "*Salmonella enterica* serotype Typhimurium DT104 antibiotic resistance genomic island I in serotype Paratyphi B." Dispatches. *Emerg Infect Dis,* Apr 2002; 8(4): 430–433

"Milkborne salmonellosis—Illinois." *MMWR,* Apr 12, 1985; 34(14): 200

Moss, M, "Peanut case shows holes in food safety net." *NY Times,* Feb 9, 2009: A1, A12

Nesbit, D et al, "Feeding sodium chlorate to livestock to kill *Salmonella* and *E. coli.*" *Agric Res,* Mar 2001; 49(3): 19

Olsen, SJ et al, "Multidrug-resistant *Salmonella* Typhimurium infections from milk contaminated after pasteurization." Dispatches. *Emerg Infect Dis,* May 2004; 10(5): 932–935

Rabatsky-Ehr, T et al, "Multidrug-resistant strains of *Salmonella enterica* Typhimurium, United States, 1997–1998." Research. *Emerg Infect Dis,* May 2004; 10(5): 795–801

Ribot, EM et al, "*Salmonella enterica* serotype Typhimurium DT104 isolated from humans, United States 1985–1990, & 1995." Research. *Emerg Infect Dis,* Apr 2002; 8(4): 387–391

Sandt, C et al, "*Salmonella* Typhimurium infection associated with raw milk & cheese consumption—Pennsylvania, 2007." *MMWR,* Nov 9, 2007; 56(44): 1161–1164

Smith, K et al, "Outbreak of multidrug-resistant *Salmonella* Typhimurium associated with rodents purchased at retail pet stores—United States, December 2003–October 2004." *MMWR,* May 6, 2005; 54(17); 429–433

Sun, M, "In search of *Salmonella's* smoking gun." *Sci,* Oct 5, 1984; 226: 30–32

—— "Desperately seeking *Salmonella* in Illinois." *Sci,* May 17, 1985; 228: 829–830

Thornley, CN et al, "First incursion of *Salmonella enterica* serotype Typhimurium DT160 into New Zealand." Dispatches. *Emerg Infect Dis,* Apr 2003; 9(4): 493–495

Török, TJ et al, "A large community outbreak of salmonellosis caused by intentional contamination of restaurant salad bars." Original Contrib. *JAMA,* Aug 6, 1997; 278(5): 389–395

Torpdahl, M et al, "Tandem repeat analysis for surveillance of human *Salmonella* Typhimurium infections." Research. *Emerg Infect Dis,* Mar 2007; 13(3): 388–394

"Update: milk-borne salmonellosis—Illinois." Epidemiol Notes Repts. *MMWR,* Apr 19, 1984; 34(15); 215–216

Villar, RG et al, "Investigation of multidrug-resistant *Salmonella* serotype Typhimurium

DT104 infection linked to raw-milk cheese in Washington State." Original Contrib. *JAMA*, May 19, 1999; 281(19): 1811–1816

Wedel, S et al, "Antimicrobial-drug susceptibility of humans & animal *Salmonella* Typhimurium, Minnesota, 1997–2003." Research. *Emerg Infect Dis*, Dec 2005; 11(12): 1899–1906

Wright, JG et al, "Multidrug-resistant *Salmonella* Typhimurium in four animal facilities." Research. *Emerg Infect Dis*, Aug 2005; 11(8): 1235–1241

Salmonella Typhi

Birkhead, GS et al, "Typhoid fever at a resort hotel in New York: a large outbreak with an unusual vehicle." *J Infect Dis*, May 1993; 167: 1228–1232

Carey, C, "Mary Mallon's Trail of Typhoid." *FDA Consumer*, June 1987: 18–20

Farbman, KS et al, "Antibacterial activity of garlic & onions: a historical perspective." *Pediat Infect Dis J*, May 1993; 12(7); 613–614

Markel, H, *Quarantine: East European Jewish Immigrants & the New York City Epidemics of 1892*. Baltimore, MD: Johns Hopkins U Press, 1997

McNeil, Jr. DG, "The deadly trails of Typhoid Mary." *NY Times*, Apr 15, 2003: F6

Roumagnac, P, "Evolutionary history of *Salmonella* Typhi." Repts. *Sci* Nov 24, 2006; 314: 1301–1304

Thayer, J et al, "Typhoid fever—Skagit County, Washington." Epidemiol Notes Repts. *MMWR*, Oct 26, 1990; 39(42); 749–751

Wersan, G, "The truth (for a change) about Typhoid Mary." *MD*, Sept 1985: 69–73

Chapter 4

Acheson, D, "*Escherichia coli*," Clin Perspect. *Fd Qual*, May 1999, Part 1, 44–46; June–July 1999; Part II: 54–56

Alexander, ER et al, "*Escherichia coli* O157:H7 outbreak linked to commercially distributed dry-cured salami—Washington & California, 1994." *MMWR*, Mar 10, 1995; 44(9); 157–160

Archer, DL, "*E. coli* O157:H7—searching for solutions." Fd Tech Back Page. *Fd Tech*, Oct 2000: 142

Banatvala, N et al, "Meat grinders & molecular epidemiology, two supermarket outbreaks of *Escherichia coli* O157:H7 infection." *J Infect Dis*, Feb 1996; 173(2); 480–483

Bell, BP et al, "A multistate outbreak of *Escherichia coli* O157:H7-associated bloody diarrhea & hemolytic uremic syndrome from hamburger: the Washington experience." *AMA*, Nov 2, 1994; 272(17); 1349–1353

Belongia, EA, "Transmission of *Escherichia coil* O157:H7 infection in Minnesota child day-care facilities." *JAMA*, Feb 17, 1993; 269(7); 883–888

Bender, JB et al, "Surveillance for *Escherichia coli* O157:H7 infection in Minnesota by molecular subtyping." *N Engl J Med*, Aug 7, 1997; 337(6); 388–394

Benoit, V et al, "Foodborne outbreaks of enterotoxigenic *Escherichia coli*—Rhode Island & New Hampshire, 1993." Emerg Infect Dis. *MMWR*, Feb 11, 1994; 43(5); 81; 87–89

Bergmire-Sweat, D et al, "*Escherichia coli* O157:H7 outbreak among teenage campers—Texas, 1999." *MMWR*, Apr 21, 2000; 49(15); 321–324

Besser, RE et al, "An outbreak of diarrhea & hemolytic uremic syndrome from *Escherichia coli* O157:H7 in fresh-pressed apple cider." Original Contrib. *JAMA*, May 5, 1993; 269(17); 2217–2220

Bettelheim, KA, "Enterohaemorrhagic *E. coli*—a review."*Internatl Fd Hyg*, 1999,Vol 7(5); 7, 9

Boeckman, A, "Warning label now required on non-pasteurized juices." *Fd Drug Pkging*, Aug 1998: 6

Boyce, TG et al, "*Escherichia coli* O157:H7 & the hemolytic-uremic syndrome." *N Engl J Med*, Aug 10, 1995; 333(6); 364–368

Brandt, JR et al, "*Escherichia coli* O157:H7-associated hemolytic-uremic syndrome after ingestion of contaminated hamburgers." *J Pediat*, Oct 1994; 4: 519–526

Breuer, T et al, "A multistate outbreak of *Escherichia coli* O157:H7 infections linked to alfalfa sprouts grown from contaminated seeds." Research. *Emerg Infect Dis*, Nov–Dec 2001; 7(6): 977–982

Brook, MG & BA Bannister, "Diarrhoea-causing *Escherichia coli*." *Digest Dis*, July–Oct 1993; 11(4–5); 288–297

Bryan, C, "*E. coli* inquiry calls for stricter laws on selling meat." *Br Med J*, Jan 25, 1997; 314(7076); 249

Buchanan, R & MP Doyle, "Foodborne disease significance of *Escherichia coli* O157:H7 & other enterohemorrhagic *E. coli*." Sci Status Summ, Inst Fd Tech Expert Panel Fd Safety & Nutr. *Fd Tech*, Oct 1997: 69–76

Burns, F, "Elusive *E. coli*." In the lab. Pathogen Detection. *Fd Qual*, Apr–May 2006: 46–48

Calvin, L, "Outbreak linked to spinach forces reassessment of food safety practices." Feature. *Amber Waves*. ERS, USDA, June 2007: 24–31

Cameron, AS, "Community outbreak of hemolytic uremic syndrome attributable to *Escherichia coli* 0111:NM—South Australia, 1995." *MMWR*, July 28, 1995: 550–551, 557–558

Cannon, M et al, "Outbreak of *Escherichia coli* O157:H7 infection—Georgia & Tennessee, June 1995." *MMWR* Mar 29, 1996; 45(12); 249–251

Carter, AO, "A severe outbreak of *Escherichia coli* O157:H7-associated hemorrhagic colitis in a nursing home." *N Engl J Med*, Dec 10, 1987; 317(24); 1496–1500

Cieslak, PR et al, "Hamburger-associated *Escherichia coli* O157:H7 infection in Las Vegas: a hidden epidemic." *Am J PH*, Feb 1997; 87(2); 176–180

Cliver, DO, "Uncowed by *E. coli*." News Analy. Sci Communicat. *Fd Tech*, Dec 1997: 18

Coghlan, A, "Killer strain raises urgent questions." *New Scientist*, Jan 25, 1997; 153(2066); 7

"Coleman blames antibiotic use in cattle for *E. coli* outbreak." *Fd Chem News*, Feb 15, 1993: 74–75

Como-Sabetti, K, "Outbreaks of *Escherichia coli* O157:H7 infections associated with eating alfalfa sprouts (Michigan & Virginia, June–July 1997, *MMWR*, Aug 1997; 46(32); 741–744

Davis, M et al, "Update: multistate outbreak of *Escherichia coli* O157:H7 infections from hamburgers—Western United States, 1992." *MMWR*, 1993; 4, 258–263, reprinted in *JAMA*, May 5, 1993; 269(17); 2194–2196

—— "Outbreaks of *Escherichia coli* O157:H7 associated with petting zoos—North Carolina, Florida, & Arizona, 2004–2005." *MMWR*, Dec 23, 2005; 54(50); 1277–1280

Dern, A, "Broken lettuce cells allow *E. coli* O157:H7 to become internalized." *Fd Chem News*, Apr 20, 1998: 5–6

Durch, J et al, "Outbreak of *Escherichia coli* O157:H7 infections associated with eating fresh cheese curds—Wisconsin, June 1998." *MMWR*, Oct 13, 2000; 49(40); 911–913

"*E. coli* O157:H7 at a glance." *Fd News for Consumers* [FSIS, USDA] Summer 1993; 19(3); Suppl 5: 5

"*Escherichia coli* O157:H7 infections associated with eating a nationally distributed commercial brand of frozen ground beef patties & burgers—Colorado, 1997." *MMWR*, Aug 22, 1997; 46(33); 777–778

"*Escherichia coli* update: *E coli* O157:H7." *FSIS Background*, USDA, May 1993: 1–4

Estrada-Garcia, T et al, "Drug-resistant diarrheogenic *Escherichia coli*, Mexico." Dispatches. *Emerg Infect Dis*, Aug 2005; 11(8); 1306–1308

Featherstone, C, "*Escherichia coli* O157:H7: superbug or mere sensation?" *Lancet*, Mar 29, 1997; 349(9056); 930

Feder, I et al, "Isolation of *Escherichia coli* O157:H7 from intact colon fecal samples of swine." Dispatches. *Emerg Infect Dis*, Mar 2003; 9(3); 380–383

"Fermentation destroys *E. coli* O157:H7 in cider, researchers find." *Fd Chem News*, Feb 10, 1997: 38–39

Finelli, L et al, "Enhanced detection of sporadic *Escherichia coli* O157:H7 infections—New Jersey, July 1994." *MMWR*, June 9, 1995; 44(22); 417–421

Flores, A, "New ways to control *E. coli* in weaned pigs." *Agric Res*, Mar 2004: 9

Fogarty, J et al, "Illness in a community associated with an episode of water contamination with sewage." *Epidemiol Infect*, Apr 1975; 114(2); 289–295

"Food safety & quality." *Quarterly Rept Selected Research Projects* [ARS, USDA], July 1–Sept 30, 1998: 6

Frost, B et al, "*Escherichia coli* O157:H7 outbreak at a summer camp—Virginia, 1994." *MMWR*, June 9, 1995; 44(22); 419–421

FSIS [Food Safety & Inspection Service] "Pilot test protocol for *E. coli* O157:H7 on beef carcasses." FSIS, USDA. Text. *Fd Safety Rept*, Apr 28, 1999; 1(14); 409–410

Foulke, JE, "How to outsmart dangerous *E. coli* strain." *FDA Consumer*, Jan–Feb 1994: 7–11

Francis, BJ, "Update: gastrointestinal illness associated with imported semi-soft cheese." *MMWR*, Jan 20, 1984; 33(2); 16; 22

Gill, CJ et al, "Risk of hemolytic uremic syndrome from antibiotic treatment of *Escherichia coli* O157:H7 colitis." Lett. *JAMA*, Dec 25, 2002; 288(24); 3110–3111

Goldwater, PN & KA Bettelheim, "An outbreak of hemolytic uremic syndrome due to *Escherichia coli* O157:H7: or was it?" Lett. *Emerg Infect Dis*, Apr–June 1996; 2(2); 153–154

Gomes, T et al, "Emerging enteropathogenic *Escherichia coli* strains." Dispatches. *Emerg Infect Dis*, Oct 2004; 10(10); 1851–1855

Gordenker, A, "KFC restaurants switch to fresh-cut coleslaw following *E. coli* O157:H7 illnesses." *Fd Chem News*, Aug 30, 1999: 15–16

Grady, D, "Quick-change pathogens gain an evolutionary edge." Microbiol. *Sci*, Nov 15, 1996; 274: 1081

Griffin, PM & RV Tauxe, "The epidemiology of infections caused by *Escherichia coli* O157:H7, other enterohemorrhagic *E. coli* & the associated hemorrhagic uremic syndrome." *Epidemiol Rev*, 1991; 13: 60–98

Guest, R, "Four die in food poisoning outbreak in Japan." *Br Med J*, July 1996; 313(705); 187

Gupta, Amita et al, "*Escherichia coli* O157:H7 cluster evaluation." Dispatches. *Emerg Infect Dis*, Oct 2004; 10(10); 1856–1858

Haack, JP et al, "*Escherichia coli* O157:H7 exposure in Wyoming & Seattle: serologic evidence of rural risk." Research. *Emerg Infect Dis*, Oct 2003; 9(10); 1226–1230

Hamano, S et al, "Neurological manifestations of hemorrhagic colitis in the outbreak of *Escherichia coli* O157:H7 infection in Japan. *Acta Paediatrica*, May 1993,Vol 82(1); 454–458

Hancock, DD et al, "The prevalence of *Escherichia coli* O157:H7 in dairy & beef cattle in Washington State." *Epidemiol Infect*, Oct 2, 1994; 113(2); 199–207

Herwaldt, Barbara L, "Waterborne-disease outbreaks, 1988–1990." CDC Surveill Summ, *MMWR*, 1991; 40(SS–3); 1–13

Hilborn, ED et al, "A multistate outbreak of *Escherichia colii* O157:H7 infections associated with consumption of mesclun lettuce." *Arch Intern Med*, 1999; 159: 1758–1764

Hooton, TM et al, "*Escherichia coli* bacteriuria & contraception method."*JAMA*, Jan 2, 1991; 265(1); 64–69

"Industry protocol targets carcasses to test for *E. coli* O157:H7, verify controls." Meat. *Fd Safety Rept*, Apr 28, 1999; 1(14); 386

"Industry warns of 'out of control' recalls, shutdown from expanding policy on *E. coli*." Meat. *Fd Safety Rept*, Mar 24, 1999; 1(9); 266–267

Keen, JE, "Shiga-toxigenic *Escherichia coli* O157:H7 in agricultural fair livestock, U.S. Research." *Emerg Infect Dis*, May 2006; 12(5); 780–786

Keene, WE et al, "A swimming-associated outbreak of hemorrhagic colitis caused by *Escherichia coli* O157:H7 & *Shigella sonnei*." *N Engl J Med*, 1994; 331: 579–584

—— "An outbreak of *Escherichia coli* O157:H7 infections traced to jerky made from deer meat." Brief Rept. *JAMA*, Apr 16, 1997; 277(15); 1229–1231

Kluger, J, "Anatomy of an outbreak." *Time*, Aug 3, 1998: 56–62

Kudaka, J, "*Escherichia* coli O157:H7 infections associated with ground beef from a U.S. military installation—Okinowa, Japan, February 2004." *MMWR*, Jan 21, 2005: 40–41

"Lawsuit blames apple juice maker for illnesses from *E. coli* infection." Wash. *Fd Safety Rept*, Apr 28, 1999; 1(14); 405

Le Clerc, JE et al, "High mutation frequencies among *Escherichia coli* & *Salmonella* pathogens. Repts. *Sci*, Nov 15, 1996; 274: 1208–1211

Le Jeune, JT et al, "Human *Escherichia coli* O157:H7 genetic marker in isolates of bovine origin." Dispatches. *Emerg Infect Dis*, Aug 2004; 10(8); 1482–1485

"Lettuce fingered as culprit in Idaho *E. coli* outbreak." *Fd Chem News*, July 15, 1996: 24–25

"Lettuce was source of Montana *E. coli* outbreak, CDC." *Fd Chem News*, Aug 14, 1995: 34–35

Lewis, R, "The bugs within us." *FDA Consumer*, Sept 1992: 37–42

Ludwig, K et al, "Outbreak of *Escherichia coli* O157:H7 infection in a large family." *Europ J Clin Microbiol Infect Dis*, Mar 1997; 16(3); 238–241

MacDonald, KL et al, "*Escherichia coli* O157:H7, an emerging gastrointestinal pathogen." *JAMA*, May 5, 1993; 269(17); 2264

MacDonald, KL & MT Osterholm, "The emergence of *Escherichia coli* O157:H7 infection in the United States, the changing epidemiology of foodborne diseases." *JAMA*, May 5, 1993; 269(17); 2264–2266

Maki, DG & N Safdar, "Risk of hemolytic uremic syndrome from antibiotic treatment of *Escherichia coli* O157:H7." Lett. *JAMA*, Dec 25, 2002; 288(24); 3112

Marks, S & T Roberts, "*E. coli* O157:H7 ranks as the fourth most costly foodborne disease." *Fd Rev*, Sept–Dec 1993: 51–59

McCarthy M & DF Splittstoesser, "Reducing risk of *E. coli* in apple cider." *Fd Tech*, Dec 1996; 50(12); 174

McDonough, S, "Foodborne outbreak of gastroenteritis caused by *Escherichia coli* O157:H7—North Dakota, 1990." *MMWR*, Sept 26, 1991; 40(16); 265–267

Mead, P, "Focus: *Escherichia coli* O157:H7 & diarrhea-associated hemolytic uremic syndrome (D+HUS) in Foodnet sites." Q/A with Paul Mead. *The Catchment* CDC, Fall 1998: 1, 3

Mermelstein, NH, "Controlling *Escherichia coli* O157:H7 in meat." *Fd Tech*, Apr 1993: 90–91

—— "High interest in testing for *E. coli* O157:H7." *Fd Tech*, Aug 1994: 100

Moore, K et al, "Outbreak of acute gastroenteritis attributable to *Escherichia coli* serotype O104:H21—Helena, Montana 1994." *MMWR*, July 14, 1995; 44(27): 501–503

Morgan, D et al, "Verotoxin producing *Escherichia coli* O157:H7 infection associated with the consumption of yoghurt." *Epidemiol Infect*, Oct 1993; 111(2); 181–187

Nataro, JP et al, "Enteroaggregative *Escherichia coli*." Synopses. *Emerg Infect Dis*, Apr–June 1998; 2(2): 251–261

Nathan, R "Japan's *E. coli* outbreak elicits fear, anger." *Nature Med*, Sept 1996; 2(9); 956

Nöel, JM & EC Boedker, "Enterohemorrhagic *Escherichia coli*: a family of emerging pathogens." *Digest Dis*, Jan–Apr 1997; 15(1–2): 67–91

Olson, SJ et al, "A waterborne outbreak of *Escherichia coli* infections & hemolytic uremic syndrome: implications for rural water systems." Research. *Emerg Infect Dis*, Apr 2002; 8(4): 370–375

Omaye, ST, "Shiga-toxin producing *Escherichia coli*: another concern." News Analy. Regulatory Impact. *Fd Tech*, May 2001: 26

"Ongoing multistate outbreaks of *Escherichia coli* serotype O157:H7 infections associated with consumption of fresh spinach—United States, September 2006." *MMWR*, Sept 29, 2006; 55(38): 1045–1046

Ostroff, SM et al, "Infections with *Escherichia coli* O157:H7 in Washington State, the first year of statewide disease surveillance." Original Contrib. *JAMA*, July 21, 1989; 262(3): 355–359

—— "Surveillance of *Escherichia coli* O157:H7 isolation & confirmation, United States, 1988." Suppl. *MMWR*, 1991; 40(SS–1): 1–6

"Outbreak of *Escherichia coli* O157:H7 infections associated with drinking unpasteurized commercial apple juice—British Columbia, California, Colorado, and Washington, October 1996." *MMWR*, 1996; 45(44): 975

Pargas, N, "Oxytetracycline injection increases O157:H7 shedding in juvenile cattle." *Fd Chem News*, Aug 24, 1998: 11–12

Perry, SM et al, "Hemorrhagic colitis in child after visit to farm visitor centre." Lett. *Lancet*, Aug 26, 1995; 346(8974): 572

Phan, Q et al, "Laboratory-confirmed non-O157:H7-shiga toxin-producing *Escherichia coli*—Connecticut, 2000–2005." *MMWR*, Jan 19, 2007; 56(2): 29–31

Planck, N, "Leafy green sewage." Op-Ed Contributor, *NY Times*, Sept 21, 2006

"Preliminary report: foodborne outbreak of *Escherichia coli* O157:H7 infections from hamburgers—western United States, 1993." Epidemiol Notes Repts. *MMWR*, Feb 5, 1993; 42(4): 85–86

Raloff, J, "Sponges & sinks & rags, oh my! Where microbes lurk and how to rout them." *Sci News*, Sept 14, 1996: 172–173

Rangel, JM et al, "Epidemiology of *Escherichia coli* O157:H7 outbreaks, United States, 1982–2002." Research. *Emerg Infect Dis*, Apr 2005; 11(4): 603–609

Robins-Browne, RM, "Enterohaemorrhagic *Escherichia coli:* an emerging food-borne pathogen with serious consequences. " *Med J Austral*, May 1995; 162(10): 511–512

Roper, William L, "Diseases transmitted through the food supply." [CDC] *Fed Reg*, Sept 8, 1992; 57(174): 40917

Sack, RB, "Enterohemorrhagic *Escherichia coli.*" *N Engl J Med*, Dec 10, 1987; 317(24): 1535–1537

Schubert, C, "Busting the gut busters, virulent *E. coli* are revealing some weaknesses." *Sci News*, Aug 4, 2001: 74–76

Semanchek, J & D Golden, "Survival of *Escherichia coli* O157:H7 during fermentation of apple cider." *J Fd Prot*, Dec 1996; 59(12): 1256–1259

Shefer, AM et al, "A cluster of *Escherichia coli* O157:H7 infections with the hemolytic uremic syndrome & death in California: a mandate for improved surveillance." *West J Med*, July–Aug 1996; 165(1–2): 15–19

Smith, HR et al, "Enteroaggregative *Escherichia coli* & outbreaks of gastroenteritis in UK." Lett. *Lancet*, Sept 13, 1997; 350(9080): 814–815

Stanley, Doris, "Induced heat resistance in *E. coli.*" *Agric Res*, July 1998: 21

Taormina, PJ et al, "Infections associated with eating seed sprouts: an international concern." Synopses. *Emerg Infect Dis*, Sept–Oct 1999; 5(5): 626–634

Tarr, PI, "Risk of hemolytic uremic syndrome from antibiotic treatment of *Escherichia coli* O157:H7 colitis." Lett. *JAMA*, Dec 25, 2002; 288(24): 3112

Tilden, Jr., J et al, "A new route of transmission for *Escherichia coli* infection from dry fermented salami." *Am J PH,* Aug 1996; 86(8): 1142–1145

Trilling, EL, "*E coli* can contaminate lettuce via soil, irrigation water, study says." *Fd Chem News,* Jan 21, 2003: 26–27

Turney, C et al, "*Escherichia coli* O157:H7 outbreak linked to home-cooked hamburger—California, July 1993." *MMWR,* Apr 1, 1994; 43(12): 213–216

Voeckler, R, "Foodborne illness problems more than enteric." Med News. *JAMA,* Jan 5, 1994; 271(1): 8–9; 11

—— "New strategies aimed at *E. coli* O157:H7." *JAMA,* Aug 17, 1994; 272(7): 503

—— "Panel calls *E. coli* screening inadequate." Med News Perspect. *JAMA,* Aug 17, 1994; 272(7): 501

Wachsmuth, IK, "*Escherichia coli* O157:H7—harbinger of change in food safety—tradition in the industrialized world." New Analy. Sci Communic. *Fd Tech,* Oct 1997: 26

Wallace, RB & ST Donta, "Antibody to *Escherichia coli*-enterotoxin in meat-packing workers." Pub Hlth Brief. *Am J PH,* Jan 1978; 68(1): 68–70

Warner, E, "Importance of culture confirmation of shiga toxin-producing *Escherichia coli* infection as illustrated by outbreaks of gastroenteritis—New York & North Carolina, 2005." *MMWR,* Sept 29, 2006; 55(38): 1042–1045

Warrner, M et al, "Lake-associated outbreak of *Escherichia coli* O157:H7—Illinois 1995." *MMWR,* May 31, 1996; 45(21): 437–439

White, DG & PA Bradford, "Expanded spectrum cephalosporin resistance in *E. coli* isolates associated with bovine calf diarrheal disease." *FDA Vet,* Jan–Feb 2000; 15(1): 4–5

Wong, CS & JR Brandt, "Risk of hemolytic uremic syndrome from antibiotic treatment of *Escherichia coli* O157:H7 colitis." Lett. *JAMA,* Dec 25, 2002; 288(24): 3111

Chapter 5

Acheson, D, "*C. jejuni* infection & the link with Guillain-Barré Syndrome."*Fd Qual,* May–June 2000: 47–49

Allos, BM, "Association Between *Campylobacter* infection and Guillain-Barré Syndrome. Suppl. *J Infect Dis,* 1997; 108: s125–s128

Altekruse, SF et al, "*Campylobacter jejuni*—an emerging foodborne pathogen. Perspect. *Emerg Infect Dis,* Jan–Feb 1999; 5(1): 28–35

"Antibiotic-resistant bacteria common in chicken, study says." New Bites. *Fd Proc,* Jan 2003:12

"Biological control could reduce food safety problems of poultry." Sc Agric. *Sci News,* U Wisconsin, Madison, Wis, Jan 1991

Beers, A, "Campylobacter tops illness list." *Fd Chem News,* June 15, 1998: 8–9

Blaser, MJ, "*Campylobacter* infections, a leading cause of acute diarrhea." Hospital. *Drug Ther,* Jan 1984: 62a–62g; 62i; 62k

Blaser, MJ et al, "*Campylobacter* enteritis—Colorado." *MMWR,* July 7 1978; 226: 231

Bolton, CF, "The changing concepts of Guillain-Barré Syndrome." *N Engl J Med*, Nov 23, 1995; 333(21): 1415–1417

Breeling, JL, "Newly recognized bacterial causes of infectious diarrhea." *Infect Dis Pract*, Jan 1989; 12(4): 1–7

Buzby, JC. et al, "Savings from reducing *Campylobacter* in food could total up to $5.6 billion per year." *Summary of Report*, ERS, USDA, 1997

—— "Estimated Annual Costs of *Campylobacter*-Associated Guillain-Barré Syndrome." *Agric Eco* Rept No 756, USDA, July 1997

"*Campylobacter* appears to be major cause of Guillain-Barré Syndrome." *Fd Chem News*, June 3, 1996, 3–5

Campylobacter Backgrounder. FSIS, USDA, Fd Safety Ed Commun Staff, Nov 1997

"*Campylobacter* infections widespread; No. 2 cause of bacterial diarrhea." *Med Wrld News for Psychiatrists*, Nov 29, 1984: 36

"*Campylobacter* outbreaks associated with certified raw milk products—California." Epidemiol Notes Repts. *MMWR*, Oct 5, 1984; 33(39): 562

"*Campylobacter* outbreaks associated with raw milk provided in a dairy tour—California." Epidemiol Notes Repts. *MMWR*, May 16, 1986; 35(19): 311–312

Campylobacter—Questions & Answers. FSIS Backgrounder. FSIS, USDA, May 1991; revised Aug 1994

"*Campylobacter* reported in 42% of raw chickens in survey." *Fd Chem News*, Sept 23, 1991: 43

"*Campylobacter*: research advances in sourcing the problem." Inside Microbiol. Interview: Nelson A Cox. *Fd Safety Mag*, Oct–Nov 2001; 17–20, 43–44

"Campylobacteriosis associated with raw milk consumption—Pennsylvania." Epidemiol Notes Repts. *MMWR*, July 8, 1983; 32(26): 327–328, 344

"Chronic diarrhea associated with raw milk consumption—Minnesota." Epidemiol Notes Repts. *MMWR*, Sept 21, 1984; 33(37): 521–522, 527–528

Clark, CG et al, "Characterization of waterborne outbreak-associated *Campylobacter jejuni*, Walkerton, Ontario." Research. *Emerg Infect Dis*, Oct 2003; 9(10): 1232–1241

Coker, A et al, "Human campylobacteriosis in developing countries." Synopses. *Emerg Infect Dis*, Mar 2002; 8(3): 237–243

Cooper, R et al, "*Campylobacter jejuni* enteritis mistaken for ulcerative colitis." *J Family Pract*, 1991; 34(3): 357; 361–362

De Bois, MHW et al, "Pancreatitis associated with *Campylobacter jejuni* infection: diagnosis by ultrasonography." *Br Med J*, 1989; 298: 1004

Deibel, KE & GJ Banwart, "The effect of oregano, sage & ground cloves on *Campylobacter fetus* ssp. jejuni." Dept of Microbiol, *Ohio State U*, June 23, 1982

Dilya, M et al, "An outbreak of *Campylobacter* infection associated with the consumption of unpasteurized milk at a large festival in England." *Europ J Epidemiol*, Oct 1994; 10(5); 581–585

Doussard, M, "*Campylobacter* passes from one generation to next in broilers, study finds, USDA." *Fd Chem News*, Mar 6, 2000, 10

Enders, U et al, "The spectrum of immune responses to *Campylobacter jejuni* & glycoconjugates in Guillain-Barré Syndrome & in other neuroimmunological disorders." *Annals Neurol*, 1993; 34, 136–144

Escartin, EP, "Survival of *C. jejuni* on sliced watermelon & papaya." *J Fd Prot*, Feb 1994; 57, 166–168

Espinoza, M, "Infectious bursal disease boosts *Campylobacter* numbers in chickens." *News Release*. Ohio State University Extension, Wooster, Ohio, Dec 1, 2003

Evans, MR et al, "A milk-borne *Campylobacter* outbreak following an educational farm visit." *Epidemiol Infect*, Dec 1996; 117(3): 457–462

—— "Hazards of healthy living: bottled water & salad vegetables as risks factors for *Campylobacter* infections." Research. *Emerg Infect Dis*, Oct 2003; 9(10): 1219–1224

Fujimoto, S, "Guillain-Barré Syndrome & *Campylobacter jejuni* infection." Lettr. *Lancet*, 1990; 335: 1350

Gallagher, P et al, "Acute pancreatitis associated with campylobacter infection." *Br J Surg*, 1981; 68: 383

Gallay, A, "*Campylobacter* antimicrobial drug resistance among humans, broiler chickens, & pigs, France." Research. *Emerg Infect Dis*, Feb 2007; 13(2): 259–266

Ginsberg, MM et al, "*Campylobacter* sepsis associated with 'nutritional therapy'—California." *MMWR*, June 26, 1981; 30(24): 294–295

Graves, TK et al, "Outbreak of *Campylobacter* enteritis associated with cross-contamination of food—Oklahoma, 1996." *MMWR*, Feb 27, 1998; 47(27): 129–131

Gruenewald, R et al, "Serologic evidence of *Campylobacter jejuni/coli* enteritis in patients with Guillain-Barré Syndrome." *Arch Neurol*, Oct 1991; 48: 1080–1082

Guillain-Barré Syndrome Fact Sheet. Natl Inst Neurol Dis Stroke, NIH, NIH Publ No 88–2902; rev. Nov 1997

Hald, B et al, "Flies & *Campylobacter* infection of broiler flocks." Dispatches. *Emerg Infect Dis*, Aug 2004; 10(8): 1490–1492

Hart, K, "High *Campylobacter* levels found in organic chickens." Research. *Fd Chem News*, Oct 8, 2001: 27

Hileman, B, "Poultry antibiotics pose human threat." *Chem Engineer News*, Nov 6, 2000: 11

—— "FDA bans veterinary drug, Baytril antibiotic, used in poultry, causes resistant bacteria to emerge." News Wk. Regulations. *Chem Engineer News* Aug 8, 2005: 16

Hingley, A, "*Campylobacter*, low profile bug is food poisoning leader." *FDA Consumer*, Sept–Oct 1999: 14–17

Hood, AM et al, "The extent of surface contamination of retailed chicken with *Campylobacter jejuni* serogroups." *Epidemiol Infect* 1988; 100: 17–25

Iovine, NM & MJ Blaser, "Antibiotics in animal feed & spread of resistant *Campylobacter* from poultry to humans." Comment. *Emerg Infect Dis*, June 2004; 10(6): 1158–1159

"Isolation of *Campylobacter jejuni* from raw milk." *Appl Environ Microbiol*, Aug 1983: 459–462

Jones, IG & M Roworth, "An outbreak of *Escherichia coli* O157:H7 & campylobacteriosis associated with contamination of a drinking water supply." *Pub Hlth,* Sept 1996; 110(5): 277–282

Leslie, M, "A gut germ goes AWOL." Meeting Briefs. Am Soc Cell Biol. *Sci,* Dec 22, 2006; 314: 1865

Marty, AT et al, "Inflammatory abdominal aortic aneurysm infected by *Campylobacter fetus.*" *JAMA,* Mar 4, 1983; 249(9): 1190–1192

McCarthy, N & J Giesecke, "Incidence of Guillain-Barré Syndrome following infection with *Campylobacter jejuni.*" *Am J Epidemiol,* Mar 15, 2001; 153: 610–614

Mertz, H et al, "Diagnosis of *Campylobacter pylori* gastritis." *Digest Dis Sci,* 1991; 35: 1–4

Murphy, J, "Store-bought chickens laden with *Campylobacter.*" *Fd Chem News,* June 1998: 12–13

Nachamkin, I, "*Campylobacter* enteritis & the Guillain-Barré Syndrome." *Curr Infect Dis Repts,* 2001; 3: 116–122

Nichols, GL, "Fly transmission of *Campylobacter.*" Perspect. *Emerg Infect Dis,* Mar 2005; 11(3): 361–364

Orr, KE et al, "Direct milk excretion of *Campylobacter jejuni* in a dairy cow causing cases of human enteritis." *Epidemiol Infect,* Feb 1995; 114(1): 15–24

Osvath, R, "*Campylobacter* infections on the rise; food a major cause." Interagency. *Fd Chem News,* Mar 11, 2002: 10

"Outbreak of *Escherichia coli* O157:H7 & *Campylobacter* among attendees of the Washington County Fair—New York, 1999." Pub Hlth Dispatch. *MMWR,* Sept 17, 1999; 48(36): 803–804

Park, CE & GW Sanders, "Occurrence of thermotolerant *Campylobacters* in fresh vegetables sold at farmers' outdoor markets & supermarkets." *Canad J Microbiol,* Apr 1992; 38(4): 313–316

Pennesi, E, "First food-borne pathogen sequenced." News Wk. Microb Genomics. *Sci,* Feb 26, 1999; 283: 1243

Peterson, MC, "Clinical aspects of *Campylobacter jejuni* infections in adults. "Conferences Rev. *West J Med,* Aug 1994; 161(2): 148–152

Phillips, CA, "Bird attacks on milk bottles & *Campylobacter* infection." Lett. *Lancet,* Aug 5, 1995; 346 (971): 386

"Premature labor & neonatal sepsis caused by *Campylobacter fetus,* subsp. *fetus*—Ontario." Internatl Notes. *MMWR,* Aug 31, 1984; 33(34): 483–484, 489

Puylaert, J et al, "*Campylobacter* ileocolitis mimicking acute appendicitis: differentiation with graded-compression US [ultrasound]." *Radiol,* 1988; 166: 737–740

"Raw milk tied to bacterial infection." *Am Med News,* Jan 11, 1986: 22

Rees, JH et al, "*Campylobacter jejuni* infections & Guillain-Barré Syndrome." *N Engl J Med,* Nov 23, 1995; 333(21): 1374–1379

Schonberg-Norio, D et al, "Swimming & *Campylobacter* infections." Dispatches. *Emerg Infect Dis,* Aug 2004; 10(8): 1474–1477

Shandera, Wayne X et al, "An outbreak of bacteremic *Campylobacter jejuni* infection." *Mt. Sinai J Med,* Jan 1992; 5(1): 53–56

Shoenfeld, Y et al, "Guillain-Barré as an autoimmune disease." *Intern Arch Allerg Immunol,* 1996; 109: 318–326

Smith, G & MJ Blaser, "Fatalities associated with *Campylobacter jejuni* infections." *JAMA,* May 17, 1985; 253(19): 2873–2875

Sorville, F et al, "Bondage, dominance, irrigations, & *Aeromonas hydrophila:* California dreamin'." Lett. *JAMA,* Feb 3, 1989; 261(5): 697–698

Southern, JP et al, "Bird attack on milk bottles possible mode of transmission of *Campylobacter jejuni* to man." *Lancet,* Dec 8, 1990; 336(8728): 1425–1427

Stehr-Green, J et al, "*Campylobacter* enteritis—New Zealand, 1990."Internatl Notes, *MMWR,* Feb 22, 1991; 40(7): 116–117, 123

Tam, Clarence C et al, "Incidence of Guillain-Barré Syndrome among patients with *Campylobacter* infection: a general practice research database study." *J Infect Dis,* 2006; 194: 95–97

—— "Influenza, *Campylobacter* & *Mycoplasma* infections, & hospital admissions for Guillain-Barré Syndrome, England." Research. *Emerg Infect Dis,* Dec 2006; 12(12): 1880–1886

Tauxe, RV, "Epidemiology of *Campylobacter jejuni* infections in the United States & other industrial nations." in *Campylobacter jejuni: Current & Future Trends,* eds. J Nachamkin, MJ Blaser and LS Tompkins. Wash, DC: Am Soc Microbiol, 1992: 9–12

Taylor, DN et al, "*Campylobacter* enteritis from untreated water in the Rocky Mountains." *Annals Intern Med,* July 1983; 99: 38–40

Ternhag, A et al, "Short- and long-term effects of bacterial gastrointestinal infections." *Emerg Infect Dis,* Jan 2008; 14(1): 143–148

Thomas, C et al, "*Campylobacter*—the next challenge." *Internatl Fd Hyg,* 1995 Vol 6(5): 5–7

Thompson, S et al, *Draft Risk Assessment on the Human Health Impact of Fluoroquinolone Resistant Campylobacter Associated with Consumption of Chicken.* CDC/USDA Natl Chicken Council/US Census Bureau/U of Penn Med Center. Rev. Feb 9, 2000.

Tiehan, W et al, "Waterborne *Campylobactor* gastroenteritis—Vermont." Epidemiol Notes Repts. MMWR, June 23, 1978; 27(25): 208

Tosh, FE et al, "Outbreak of *Campylobacter* enteritis associated with raw milk—Kansas." *MMWR,* May 15, 1981; 31(18): 218–220

Tracz, DM et al, "pVir & bloody diarrhea in *Campylobacter jejuni* enteritis." Research. *Emerg Infect Dis,* June 2005; 11(6): 838–843

Vellinga, A & F van Loock, "The dioxin crisis as experiment to determine poultry-related *Campylobacter* enteritis." Research. *Emerg Infect Dis,* Jan 2002; 8(1): 19–22

Welbourn, JL, "*Campylobacter:* no longer the 'quiet pathogen'." *Fd Test Analy,* June–July 1998: 20–22

Wheelock, V, "Cheese—the case for raw milk." *Internatl Fd Hyg,* July 1998; 8(7): 21–23

Wilson, IG & JE Moore, "Presence of *Salmonella* ssp. & *Campylobacter* ssp. in shellfish." *Epidemiol Infect,* Apr 1996; 116(2): 147–153

Windstrand, A et al, "Fresh chicken as main risk factor for campylobacteriosis, Denmark." Research. *Emerg Infect Dis,* Feb 2006; 12(2): 280–284

Wood, M, "Curtailing *Campylobacter.*" *Agric Res,* July 2001: 8–9

Chapter 6

Amur, JS, "*Shigella dysenteriae* type 1 in tourists in Cancun, Mexico." Epidemiol Notes Repts. *MMWR*, Aug 12, 1988; 37(31): 466

Arnell, B et al, "*Shigella sonnei* outbreak associated with contaminated drinking water—Island Park, Idaho, Aug 1995." *MMWR*, Mar 22, 1996; 45(11): 229–231

Black, RE et al, "Epidemiology of common-source outbreaks of shigellosis in the United States, 1961–1975." *Am J Epidemiol*, 1978; 108: 147–152

Brody, JE, "Food poisoning called shigellosis is on the rise, prompting efforts to fight it." Hlth. Personal Hlth. *NY Times*, Sept 13, 1990: B17

Butler, ME, "Five-layer dip recalled nationwide after shigellosis outbreak in three states." General. *Fd Chem News*, Jan 31, 2000: 13–14

Centers for Disease Control and Prevention, "Outbreak of *Shigella flexneri* [type] 2a infections on a cruise ship." *MMWR*, 1994; 43(35): 657.

Centofanti, M, "Just lookin' for a home, many bacteria sneak into cells via entry routes already in place." *Sci News*, Jan 6, 1996: 12–13

Cook, K et al, "A multistate outbreak of *Shigella flexneri* [type] 6 traced to imported green onions." *Presentation* 35th Intersci Conf Antimicrob Agents Chemother, San Francisco, CA, Sept 1995

—— "Increasing antimicrobial resistant *Shigella* infections in the United States." *Presentation*, 36th Intersci Conf Antimicrob Agents Chemother. New Orleans, LA Sept 1996

Crowe, L et al, "Outbreaks of *Shigella sonnei* infection associated with eating fresh parsley—United States & Canada, July–Aug 1998." *MMWR*, Apr 16, 1999; 48(14): 285–289

Cruz, RJ, "*Shigella dysenteriae* type 1—Guatemala, 1991." Internatl Notes. *MMWR*, June 28, 1991; 40(25): 421, 427–428

Davis, H et al, "A shigellosis outbreak traced to commercially distributed shredded lettuce." *Am J Epidemiol*, 1988; 128: 1312–1321

Dunn, RA et al, "Outbreak of *Shigella flexneri* linked to salad prepared at a central commissary in Michigan." Sci Contrib. *Pub Hlth Repts*, Sept–Oct 1995; 110: 580–586

Fackelmann, KA, "Football players benched by foul foods." *Sci News*, Dec 12, 1992: 407

Fewtrell, L et al, "An investigation into the possible links between shigellosis & Hepatitis A & public water supply disconnections." *Pub Hlth*, May 1997; 111(3): 179–181

"Four *Shigella* cases traced to restaurant oysters in Texas." *Fd Chem News*, Feb 22, 1993, 35

Frost, JA et al, "An outbreak of *Shigella sonnei* infection associated with consumption of iceberg lettuce." *Emerg Infect Dis*, Jan 1995; 1(1): 26–29

Gessner, BD & M Beller, "Moose soup shigellosis in Alaska." *West J Med*, May 1994; 160(5): 430–433

Groseclose, S et al, *Summary of Notifiable Diseases—United States, 2000*. CDC, June 14, 2002; 49(53): 64–65

—— *Summary of Notifiable Diseases: United States, 2001*. *MMWR*, May 2003; 50(53): 72–73

Gupta, A et al, "Laboratory-confirmed shigellosis in the United States 1989–2002: epidemiologic trends & patterns." *Clin Infect Dis*, 2004; 38: 1372–1377

Hartley, DM et al, "Shigellosis & cryptosporidiosis, Baltimore, Maryland." Lett. *Emerg Infect Dis*, July 2006; 12(7): 1164–1165

Hedberg, CW, "An international foodborne outbreak of shigellosis associated with a commercial airline." *JAMA*, Dec 9, 1992; 268(22): 3208–3212

Hewitt, SM et al, "Surveillance for foodborne-disease outbreaks—United States, 1993—1997." Suppl. *MMWR*, May 17 2000; 49(SS1): 57

Hoge, CW et al, "Emergence of Nalidixic acid resistant *Shigella dysenteriae* type 1 in Thailand: an outbreak associated with consumption of a coconut milk dessert." *Internatl J Epidemiol*, Dec 1995; 24(6): 1228–1232

Kapperud, G et al, "Outbreak of *Shigella sonnei* infection traced to imported iceberg lettuce." *J Clin Microbiol*, 1995; 33: 609–614

Keene, WE et al, "A swimming-associated outbreak of hemorrhagic colitis caused by *E. coli* O157:H7 & *Shigella sonnei*." *N Engl J Med*, Sept 1, 1994; 331(9): 579–583

Kimura, AC et al, "Multistate shigellosis outbreak & commercially prepared food, United States." Dispatches. *Emerg Infect Dis*, June 2004; 10(6): 1147–1149

Klausner, JD et al, "*Shigella sonnei* outbreak among men who have sex with men—San Francisco, 2000–2001." *MMWR*, Oct 26, 2001; 50(42): 922–926

Kolavic, SA et al, "An outbreak of *Shigella dysenteriae* type 2 among laboratory workers due to intentional contamination." In Issue. *JAMA*, Aug 6, 1997; 278(5): 396–398

Kolenz, M et al, "Shigellosis in child day care centers—Lexington-Fayette County, Kentucky, 1991." *MMWR*, June 26, 1992; 41(25): 440–442

Lohff, CJ et al, "Shigellosis outbreak associated with an unchlorinated fill-and-drain wading pool —Iowa, 2001." *MMWR*, Sept 21, 2001; 50(37): 797–800

Longfield, L, "Hospital-associated outbreak of *Shigella dysenteriae* type 2—Maryland." *MMWR*, May 21, 1983; 32(19): 251–252

MacCormack, JN et al, "Nationwide dissemination of multiple resistant *Shigella sonnei* following a common-source outbreak." Epidemiol Notes Repts. *MMWR*, Oct 2, 1987; 36(38): 633–634

Martin, DL et al, "Contaminated produce—a common source for two outbreaks & *Shigella*-gastroenteritis." *Am J Epidemiol*, 1986; 124: 299–305

McNabb, SJN et al, "Summary of notifiable diseases—United States, 2005." *MMWR*, Mar 30, 2007 for 2005; 54(53): 13–14

Mølbak, K et al, "Outbreak in Denmark of *Shigella sonnei* infections related to uncooked 'baby maize' imported from Thailand." *Eurosurveill Wkly*, 1998; 2(33): 1171

Morgan, O et al, "*Shigella sonnei* outbreak among homosexual men, London." Lett. *Emerg Infect Dis*, Sept 2006; 12(9): 1458–1460

Obiesie, N et al, "Outbreak of multi-drug resistant *Shigella sonnei* gastroenteritis associated with day care centers—Kansas, Kentucky & Missouri, 2005." *MMWR*, Oct 6, 2006; 55(39): 1069–1071

"Outbreak of *Shigella sonnei* infections associated with eating a nationally distributed dip—

California, Oregon & Washington, Jan 2000." Pub Hlth Dispatch. *MMWR,* Jan 28, 2000; 49(3): 60–61

Pate, C et al, "Community outbreak of shigellosis—United States." Curr Trends. *MMWR,* Aug 3, 1990; 39(30): 509–515

Reeve, G et al, "An outbreak of shigellosis associated with the consumption of raw oysters." *N Engl J Med,* July 27, 1989; 324(4): 224–227

Schulman, SK, "Multistate outbreak of *Shigella sonnei* gastroenteritis—United States." Epidemiol Notes Repts. *MMWR,* July 17, 1987; 36(27): 448–449

"*Shigella flexneri* serotype 3 infections among men who have had sex with men —Chicago, Illinois, 2003–2004." *MMWR,* Aug 26, 2005; 54(33): 820–822

"Shigellosis—North Carolina." Epidemiol Notes Repts. *MMWR,* July 17, 1987; 36(27): 449–450

"Shigellosis outbreak traced to shredded lettuce in restaurants." *Fd Chem News,* Sept 14, 1987: 8–9

Tauxe, RV et al, "The persistence of *Shigella flexneri* in the United States: increasing role of adult males." *Am J Pub Hlth,* 1988; 78: 1432–1435

"Ten leading nationally notifiable infectious diseases—United States, 1995." *MMWR,* Oct 18, 1996; 45(41): 883–884

Totaro, J et al, "Day care-related outbreaks of rhammose-negative *Shigella sonnei*—six states, June 2001–Mar 2003." *MMWR,* Jan 30, 2004; 53(3): 60–63

Travis, J, "Swallowing *Shigella,* can bacteria that cause food poisoning deliver oral DNA vaccines?" *Sci News,* May 11, 1996: 302–303

Zajdowicz, T, "Epidemiologic & chemical aspects of shigellosis in American forces deployed to Saudi Arabia." *South Med J,* 1993; 86: 647–650

Chapter 7

Abter, E, "Ocular toxoplasmosis." Lett. *JAMA,* Aug 3, 1994; 272(5): 356

Angier, N, "In parasite survival, ploys to get help from a host." Basics. *NY Times,* June 26, 2007: D7

Bahia-Oliveira, LMG et al, "Highly endemic, waterborne toxoplasmosis in North Rio de Janero State, Brazil." Research. *Emerg Infect Dis,* Jan 2003; 9(1): 55–62

Benenson, MW et al, "Oocyst-transmitted toxoplasmosis associated with ingestion of contaminated water." *N Engl J Med,* 1982; 307: 666–669

Berdoy M et al, "Fatal attraction in rats infected with *Toxoplasma gondii.*" *Proceedings of the Royal Society: Biological Sciences,* Aug 7, 2000; 267: 1591–1594

Bliss, R, "Assessing the risk: retail meat analyzed." *Agric Res,* Feb 2007: 22

Bower, B, "Sickness & schizophrenia, psychotic ills tied to previous infections. *Sci News,* Jan 24, 2008: 53–54

Bowie, WR et al, "Outbreak of toxoplasmosis associated with municipal drinking water." The BC [British Columbia] Toxoplasmosis Investigation Team. *Lancet,* 1997; 350: 173–177

"Congenital toxoplasmosis may go undiagnosed, Finnish researcher says." *Fd Chem News,* Oct 28, 1996: 12

Connor, E et al, "Central nervous system toxoplasmosis mimicking a brain abscess in a compromised pediatric patient." *Pediat Infect Dis,* 1984; 3: 552–555

Daffos, F, "Prenatal management of 746 pregnancies at risk for congenital toxoplasmosis." *N Engl J Med,* 1988; 318: 271–275

Dubey, JP, "Tracking *Toxoplasma* in feed & food." Sci Update. *Agric Res,* Nov 2002: 23

Dunn, PJ, "Chronic fatigue syndrome." The Doctor's Corner. *Nutrition for Optimal Health News,* Spring 1992; 17(2): 2–4

Edwards, KR et al, "Central nervous system lymphomas versus toxoplasmosis in a patient with AIDS." Corresp. *N Engl J Med,* Dec 10, 1987; 317(24): 1540

Flegr J et al, "Correlation of duration of latent *Toxoplasma gondii* infection with personality changes in women." *Biological Psychology,* May 1 2000; 53(1): 57–68

Folkenberg, J, "Pet ownership, risky business." *FDA Consumer,* Apr 1990: 29

Frenkel, JK, "Toxoplasmosis testing during pregnancy." Lett. *JAMA,* Jan 9, 1991; 265(2): 211

Grigg, ME et al, "Success & virulence in *Toxoplasma* as the result of sexual recombination between two distinct ancestries." Repts. *Sci,* Oct 5, 2001; 294: 161–165

Hay, SM, "The cat/pig toxoplasmosis connection." *Agric Res,* Feb 1996: 8–9

Heukelbach, J et al, "Waterborne toxoplasmosis, Northeastern Brazil." Dispatches. *Emerg Infect Dis,* Feb 2007; 13(2): 287–289

Holliman, RE et al, "*Toxoplasma* infection in the elderly." Infect Dis. *Geriat Med Today,* Apr 1986; 5(4): 97–102

"Information in Zoonoses: 2. Toxoplasmosis." *FDA Vet,* May–June 1990; 5(3): 7

Jacobs, L et al, "A survey of meat samples from swine, cattle, & sheep for the presence of encysted *Toxoplasma*." *J Parasitol,* 1960; 46: 23–28

Jennel, D et al, "What is known about the prevention of congenital toxoplasmosis?" *Lancet,* 1990; 336: 359–361

Joiner, KA et al, "*Toxoplasma gondii:* fusion competence of parasitophorus vacuoles in Fc receptor transfected fibroblasts." Research Article. *Sci,* Aug 10, 1990; 249: 641–646

Jones, JL et al, "*Toxoplasma gondii* infections in the United States, 1999–2000." Synopses. *Emerg Infect Dis,* Nov 2003; 9(11): 1371–1374

—— "Recently acquired *Toxoplasma gondii* infections, Brazil." Research. *Emerg Infect Dis,* Apr 2006; 12(4): 582–586

"Just one *Toxoplasma gondii* parasite infects pigs." *Quarterly Report of Selected Research Projects,* ARS USDA, July–Sept 1995: 7

Kean, BH et al, "An epidemic of acute toxoplasmosis." *JAMA,* 1969; 208: 1002–1004

Kim, K et al, "Gene replacement in *Toxoplasma gondii* with chloramphenicol acetyltransferase as selectable marker." *Sci,* Nov 5, 1993; 262: 911–914

Leech, JH et al, eds, *Contemporary Issues in Infectious Diseases. Parasitic Infections* (Vol 7); NY, NY: Churchill Livingstone, 1988

Lopez, A et al, "Preventing congenital toxoplasmosis." *MMRW,* Mar 31, 2000; 49(RR-2): 57–68

Lou P et al, "Ocular toxoplasmosis in three consecutive siblings." *Archives of Ophthalmology,* Apr 1978; 96(4): 613–614)

Luft, BJ et al, "Outbreak of central nervous system toxoplasmosis in Western Europe & North America." *Lancet* (I), Apr 9, 1983: 781–784

Luft, BJ & JS Remington, "Toxoplasmic encephalitis in AIDS." *Clin Infect Dis,* 1992; 15: 211–222

Marcus, LC, "Preventing & treating toxoplasmosis." *Drug Ther,* Mar 1983: 81–96

Maurin, M et al, "*Toxoplasma gondii* prevalence, United States." Lett. *Emerg Infect Dis,* Apr 2007; 13(4): 656–657

McBride, J, "Giving pork a new image." *Agric Res,* Aug 2000: 18–19

—— "Defining risk from meatborne parasites." *Agric Res,* May 2002: 20–21

Meissner, M et al, "Role of *Toxoplasma gondii* myosin A in powering parasite gliding & host cell invasion." Repts, *Sci,* Oct 25, 2002; 298: 837–840

Moorthy, RS et al, "Progressive ocular toxoplasmosis in patients with acquired immunodeficiency syndrome. *Am J Opthalmol,* 1993; 115: 742–747

Moura, Lenildo de et al, "Waterborne toxoplasmosis, Brazil: from field to gene." Dispatches. *Emerg Infect Dis,* Feb 2000; 12(2): 326–329

Mullens, A, "I think we have a problem in Victoria: MDs respond quickly to toxoplasmosis outbreak in BC [British Columbia]." *Can Med Assoc J,* June 1996; 154(11): 1721–1724

Murrell, RD, "Parasites: the problems persist." Forum. *Agric Res,* Dec 1996: 2

Niebuhr D et al, "Selected infectious agents and risk of schizophrenia among U.S. military personnel." *American Journal of Psychiatry,* Jan 2008; 165:99–106

Nordin, BEC et al, "Central nervous system toxoplasmosis & hemolytic uremic syndrome." Corresp. *N Engl J Med,* Dec 10, 1987; 317(24): 1540–1541

"Nurse group warns of toxoplasmosis. *Am Med News,* Feb 1, 1985: 28

Nussenblatt, RB et al, "Ocular toxoplasmosis, an old disease revisited." *JAMA,* Jan 26, 1994; 271(4): 304–307

Paradisi, F et al, ""Is fast food toxo-food?" Corresp. *N Engl J Med,* Oct 24, 1985; 313: 1092

"Parasites favor boys?" Constance Holden, Random Samples. Constance Holden, ed. *Sci,* Oct 20, 2006: 314(5798): 395

Pons, JC et al, "Congenital toxoplasmosis: mother-to-fetus transmission of pre-pregnancy infection." *Presse Med,* 1995; 24: 179–182

Porter, SB & MA Sande, "Toxoplasmosis of the central nervous system in the acquired immunodeficiency syndrome." *N Engl J Med,* 1992; 237: 1643–1648

"Primary toxoplasmosis in pregnancy a threat to fetus." *Med Trib,* July 27, 1983: 2

Raloff, J, "Another hazard in undercooked pork." *Sci News,* July 19, 1986: 37

—— "Lethal look-alike unmasked, examined." *Sci News,* July 29, 1989: 71

Remington, JS, "Routes of contagion for toxoplasmosis." Q/A. *Med Aspects Human Sexuality,* Sept 1984; 18(9): 17

Rhoden, WC, "Ashe says he has AIDS from a transfusion." *NY Times,* Apr 8, 1992: B1

Roberts, T et al, "Estimating income losses & other preventable costs caused by congenital toxoplasmosis in people in the U.S." *J Am Vet Med Assoc,* 1990; 196: 249–256

Rovner, S, "Pet-borne illnesses & unsuspecting owners." Healthtalk. *Wash Post Health,* July 17, 1990: 11

Sachs, JJ, "Transmission of toxoplasmosis in the family." Q/A. *Med Aspects Human Sexuality,* July 1985; 19(7): 16

Saeij, JPJ et al, "Polymorphic secreted kinases are key virulence factors in toxoplasmosis." Repts. *Sci,* Dec 15, 2006; 314:1780–1783

Segal, M, "Parasitic invaders & the reluctant human host." *FDA Consumer,* July–Aug, 1993: 7–13

Shanks, G et al, "*Taxoplasma* encephalitis in an infant with acquired immunodeficiency syndrome." *Pediat Infect Dis,* 1987; 6: 70–71

Skolnick, AA, "Obtaining drug for AIDS-related toxoplasmosis." *JAMA,* Mar 3, 1993; 269(9): 1086

Su, C et al, "Recent expansion of *oaxoplasma* through enhanced oral transmission." Repts. *Sci,* Jan 17, 2003; 299: 414–416

Suzuki, Y et al, "Interferon-(: the major mediator of resistance against *Taxoplasma gondii.*" Repts. *Sci,* Apr 22, 1988; 2401: 516–518

Taylor, S et al, "A secreted serine-threonine kinase determines virulence in the eukaryotic pathogen *Toxoplasma gondii.*" Repts. *Sci,* Dec 15, 2006; 314: 1776–1780

"*Toxoplasma gondii* costs seen outstripping other diseases." *Fd Chem News,* Nov 8, 1993: 15

"Toxoplasmosis widespread, costly, researcher says." *Fd Chem News,* Dec 20, 1993: 30

"Update: availability of sulfadiazine—U.S." Notice to Readers. *MMWR,* Feb 12, 1993; 42(5): 105

Vendrell, JP et al, "In-vitro synthesis of antibodies to *Toxoplasma gondii* by lymphocytes from HIV-1-infected patients." Short Repts. *Lancet,* July 3, 1993; 342: 22–23

Vogel, G, "Parasites shed light on cellular evolution." Cell Biology. *Sci,* Mar 7, 1997; 275: 14–22

Vyas A et al, "Behavioral changes induced by *Toxoplasma* infection of rodents are highly specific to aversion of cat odors." *Proceedings of the National Academy of Sciences,* Apr 2, 2007; 104(15): 6442–6447

Wallace, MR et al, "Cats & toxoplasmosis risk in HIV-infected adults." Brief Rept. *JAMA,* Jan 6, 1993; 269(1): 76–77

Wallon, M et al, "Congenital toxoplasmosis, assessment of prevention policy." *Presse Med,* 1994; 23: 1467–1470

Weinman, D et al, "Toxoplasmosis in man & swine—an investigation of the possible relationship." *JAMA,* 1956; 161: 229–232

Weisburd, S, "Prenatal toxoplasmosis tests: medical advances, backward policy?" *Sci News*, Feb 13, 1988; 133: 102–103

Williams, RD, "Healthy pregnancy, healthy baby." *FDA Consumer*, Mar–Apr 1999: 18–22

Work, K, "Toxoplasmosis with special reference to transmissions & life cycle of *Toxoplasma gondii*." *Acta Pathol Microbiol Immunol Scand* (B), 1971; Suppl 221: 1–51

Zimmer, C, "Parasites make scaredy-rats foolhardy." Evolution. *Sci*, July 28, 2000; 289: 525

—— "A common parasite's strongest asset: it's stealth." *NY Times*, June 20, 2006: F6

Chapter 8

Altman, LK, "Cheese microbe underscores mystery." The Doctor's World. *NY Times*, July 2, 1985: C3

Anderson, G et al, "Update: foodborne listeriosis in United States, 1988–1990." Epidemiol Notes Repts. *MMWR*, Apr 17, 1992; 41(15): 251–258

Aronin, S et al, "*Listeria monocytogenes* Rhombencephalitis in a patient on immunosuppressive therapy." *Conn Med*, Nov 1992; 56(1): 620

Aureli, P et al, "An outbreak of febrile gastroenteritis associated with corn contaminated by *Listeria monocytogenes*." *N Engl J Med*, 2000; 342: 1236–1241

Bader, JM, "Listeriosis epidemic." *Lancet*, Sept 4, 1993; 342(8871): 607

Barnes, R et al, "Listeriosis associated with consumption of turkey franks." Epidemiol Notes Repts. *MMWR*, Apr 21, 1989; 38(15): 267–268

Barry, B, "The Listeria control game plan: where are we now?" *Fd Safety Mag*, June–July 2007: 36–38, 40, 42–44, 46–47

Berger, A, "Cheese please but don't chill it." *New Scientist*, June 10, 1995; 146 (1981): 5

Bernard, DT & VN Scott, "*Listeria monocytogenes* in meats; new strategies are needed." Back Page. *Fd Tech*, Mar 1999: 1241

Beverly, RL & ME James, "Pathogenic survivors tracking *Listeria monocytogenes* on ready-to-eat meat products at freezer temperatures." *Fd Qual*, Oct–Nov 2005; 30: 32–34

Blackman, IC and Frank, JF, "Growth of *Listeria monocytogenes* as a biofilm on various food-processing surfaces." *Journal of Food Protection*, 1996; 59: 827–831

Blumenthal, D et al, "Unsanitary sandwich firm gets FDA's attention." Investigators' Repts. *FDA Consumer*, Oct 1990: 35–36

Bologna, MJ, "Grand jury investigating circumstances surrounding recent listeriosis outbreaks." Enforcement. *Fd Safety Rept*, Mar 24, 1999: 270–271

Brody, JE, "Despite strides, *Listeria* needs vigilance." Personal Health. *NY Times*, Oct 16, 2007: D8

Buchanan, RL et al, "Non-thermal inactivation models for *Listeria monocytogenes*." *J Fd Sci*, Jan–Feb 1994; 59 (1): 179–188

Burros, M, "A food-borne illness that still isn't getting the attention it deserves." Eating Well. *NY Times*, Jan 27, 1999: D5

—— *Listeria* thrives in a political hotbed." Eating Well. *NY Times*, Oct 30, 2003: D6

—— "Experts concerned about return of deadly bacteria in cold cuts." *NY Times*, Mar 14, 1999; NE 1: 23

Calder, J, "*Listeria* meningitis in adults." *Lancet*, Aug 2, 1997; 350(9074): 307

"Can shipping conditions influence your *Listeria* test results?" *Fd Safety Mag*, Apr–May 2005: 46

Carey, C et al, "*Listeria* a la mode." Investigators' Repts. *FDA Consumer*, Feb 1989: 43

Ciesielski, Carol A, "Listeriosis in the United States 1980–1982." *Arch Intern Med*, 1988; 148: 1416–1419

"Combination meat processing plant doesn't duck *Listeria* testing." *Fd Safety Mag*, Apr–May 2005: 50

Cooke, L, "Food poisoning cases linked to DNA fingerprints." *Agric Res*, Oct 1992: 24–26

"Cornell scientists report *Listeria* persistence." *Fd Safety Mag*, Aug–Sept 2004: 11

Dalton, CB, "An outbreak of gastroenteritis and fever due to *Listeria monocytogenes* in milk." *N Engl J Med*, Jan 9, 1997; 336(2): 100–105

Datta, AR, "Probes for identifying *Listeria*." Lett. *JAMA*, Sept 22–29, 1989; 262(12): 1629

Day, D, "Add listeriosis to the list of fever, abortion causes." *Med Trib*, Oct 2, 1985: 7

Dealler, SF and Lacey RW, "Superficial microwave heating." *Nature*, Apr 5, 1990; 344: 496

Decatur, AL & DA Portnoy, "A PEST-like [pore-forming protein-listerolysis] O essential for *Listeria monocytogenes* pathogenicity." *Sci*, Nov 3, 2000; 290(5493): 992–995

"Deli items may dish up dose of *Listeria*," *FDA Consumer*, July–Aug 1992: 8–12

Donnelly, CW, "*Listeria*—an emerging food-borne pathogen." *Nutr Today*, Sept–Oct 1990; 25(5): 7–11

—— [interview with] "Getting a handle on *Listeria*." Inside Microbiol. *Fd Safety Mag*, Dec 2002–Jan 2003: 18, 20–22, 24, 26–27

—— "Controlling *Listeria*, environmental plate technology hunts down all species." In the Lab, Raw Materials. *Fd Qual*, Apr–May 2006: 50, 52, 54–55

Doyle, MP, "Should regulatory agencies reconsider the policy of zero-tolerance of *Listeria monocytogenes* in all ready-to-eat foods?" *Fd Safety Notebk*, Oct–Nov 1991: 89–91

Dunn, GA, "*Listeria* detection, isolation & confirmation." In the Lab. Lab Analysis. *Fd Qual*, Feb–Mar 2005: 46, 48, 50

Fabricant, F, "Tracking bad brie," Fd Notes. *NY Times*, Apr 16, 1986: C9

Fackelmann, KA, "When refrigerator fare turns foul." *Sci News*, Apr 18, 1992: 247

"Factors contribute to *Listeria* virulence." *Fd Prod Design*, Sept 2003: 25

Fairchild, T M & PM Foegeding, "A proposed nonpathogenic biological indicator for thermal inactivation of *Listeria*." *Appl Environ Microbiol*, Apr 1993; 59(4): 1247–1250

"FDA & FSIS issue *Listeria* health advisory." Updates. *FDA Consumer*, Nov–Dec 2002: 5

"FDA checking imported, domestic shrimp, crabmeat for *Listeria*." *Fd Chem News*, Aug 17, 1987: 15–17

"Filters hold key to preventing *Listeria* contamination at dairy plant." *Fd Engineer,* June 1989: 119

Finlay, BB, "Cracking *Listeria*'s password." Perspectives: Microbiol. *Sci,* June 1, 2001; 292 (5522): 1665–1667

"Firms in Canada, U.S., remove products that may contain *Listeria,* USDA announces." Recalls. *Fd Safety Rept,* Feb 10, 1999: 81

Fleming, DW, "Pasteurized milk as a vehicle of infection in an outbreak of listeriosis." *N Engl J Med,* 1985; 312: 404–407

Floyd, B, "Increasing *Listeria* awareness." Tech Support. *Fd Prod Design,* May 2005: 93–97

Foodborne Listeriosis. Proceedings of Problems of Foodborne Listeriosis. European Symposium, Wiesbaden, Fed Rep Germany, Sept 7, 1968. Lancaster, PA: Technomic Pub, 1990

"Food Safety." Updates. *FDA Consumer,* Sept–Oct 1998: 4

Forgey, R, "The return of *Listeria,* recent outbreaks cause renewed interest." Inside Microbiol. *Fd Test Analysis,* June–July 1999; 10: 12

Foulke, JE, "Fish firm ordered to clean up." *FDA Consumer,* Jan–Feb 1993: 30–31

"FSIS adopts scanning method for *Listeria monocytogenes.*" *Fd Safety Mag,* June–July 2002: 32

"FSIS strengthens regulations to reduce *Listeria monocytogenes* in ready-to-eat meat & poultry products." *Fd Safety Mag,* June–July 2003: 8

Gale, SF, "Beating *Listeria:* Specialty Brand's aggressive approach." Case Studies Fd Protection. *Fd Safety Mag,* Dec 2003–Jan 2004: 30–32

Gall, K [interview with] "Industry collaboration advances *Listeria* control in RTE [ready-to-eat] seafood plants." *Fd Safety Mag,* Aug–Sept 2005: 52, 54, 63–64

Gellin, BG & CV Broome, "Listeriosis." State of the Art/Review. *JAMA,* Mar 3, 1989; 261(9): 1313–1320

Gillespie, IA, "Changing pattern of human listeriosis, England & Wales 2001–2004." *Emerg Infect Dis,* Sept 2006; 12(9): 1361–1366

Glaser, P et al, "Comparative genomics of *Listeria* species." Repts. *Sci,* Oct 26, 2001; 294 (5543): 849–852

Gombas, DE et al, "Survey of *Listeria monocytogenes* in ready-to-eat foods." *J Fd Protect,* Apr 2003; 66: 559–569

Goulet, V et al, "Effect of prevention measures in incidence of human listeriosis, France, 1987–1997." Research. *Emerg Infect Dis,* Nov–Dec 2001; 7(6): 983–988

Grinstead, Dale, "The reputation drain, *Listeria* lurks in store drains & can damage store image if not controlled properly." In the Lab. Raw Materials. *Fd Qual,* Feb–Mar 2007; 42: 44

Hardy, J et al, "Extracellular replication of *Listeria monocytogenes* in the marine gall bladder" Repts. *Sci,* Feb 6, 2004; 303: 851–853

Henkel, J, "Sandwich maker enjoined." Investigators' Repts. *FDA Consumer,* Oct 1993: 37–38

Hernández, D, "6 in New York region die of listeriosis, a food-borne illness." New York Rept. *NY Times,* Sept 17, 2002: B1

Higgins, KT, "Pasteurization in a flash, a burst of steam & a jigger of bactericide in a high-speed packaging machine might provide hot-dog packers with a *Listeria monocytogenes*-silver bullet." Engineer R&D. *Fd Engineer*, Jan 2007: 167–168

Ho, JL et al, "An outbreak of Type 4b *Listeria monocytogenes* infection involving patients from eight Boston hospitals." *Arch Intern Med*, Mar 1986; 146: 520–524

Hunter, BT, "Listeriosis." *Consumers' Research Mag*, Nov 1991: 8–9

Hurd, S et al, "Multistate outbreak of listeriosis—United States, 2000." *MMWR*, Dec 22, 2000; 49(50): 1129–1130

Iwanicki, S, "Fighting *Listeria*." Tech Support, *Fd Prod Design*, Mar 2007: 81–82, 87

James, SM et al, "Listeriosis outbreak associated with Mexican-style cheese—California." Epidemiol Notes Repts. *MMWR*, June 21, 1985; 34(24): 357–359

Johnson, JL et al, "*Listeria monocytogenes* & other *Listeria ssp.* in meat & meat products. A review." *J Fd Protect*, Dec 1989; 52(12): 81

Joy, D, "New rules on reporting contamination." Regulatory Issues. *Fd Proc*, Nov 2007: 13

"Key steps to a total *Listeria* testing solution." *Fd Safety Mag*, Apr–May 2005: 46

Kim, KT et al, "Heating & storage conditions affect survival & recovery of *Listeria monocytogenes* in ground pork." *J Fd Sci*, Jan–Feb 1994; 59(1): 30–32

Kraft, AA, *Psychrotrophic Bacteria & Foods: Disease & Spoilage*. Boca Raton, FL: CRC Press, 1992

La Budde, RA, "Ready-to-eat finished product sample & test plan for *Listeria monocytogenes*." Inside Microbiol. *Fd Test Analysis*, Oct–Nov 1999: 14–16

Lambert, V, "Contaminated crab meat cleanup." *FDA Consumer* Apr 1993: 36–37

Lauer, WF. "Detecting *Listeria monocytogenes*." News Notes. *Fd Qual*, Sept–Oct 2003: 8

Lawrence, LM et al, "Development of a random amplification of polymorphic DNA typing method for *Listeria monocytogenes*." Notes. *Appl Environ Microbiol*, Sept 1993; 59(9): 3117–3119

Lecos, C, "FDA, FSIS Statement on CDC *Listeria* study." *Talk Paper*, Rockville, MD: FDA, Apr 14, 1992

Lecuit, M et al, "A transgenic model for listeriosis: role of internalin in crossing the intestinal barrier." Repts. *Sci*, June 1, 2001; 292 (5522): 1722–1725

Liewen, MB & NW Plautz, "Occurrence of *Listeria monocytogenes* in raw milk in Nebraska." *J Fd Protect*, Nov 1988; 51(11): 840

"*Listeria*." New Analysis. *Fd Tech*, Dec 2003: 8

"*Listeria* action plan, risk assessment released for comments." In the News. *Inside Lab Manage*, Mar–Apr 2001: 7

"*Listeria* getting out of hand." *Fd Qual*, Sept–Oct 2002: 12–13

Listeria guidelines for industry. USDA, FSIS, May 1999

Listeria monocytogenes. FSIS Background. Wash, DC: USDA, Mar 1992

"*Listeria* sequence completed." *Fd Prod Design*, Aug 2001: 21

Lowe, DS, "Minimizing microbes on fresh-cut foods." *Agric Res,* June 1999: 10–12

Manning, T, "*Listeria monocytogenes:* know your enemy. We have seen the enemy & it is our coolers. And our drains." Safety & Sanit. Sanit Tech. *Fd Qual,* Feb–Mar 2004: 79–80, 82

Mascola, L et al, "Listeriosis: a previously unreported medical complication in women with multiple gestations." *Am J Obstet Gynecol,* May 1994; 170(5): Part I, 1328–1332

McCarthy, SA, "Attachment of *Listeria monocytogenes* to chitin & resistance to biocides." *Fd Tech,* Dec 1992: 84–87

McGee, H, "Tainted cheeses: how dangerous?" *NY Times,* Aug 27, 1986: C13

McGinnis, L, "New methods for detecting *Listeria.*" *Agric Res,* Oct 2006: 13

"Meat industry groups issue guidance on *Listeria* in ready-to-eat products. *Listeria. Fd Safety Rept,* Apr 28, 1999: 387–388

Miller, RK & GR Acuff, "Sodium lactate affects pathogens in cooked beef." *J Fd Sci,* Jan–Feb 1994; 59(1): 15–19

Mitchell, M, "The evaluation of novel antimicrobial ingredients in maintaining the safety & shelf-life of refrigerated foods." *Fd Safety Mag,* Apr–May 2006: 58, 60, 62–65

"Mousing out pathogens." Sci Technol Concentrates. *Chem Engineer News,* June 11, 2007: 29

Myers, ER et al, "Sodium chloride, potassium chloride, & virulence in *Listeria monocytogenes.*" *Appl Environ Microbiol,* July 1993; 59(7): 2082–2086

Nickelson, N & CW Schmidt, "Taking the hysteria out of *Listeria:* the mechanisms of *Listeria* & strategies to find it." *Fd Qual,* Apr 1999: 28, 30–32, 34, 36–38

Nightingale, SL, "Efforts to prevent foodborne listeriosis." From FDA. *JAMA,* July 8, 1992; 268(2): 180

O'Donnell, CD, "Solving salad bar *Listeria.*" R & D Horizons. *Prep Fds,* May 1993: 45–46

Ohr, LM, "Building a safety net for meats." Info Ingred Challenges. Fd Foundations. *Prep Fds,* June 2002: 55–56, 58

"Outbreak of listeriosis—Northeastern United States, 2002." Pub Health Dispatch. *MMWR,* Oct 23, 2002; 51(42): 950–951

"Pasteurized milk a culprit in disease." *Sci News,* Mar 2, 1985: 141

Pennisi, E, "*Listeria* enlists host in its attack." Microbiol. *Sci,* Nov 3, 2000; 290: 915–916

Perl, P, "Packaged poison, why did regulations act so slowly in a deadly case of food contamination?" Wkly Ed. *Wash Post,* Jan 24, 2000: 6–10

Pinner, RW et al, "Role of foods in sporadic listeriosis. II. Microbiologic & epidemiologic investigation." *JAMA,* Apr 1992; 267(15): 2046–2050

Preventing Foodborne Listeriosis. Background. Wash, DC: USDA/FSIS/DHHS/FDA, Mar 1992, rev Apr 1992

Rado, C, "Preventing *Listeria* contamination in foods." *FDA Consumer,* Jan–Feb 2004: 10–11

Raupe, B, "Modern production methods increase risk of *Listeria* problem, scientist says." Listeria. *Fd Safety Rept,* May 6, 1999: 428

"Research on *Listeria monocytogenes.*" *FDA Drug Bull,* Oct 1987: 28

Rouhi, M, "Breaching the intestinal wall, pathogen crosses intestinal barrier with help from a surface protein." News of Wk. Sci. *Chem Engineer News*, June 4, 2001: 13

Roy, B et al, "Biological inactivitation of adhering *Listeria monocytogenes* by *Listeria*-phages & a quaternary ammonium compound." *Appl Environ Microbiol*, Sept 1993; 59(9): 2914–2917

Ryser, ET et al, *Listeria, Listeriosis & Food Safety*. NY, NY: Marcel Dekker, 1991

Saguy, I, "Simulated growth of *Listeria monocytogenes* in refrigerated foods stored at variable temperatures." *Fd Tech*, Mar 1992: 69–71

Salamina, G et al, "A foodborne outbreak of gastroenteritis involving *Listeria monocytogenes*" *Epidemiol Infect*, Dec 1996; 117(3): 429–436

Schaack, MM et al, "Survival of *Listeria monocytogenes* in refrigerated cultured milks & yogurts." *J Fd Protect*, Nov 1988; 51(11): 848

Schildhouse, J et al, "Reducing *Listeria* risk." News. *Fd Prod Design*, Apr 2001: 25–26

Schlech, III, WF, "Listeriosis, new pieces to an old puzzle." Lett. *Arch Intern Med*, Mar 1986; 146(3): 459–460

—— "Expanding the horizons of foodborne listeriosis." *JAMA*, Apr 15, 1992; 267(15): 2081–2082

—— "*Listeria* gastroenteritis—old syndrome, new pathogen." Ed'al. *N Engl J Med*, Jan 9, 1997; 336(2): 130–132

Schuchat, A et al, "Role of foods in sporadic listeriosis. I. Case-control study of dietary risk factors." Orig Contrib. *JAMA*, Apr 15, 1992; 267(15): 2041–2050

"Scientists design *Listeria* sensor." *Fd Prod Design*, Dec 2004: 29

Siegman-Igra, Y et al, "*Listeria monocytogenes* infection in Israel & review of cases worldwide." Research. *Emerg Infect Dis*, Mar 2002; 6(3): 305–310

Silverman, J, "Virulence differences exist among strains of *Listeria*, New York research concludes." Research. *Fd Safety Rept*, Feb 24, 1999: 139–140

—— "*Listeria* action plan, new technologies needed to address health concern, officials say." News. *Fd Safety Rept*, Feb 17, 1999: 101–102

—— "USDA Advisory Group recommends methods for tracking, analyzing *Listeria*," News. *Fd Safety Rept*, Mar 3, 1999: 163–164

Skinner, KJ, "*Listeria*, battling back against one 'tough bug.'" *FDA Consumer*, Aug 1988: 12–15

Smith, S, "Mass. Dairy shuts after product is linked to 2 deaths." *Boston Globe*, Dec 28, 2007: A1

Snelling, AM et al, "The survival of *Listeria monocytogenes* on fingertips & factors affecting elimination of the organism by handwashing & disinfection." *J Fd Protect*, May 1991; 54(5): 343–348

Stapleton, S, "Perils of food poisoning, outbreaks of illness from foodborne organisms such as *Listeria* highlight physicians' role in the public health response." Health Sci. *Am Med News*, Mar 22–29, 1999: 35

Swanson, KMJ, "*L. monocytogenes* challenge study 'How to' guidelines." Testing. *Fd Safety Mag*, Apr–May 2005: 12, 14–17

Sweintek, B, "Symposium: *Listeria monocytogenes.*" *Prep Fds*, Sept 1999: 48

Tappero, JW et al, "Reduction in the incidence of human listeriosis in the U.S.: Effectiveness of prevention efforts." *JAMA*, Apr 12, 1995; 273(14): 1118–1122

"Three cheese industry executives jailed over *Listeria* deaths from their products." *Fd Safety Rept*, June 2, 1999: 548–549

"Tyson Foods recalls frozen burritos because of possible contamination." Recalls. *Fd Safety Rept*, Feb 17, 1999: 111

"Update: listeriosis & pasteurized milk." Epidemiol Notes Repts. *MMWR*, Dec 15, 1988; 37(49): 764–766

"Update: Multistate outbreak of listeriosis—United States, 1998–1999." *MMWR*, Jan 8, 1999; 47(51–52): 1117–1118

Voelker, R, "Listeriosis outbreak prompts action—finally." Med News Perspect. *JAMA*, Dec 4, 2002; 288(21): 2675–2676

Wickelgren, I, "Lethal *Listeria* surfaces on fresh vegetables." *Sci News*, Aug 19, 1989, 169

Williams, M et al, "Special report: *Listeria*, 12 deaths, 79 illnesses traced to meat from Michigan Sara Lee plant." *Fd Safety Rept*, Jan 27, 1999: 32–33

Wolski, M, "Kohler Mix Specialties recalls reduced fat milk made for Land O' Lakes." Recalls. *Fd Safety Rept*, Feb 10, 1999: 80–81

Woteki, CE. "Dieticians can prevent listeriosis." For Yr Info. *J Am Diet Assoc*, Mar 2001: 285

Wong, HC et al, "Incidence & characterization of *Listeria monocytogenes* in foods available in Taiwan." *Appl Environ Microbiol*, Oct 1990; 56(10): 3101–3104

Chapter 9

Anderson, L et al, "Norovirus activity—United States 2002." *MMWR* Jan 24, 2003; 52(3): 41–45

Aristaguieta, C et al, "Multistate outbreak of viral gastroenteritis associated with consumption of oysters—Apalachicola Bay, Florida, December 1994–January 1995." Epidemiol Notes Repts. *MMWR*, Jan 20, 1995; 44(2): 37–39

Arness, M, "Norwalk-like viral gastroenteritis in U.S. Army trainees—Texas, 1998." *MMWR*, Mar 26, 1999; 48(11): 225–227

Becker, KM et al, "Transmission of Norwalk virus during a football game." *N Engl J Med*, 2000; 343: 1223–1227

Beller, M et al, "Outbreak of viral gastroenteritis due to a contaminated well, international consequences." *JAMA*, Aug 20, 1997; 278(7): 563–568

Blevins, L, "An outbreak of norovirus gastroenteritis at a swimming club—Vermont 2004." *MMWR*, Sept 3, 2004; 53(34): 793–795

Boccia, D, "Waterborne outbreak of Norwalk-like virus gastroenteritis at a tourist resort, Italy." Research. *Emerg Infect Dis*, June 2002; 8(8): 563–568

Bohm, SR et al, "Norovirus outbreak associated with ill food-service workers—Michigan, January–February 2006." *MMWR*, Nov 23, 2007; 56(46): 1212–1216

"Brief Notes." *Fd Chem News*, Jan 27, 1997, 43; Apr 7, 1997, 42; Apr 14, 1997, 29; June 15, 1998, 30; Feb 21, 2000, 31

Brown, D et al, "Outbreak of acute gastroenteritis associated with Norwalk-like viruses among British military personnel—Afghanistan, May 2002." *MMWR*, June 7, 2002; 51(22): 477–480

"CDC says routine H2O monitoring didn't detect Norwalk virus." *Fd Chem News*, July 4, 1994: 7–8

Chan, M et al, "Fecal viral load & norovirus-associated gastroenteritis." Dispatches. *Emerg Infect Dis*, Aug 2006; 12(8): 1278–1280

—— "Cell culture assay for human noroviruses." Lett. *Emerg Infect Dis*, July 2007; 13(7): 1117

Chandler, B et al, "Outreaks of Norwalk-like viral gastroenteritis—Alaska & Wisconsin, 1999." *MMWR*, Mar 17, 2000; 49(10): 207–211

Cheek, JE et al, "Norwalk-like virus-associated gastroenteritis in a large, high-density encampment—Virginia, July 2001." *MMWR*, Aug 2, 2002; 51(30): 661–663

Cliver, DO, "Virus transmission via food" *IFT Scientific Status Summary. Expert Panel on Food Safety & Nutrition. Fd Tech*, Apr 1997: 71–77 [revision from Oct 1988]

"Coleslaw served at restaurant linked to Mississippi foodborne outbreak." *Fd Chem News*, Feb 5, 1996: 11

Collins, J, "Cloning of virus that causes diarrheal epidemics." *National Research Resources Reporter*, NIH, Aug 1991: 8–9

Colomba, C et al, "Norovirus & gastroenteritis in hospitalized children, Italy." *Emerg Infect Dis*, Sept 2007; 13(9): 1389–1391

Conlon, L et al, "Norwalk-like virus outbreaks at two summer camps—Wisconsin, June 2001." PH Dispatch. *MMWR*, Aug 2, 2001; 50(30): 642–643

Conrad, C et al, "Multistate outbreak of viral gastroenteritis related to consumption of oysters—Louisiana, Maryland, Mississippi, & North Carolina, 1993." Epidemiol Notes Repts. *MMWR*, Dec 17, 1993; 42(49): 945–948

Cromeans, TL, "Understanding & preventing virus transmission via foods." Sci Communications. *Fd Tech*, Apr 1997: 20

Davis, C et al, "Gastroenteritis associated with consumption of raw oysters—Florida, 1993." *MMWR*, June 24, 1994; 43(24): 446–448

Diggs, R et al, "Norovirus outbreak in an elementary school—District of Columbia, February 2007." *MMWR*, Jan 4, 2008; 56(51 & 52): 1340–1345

Du Pont, HL, "Consumption of raw shellfish—is the risk now unacceptable?" Ed'al. *N Engl J Med*, Mar 13, 1986; 314(11): 707–708

—— "Clam-associated gastroenteritis." Corresp. *N Engl J Med*, Aug 28, 1986; 315(9): 584

Enserink, M, "Gastrointestinal virus strikes European cruise ships" Infect Dis. *Sci*, Aug 11, 2006; 313: 747

Filipic, M, "Virus is top cause of food-borne illness." *Chow Line*. [News release] Wooster, Ohio: Ohio State U, Mar 3, 2002

Glasscock, S et al, "Multistate outbreak of norovirus gastroenteritis among attendees at a family reunion—Grant County, West Virginia, October 2006. *MMWR*, July 13, 2007; 56(27): 673–677

Grahame, DY et al, "Norwalk virus infection of volunteers: new insights based on improved assays." *J Infect Dis*, July 1994; 170(1): 34–43

Gunn, RA et al, "Norwalk virus gastroenteritis aboard a cruise ship: outbreak on five consecutive cruises." *Am J Epidemiol*, 1980; 112(8): 820–827

Herwaldt, BL et al, "Waterborne-disease outbreaks 1989–1990, CDC Surveillance Summaries." *MMWR*, 1991; 40(SS–3): 1–13

Hunter, BT, "Eating raw seafood." *Consumers' Research Mag*, June 1985: 8–9

—— "A foodborne viral illness." *Consumers' Research Mag*, Aug 1989: 8–9

—— "A food safety primer: the risky nature of the Norwalk virus." *Consumers' Research Mag*, July 2001: 21

Isakbaeva, ET et al, "Norovirus transmission on cruise ship." Dispatches. *Emerg Infect Dis*, Jan 2005; 11(1): 154–157

Jenkins, P et al, "Norovirus activity—United States 2006–2007." *MMWR*, Aug 24, 2007; 56(33): 842–846

Jiang, X et al, "Norwalk virus genome cloning & characterization." *Sci*, Dec 14, 1990; 250: 1580–1583

Johnston, JM, "Clam-associated gastroenteritis." Corresp. *N Engl J Med*, Aug 28, 1986; 315(9): 583

Kapikian, AZ, "Virus gastroenteritis." Grand Rounds at Clin Center NIH, Saul Rosen, ed. Section ed. *JAMA*, Feb 3, 1993; 269(5): 627–630

Karst, SM et al, "STAT1-dependent innate immunity to a Norwalk-like virus." *Sci*, Mar 7, 2003; 299: 1575–1578

Kohn, MA et al, "An outbreak of Norwalk virus gastroenteritis associated with eating raw oysters: implications for maintaining safe oyster beds." *JAMA*, Feb 8, 1995; 273(6): 466–471

Kurtzwell, P, "Critical steps toward safer seafood," *FDA Consumer*, Nov–Dec 1997: 10–14

Lambden, PR et al, "Sequence & genome organization of a human small round-structured (Norwalk-like) virus." *Sci*, Jan 22, 1993; 259: 516–519

Lee, N et al, "Fecal viral concentration & diarrhea in norovirus gastroenteritis." *Emerg Infect Dis*, Sept 2007; 13(9): 1399–1401

Le Guyader, FS et al, "Norwalk virus-specific binding in oyster digestive tissues." Research. *Emerg Infect Dis*, June 2006; 12(6): 931–936

"Louisiana oysters are recalled after 389 illnesses tied to consumption." *Fd Chem News*, Jan 13, 1997: 19–20

Mattison, K, "Human noroviruses in swine & cattle." Research. *Emerg Infect Dis*, Aug 2007; 13(8): 1184–1188

Maunula, L et al, "Norovirus outbreaks from drinking water." Research. *Emerg Infect Dis*, Nov 2005; 11(11): 1716–1721

McDonnell, S et al, "Failure of cooking to prevent shellfish-associated gastroenteritis." *Arch Intern Med,* Jan 13, 1997; 157(1): 111–116

Miller, RW, "Get hooked on seafood safety." *FDA Consumer,* June 1991: 7–11

Morse, DL et al, "Widespread outbreaks of clam- & oyster-associated gastroenteritis: role of Norwalk virus." *N Engl J Med,* 1986; 314(9): 678–681

——— "Clam-associated gastroenteritis." Corresp. *N Engl J Med,* Aug 28, 1986; 315(9): 583

"Norwalk-like virus believed cause of Canadian oyster cases." *Fd Chem News,* Aug 2, 1993, 16

"Norwalk-like viruses: public health consequences & outbreak management." *MMWR,* June 1, 2001; 50(RR9): [Recommendations & Reports]

Osvath, R, "Norwalk virus outbreaks reported in Florida—FDA." *Fd Chem News,* Jan 31, 2000: 4–5

"Outbreak of Norwalk illnesses tied to oyster harvester." *Fd Chem News,* June 27, 1994: 47–48

Papaventsis, DC et al, "Norovirus infection in children with acute gastroenteritis, Madagascar, 2004–2005." Dispatches. *Emerg Infect Dis,* June 2007; 13(6): 908–911

Parmley, MA, "Introducing the Norwalk virus." *Fd News for Consumers, USDA,* Winter 1989; 5(4): 6–7

Payne, JK et al, "Multisite outbreak of norovirus associated with a franchise restaurant—Kent County, Michigan, May 2005." *MMWR,* Apr 14, 2006; 55(14): 395–397

Prasad, B et al, "X-ray crystallographic structure of the Norwalk virus capsid." *Sci,* Oct 8, 1999; 286: 287–290

Roper, WI, "Centers for Disease Control: diseases transmitted through the food supply: *Fed Register,* Sept 8, 1992; 57(174): 40917

"Science roundup." *Chem Engineer News,* July 24, 2000: 35

Siebenga, JJ et al, "Gastroenteritis caused by norovirus GG11.4, the Netherlands, 1994–2005." Dispatches. *Emerg Infect Dis,* Jan 2007; 13(1): 144–146

Soares, CC et al, "Norovirus detection & genotyping for children with gastroenteritis, Brazil." Dispatches. *Emerg Infect Dis,* Aug 2007; 13(8): 1244–1246

Straub, TM et al, "In vitro cell culture infectivity assay for human noroviruses." Research. *Emerg Infect Dis,* Mar 2007; 13(2): 396–403

Tu, ET et al, "Norovirus G11.4 strains & outbreaks, Australia." Lett. *Emerg Infect Dis,* July 2007; 13(7): 1128–1129

Vogt, RL et al, "Clam-associated gastroenteritis." Corresp. *N Engl J Med,* Aug 28, 1986; 315(9): 582–583

Wang, QH et al, "Porcine noroviruses related to human noroviruses." Research. *Emerg Infect Dis,* Dec 2005; 11(12): 1874–1881

Warner, RD et al, "A large nontypical outbreak of Norwalk virus: gastroenteritis associated with exposing celery to nonpotable water & with *Citrobacter freundii.* Original Invest. *Arch Intern Med,* Dec 1991; 151(2): 2419–2424

Widdowson, MA et al, "Norovirus & foodborne disease, United States, 1991–2000." Research. *Emerg Infect Dis*, Jan 2005; 11(1): 95–102

—— "Are noroviruses emerging?" Comment. *Emerg Infect Dis*, May 2005; 11(5): 735–737

Chapter 10

Ahmed, HM et al, "Molecular characterization of rotavirus gastroenteritis strains, Iraqi Kurdistan." Dispatches. *Emerg Infect Dis*, May 2006; 12(5): 824–826

Ahmed, K et al, "Rotavirus G5 [6] in child with diarrhea, Vietnam." Dispatches. *Emerg Infect Dis*, Aug 2007; 13(8): 1232–1235

Ball, JM et al, "Age-dependent diarrhea induced by a rotaviral nonstructural glycoprotein," *Sci*, Apr 5, 1996; 272: 101–104

Bányai, K et al, "Emergence of serotype G12 rotaviruses, Hungary." Dispatches. *Emerg Infect Dis*, June 2007; 13(6): 916–919

Bartz, C et al, "Prevention of murine rotavirus infection with chicken egg yolk immune globulins." *J Infect Dis*, Sept 1980; 142(3): 439–444

Bernstein, DI et al, "Evaluation of rhesus rotavirus monovalent and tetravalent reassortant vaccines in US children," *JAMA*, Apr 19, 1995; 273(15): 1191–1196

Bonrud, PA et al, "Viral gastroenteritis—South Dakota & New Mexico." Epidemiol Notes Repts. *MMWR*, Feb 12, 1988; 37(5): 69–71

Bosley, MT, "Laboratory-based surveillance for rotavirus—United States, July 1996–1997." *MMWR*; 46(46): 1092–1094

Buehler, JW et al, "Laboratory based surveillance for rotavirus—United States, July 1997 June 1998." *MMWR*, Nov 20, 1998; 47(45): 978, 980

Burns, JW et al, "Protective effect of rotavirus V86-specific IgA monoclonal antibodies that lack neutralizing activity." *Sci*, Apr 15, 1996; 272: 104–107

Centers for Disease Control and Prevention, "Recommended childhood immunization schedule—United States, 1999." *MMWR*, 1999, 48:12–16; *JAMA*, Feb 17, 1999 281(1): 601–602

"Child vaccine linked to bowel obstruction." Updates. *FDA Consumer*, Nov–Dec 1999: 2

Cohen, J, "Rethinking a vaccine's risk." News Focus. *Sci*, Aug 31, 2001; 292: 1576–1577

Cormier, DP et al, "Acute infantile gastroenteritis." *Conn Hlth Bull*, 1984, 98(1); 1985, 99(1): 89–93

Cunliffe, NA et al, "Expanding global distribution of rotavirus serotype G9; detection in Libya, Kenya, & Cuba." Dispatches. *Emerg Infect Dis*, Sept–Oct 2001; 7(5): 890–892

Danovaro-Holliday, MC et al, "Rotavirus vaccine & the news media, 1987–2001." Med Media. *JAMA*, Mar 20, 2002; 287(11): 1455–1462

De Grazia, S et al, "Canine origin G3P[3] rotavirus strain in child with acute gastroenteritis." Dispatches. *Emerg Infect Dis*, July 2007; 13(7): 1091–1093

Duffy, LC et al, "The effects of infant feeding on rotavirus-induced gastroenteritis: a prospective study." *Am J PH*, 1986; 76: 259–263

Dupuis, P, "An epidemic of viral gastroenteritis in elderly people." *Presse Medicale,* 1995; 24: 356–358

Edwards, D, "Infant diarrhea in research spotlight." Biomed. *Sci News,* Oct 17, 1987: 255

Ehresman, K et al, "Intussusception among recipients of rotavirus vaccine—United States, 1998–1999." *MMWR* July 16, 1999; 48(27): 577–581

Endara, P, "Symptomatic & subclinical infection with rotavirus P[8]G9, rural Ecuador." Res. *Emerg Infect Dis,* Apr 2007; 13(4): 574–580

"F.D.A. approves vaccine for childhood diarrhea." *NY Times,* Sept 1, 1998: D3

Fischer, TK et al, "Incidence & cost of rotavirus hospitalizations in Denmark." Res. *Emerg Infect Dis,* June 2007; 13(6): 855–859

Fletcher, M, "Foodborne outbreak of group A rotavirus gastroenteritis among college students—District of Columbia, March–April 2000." *MMWR,* Dec 22, 2000; 49(50): 1131–1133

Glass, RI et al, "Rotavirus vaccines: success by reassortment?" Perspect. *Sci,* Sept 2, 1994; 265: 1389–1391

—— "New lessons for rotavirus vaccine." *Sci,* Apr 5, 1996; 272: 46–48

Gurgel, RQ et al, "Predominance of rotavirus P[4]G2 in a vaccinated population, Brazil." Dispatches. *Emerg Infect Dis,* Oct 2007; 13: 1571–1573

Harder, B, "Checkmate for a child killer? Vaccine researchers close in on rotavirus." *Sci News,* Sept 27, 2003: 204–205

"High-dose rotavirus vaccine protects kids." *Sci News,* Oct 25, 1997: 263

Ho, MS et al, "Diarrheal deaths in American children. Are they preventable?" Original Contribut. *JAMA,* Dec 9, 1988; 260(22): 3281–3285

Holzel, H et al, "An outbreak of rotavirus infection among adults in a cardiology ward." *J Infect,* 1980; 2: 33–37

Hunter, BT, "Beware of rotavirus!" *Consumers' Res Mag,* July 2001: 8–9

"Improved method for rotavirus detection in raw milk proposed." *Fd Chem News,* Oct 16, 1995: 12

Kirkwood, C et al, "Rotavirus serotype G9P[8] & acute gastroenteritis outbreak in children, Northern Australia." Res. *Emerg Infect Dis,* Sept 2004; 10(9): 1593–1600

Lambert, M et al, "An outbreak of rotavirus gastroenteritis in a nursing home for senior citizens." *Can J PH,* 1991; 82: 351–353

LeBaron, CW et al, "Annual rotavirus epidemic patterns in North America. Results of a 5-year retrospective survey of 88 centers in Canada, Mexico, & the United States." Original Contribut. *JAMA,* Aug 22–29, 1990; 264(8): 983–988

Lundgren, O et al, "Role of the enteric nervous system in the fluid & electrolyte secretion of rotavirus diarrhea." *Sci,* Jan 21, 2000; 287: 491–495

Marwick, C, "Rotavirus vaccine a boon to children." Med News Perspect. *JAMA,* Feb 18, 1998; 279(7): 489–490

Nath, G et al, "Childhood diarrhea due to rotavirus in a community." *Indian J Med Res,* 1992; 95: 259–262

"Oral rotavirus vaccine success." Hlth Agencies Update. *JAMA*, Nov 19, 1997: 1563

Parashar, UD et al, "Progress toward rotavirus vaccines." Pub Forum, Pub Hlth. *Sci*, May 12, 2006; 312: 851–852

—— "Rotavirus." Synopses. *Emerg Infect Dis*, Oct–Dec, 1998; 4(4): 561–570

—— "Global illness & deaths caused by rotavirus disease in children." Res. *Emerg Infect Dis*, May 2003; 9(5): 565–572

—— "Rotavirus & severe childhood diarrhea." Dispatches. *Emerg Infect Dis*, Feb 2006; 12 (2): 304–306

—— "Prevention of Rotavirus Gastroenteritis Among Infants & Children. Recommendations of the Advisory Committee on Immunization Practices (ACIP)." *MMWR*, Aug 11, 2006; 55(RR–12)

Pérez SI et al, "Efficacy of the rhesus rotavirus-based quadrivalent vaccine & young children in Venezuela." *N Engl J Med*, Oct 23, 1997; 337: 1181–1187

Pun, SB et al, "Detection of G12 human rotaviruses in Nepal." Dispatches. *Emerg Infect Dis*, Mar 2007; 13(3): 482–484

"Quadrivalent rhesus rotavirus vaccine effective in children." *Cortlandt Forum*, Mar 1999: 25

Rahman, M et al, "Prevalence of G2P[4] & G128[6] rotavirus, Bangladesh." Res. *Emerg Infect Dis*, Jan 2007; 13(1): 18–24

"Report on rotavirus vaccine." Updates. *FDA Consumer*, July–Aug 1993, 3–4

Roberts, L, "Rotavirus vaccines' second chance. News Focus. *Sci*, Sept 24, 2004; 305: 1890–1893

"Rotavirus Vaccine for the Prevention of Rotavirus Gastroenteritis Among Children. Recommendation of the Advisory Committee on Immunization Practices (ACIP)." MMWR, Mar 19, 1999; 48(RR–2)

"Rotavirus Surveillance—United States, 1989–1990." Natl Rotavirus Surveillance System. *MMWR*, Feb 8, 1991; 40(5): 80–81, 87

Sánchez-Fauquier, A et al, "Human rotavirus G9 & G3 as major cause of diarrhea in hospitalized children, Spain." Res. *Emerg Infect Dis*, Oct 2006; 12(10): 1536–1541

Seppa, N, "DNA vaccines for rabies, rotavirus advance." *Sci News*, Aug 8, 1998: 85

Snyder, J, "Too many deaths from diarrhea." Ed'al. *JAMA*, Dec 9, 1988; 260(22): 3329

Sternberg, S, "Chance reveals deadly rotavirus secret." *Sci News*, Apr 6, 1996: 213

Tucker, AW et al, "Cost effectiveness analysis of a rotavirus immunization program for the United States." *JAMA*, May 6, 1998; 279(17): 1371–1376

"Vaccines not immune to criticism about safety." *AMA Med News*, Aug 2, 1999; 1: 38

Wecker, J, "Costs of a rotavirus vaccine." *Sci*, Jan 28, 2005; 307: 517

Wenman, WM et al, "Rotavirus infection in adults: result of a prospective family study." *N Engl J Med*, 1979; 301: 303–306

Wickelgren, I, "How rotavirus causes diarrhea." Microbiol Dis. *Sci*, Jan 21, 2000; 287: 409, 411

"Withdrawal of rotavirus vaccine recommendation." *MMWR*, Nov 5, 1999; 48(43): 1007

Yang, J et al, "Emergence of human rotavirus Group A genotype of G9 strains, Wuhan, China." Dispatches. *Emerg Infect Dis,* Oct 2007; 13(10): 1587–1589

Chapter 11

Anderson, C, "Cholera epidemic: traced to risk miscalculation." *Nature,* Nov 28, 1991; 354(6351): 255

Anderson, I, "End of the line for deadly stowaways?" *New Scientist,* Oct 24, 1992; 136(1844): 12–13

Bailey, N et al, "Cholera associated with food transported from El Salvador—Indiana, 1994." *MMWR,* May 26, 1995; 44(20): 385–386

Barua, D and WB Greenough, eds. *Cholera. Current Topics in Infectious Diseases.* NY, Plenum Med, 1992

Beller, M et al, "Outbreak of viral gastroenteritis due to a contaminated well." Internatl Consequences. *JAMA,* Aug 20, 1997; 278(7): 563–568

Besser, RE et al, "Diagnosis & treatment of cholera in the United States: are we prepared?" Brief Rept. *JAMA,* Oct 19, 1994; 272(15): 1203–1205

——— "All *Vibrio cholera* infections are not created equal" Lett. *JAMA,* May 10, 1995; 273(18): 1417

Blake, PA et al, "Cholera—a possible endemic focus in the United States." *N Engl J Med,* 1980; 302: 305–309

Brand, S et al, "Cholera epidemic after increased civil conflict—Monrovia, Liberia, June–Sept 2003." *MMWR,* Nov 14, 2003; 52(45): 1093–1095

Chase, A, "Now it can be told: epidemiologists quietly traced U.S. cholera source." *Med Trib,* Mar 26, 1980: 6

"Cholera in 1992." *Bull WHO,* 1993; 71(5): 641

Cholera Prevention. Div Bacterial Mycotic Dis, CDC/NCID, May 1992, [brochure]

"Cholera—Update in California & the Americas." *Cal Morbid,* Nov 27, 1992; 47(48): 1

Colwell, RR, "Global climate & infectious disease: the cholera paradigm." [modified form of presentation, AAAS annual meeting 1996] *Sci,* Dec 20, 1996; 274: 2025–2031

Cooper, G et al, "Cholera associated with international travel, 1992." *MMWR,* Sept 11, 1992; 41(36): 664–667

Dalsgaard, A et al, "*Vibrio cholera* 0139 in Denmark." Lett. *Lancet,* June 24, 1995; 345(8965): 1637–1638

D'Aquino, M et al, "Lemon juice as a national biocide for disinfecting drinking water." *Bull Pan Am Hlth Org,* Dec 1994; 28(4): 324–330

Davis, BM et al, "Convergence of the secretory pathways for cholera toxin & the filamentous phage, CTXphi." Repts. *Sci,* Apr 14, 2000; 288: 333–335

Doran, M et al, "Toxigenic *Vibrio cholerae* 01 infection acquired in Colorado." Epidemiol Notes Repts. *MMWR,* Jan 20 1989; 38(2): 19–20

Eberhart-Phillips, J et al, "An outbreak of cholera from food served on an international aircraft." *Epidemiol & Infect*, Feb 1996; 116(1): 9–13

Eichold II, BH et al, "Isolation of *Vibrio cholerae* 01 from oysters—Mobile Bay, 1991–1992." Epidemiol Notes Repts. *MMWR*, Feb 12, 1993; 42(5): 91–93

Engelthaler, D, "Vibrio illnesses after hurricane Katrina—multiple states, August–September 2005." *MMWR*, Sept 23, 2005; 54(37): 928–931

Farbman, KS et al, "Antibacterial activity of garlic & onions: a historical perspective." *Pediat Infect Dis J*, July 1993; 12(7): 613–614

Faruque, SM et al, "Reemergence of epidemic *Vibrio cholerae* 0139, Bangladesh." Res. *Emerg Infect Dis*, Sept 2003; 9(9): 1116–1122

Gibbons, A, "New 3-D protein structures revealed, the shape of cholera." Res News. *Sci*, July 26, 1991; 253: 382–383

Glass, RI et al, "Epidemic cholera in the Americas." Perspect. *Sci*, June 12, 1992; 256: 1524–1525

Hanne, M et al, "Outbreak of gastrointestinal illness associated with consumption of seaweed." *MMWR*, Oct 6, 1995; 44 (39): 724–727

Helton, B et al, "Cholera on a Gulf Coast oil rig—Texas." Epidemiol Notes Repts. *MMWR*, Dec 4, 1981; 30(47): 589–590

Hempel, S, *The Strange Case of the Broad Street Pump: John Snow & the Mystery of Cholera.* Berkeley, CA: U Cal Press, 2007

Hunter, BT, "Cholera & the food supply." *Consumers' Res Mag*, Dec 1991: 8–9

Lacey, C et al, "Cholera associated with imported frozen coconut milk—Maryland, 1991." *MMWR*, Dec 13, 1991; 40(49): 844–845

Layseca, CV et al, "Cholera—Peru, 1991." Internatl Notes. *MMWR*, Feb 15, 1991; 40(6): 108–110

Mahon, BE et al, "Reported cholera in the United States, 1991–1994." *JAMA*, July 31, 1996; 276(4): 307–312

Mascola, L et al, "Cholera associated with an international airline flight, 1992." *MMWR*, Feb 28, 1992; 41: 134–135

Matthys, F et al, "Cholera outbreak among Rwandan refugees—Democratic Republic of Congo, April 1997." *MMWR*, May 22, 1998; 47(19): 389 391

Mazel, D et al, "A distinctive class of integron in the *Vibrio cholerae* genome." Repts. *Sci*, Apr 24, 1998; 280: 605–608

McFarland, L et al, "Toxigenic *Vibrio cholerae* 01 infections—Louisiana & Florida." *Epidemiol Notes Repts. MMWR*, Sept 26, 1986; 35(38): 606–607

—— "Cholera in Louisiana—update." *MMWR*, Nov 7, 1986; 25(44): 687–688

Mekalanos, J et al, "Cholera vaccines: fighting an ancient scourge." Perspect. *Sci*, Sept 2, 1994; 265: 1387–1388

Mujica, OJ, "Epidemic cholera in the Amazon: the role of produce in disease risk & prevention." *J Infect Dis*, June 1994; 169(6): 1381–1384

Ndayimirije, N et al, "Epidemic cholera." *MMWR*, June 4, 1993; 42(21): 408–409; 415–416

"New cholera vaccine in phase II trials." *Med Trib*, Dec 26, 1991, 4

Newton, S et al, "Immune response to cholera toxin epitope inserted in *Salmonella* flagellin." Repts. *Sci*, Apr 7, 1989; 244: 70–72

"Of cabbages & chlorine: cholera in Peru." Ed'al. *Lancet*, July 4, 1992; 340(8810): 20–21

"One hundred fiftieth anniversary of John Snow & the pump handle." *MMWR*, Sept 3, 2004; 53(34): 783

Pennisi, E, "Versatile gene uptake system found in cholera bacterium." Microbiol. *Sci*, Apr 24, 1998; 280: 521–522

Pereira G et al, "Surveillance for cholera—Cochabamba Department, Bolivia. January–June 1992." Internatl Notes. *MMWR*, Aug 27, 1993; 42(33): 636–639

Peterson, JW and LG Ochoa, "Role of prostaglandins & cAMP in the secretory effects of cholera toxin." Repts. *Sci*, Aug 25, 1989; 245: 857–859

Picardi, JL et al, "Cholera—Florida." Epidemiol Notes Repts. *MMWR*, Dec 10, 1980; 29(50): 601

Qadri, F et al, "Enterotoxigenic *Escherichia coli* & *Vibrio cholera* diarrhea, Bangladesh, 2004." Dispatches. *Emerg Infect Dis*, July 2005; 11(7): 1104–1107

Ragazzoni, H et al, "Cholera—New Jersey & Florida." *MMWR*, May 3, 1991; 40(17): 287–289

Ribi, HO et al, "Three-dimensional structure of cholera toxin penetrating a lipid membrane." Res Articles. *Sci*, Mar 11, 1988; 239: 1272–1276

Rice, EW et al, "Chlorine & survival of 'rugose' *Vibrio cholerae*." Lett. *Lancet*, Sept 19, 1992; 340(8821): 740

"Risk of cholera transmission by foods." *Bulletin of the Pan American Health Organization*, 1991; 25(3): 274–277

Roman, R et al, "Cholera (New York, 1991." Epidemiol Notes Repts. *MMWR*, Aug 2, 1991; 40(30): 516–518

Salim, A et al, "*Vibrio cholerae* pathogenic clones." Dispatches. *Emerg Infect Dis*, Nov 2005; 11(11): 1758–1760

Sinkala, M et al, "Cholera epidemic associated with raw vegetables—Lusake, Zambia, 2003–2004." *MMWR*, Sept 3, 2004; 53(34): 783–786

Straif-Bourgeois, S et al, "Two cases of toxigenic *Vibrio cholerae* 01 infection after Hurricanes Katrina & Rita—Louisiana, October 2005." *MMWR*, Jan 20, 2006; 55(2): 31–32

Swerdlow, DL, "Cholera in the Americas, guidelines for the clinician." Special Communication. *JAMA*, Mar 18, 1992; 267(11): 1495–1499

Swerdlow, DL et al, "Waterborne transmission of epidemic cholera in Trujillo, Peru: lessons for a continent at risk." *Lancet*, July 4, 1992; 340(8810): 28–33

Tauxe, RV and PA Blake, "Epidemic cholera in Latin America." Lett from Peru. *JAMA*, Mar 11, 1992; 267(10): 1388–1390

Tormey, M et al, "Imported cholera associated with a newly described toxigenic *Vibrio cholerae* 0139 strain—California, 1993." Emerg Infect Dis, *MMWR*, July 9, 1993; 42(26): 501–503

"Update: Cholera—Western Hemisphere, 1991." *MMWR*, Dec 13, 1991; 40(49): 860

"Update: Cholera—Western Hemisphere, 1992." Current Trends. *MMWR*, Sept 11, 1992; 41(36): 667–668

"Update: Cholera—Western Hemisphere, 1992." Internatl Notes. *MMWR*, Feb 12, 1993; 42(5): 89–91

"Update: Cholera—Western Hemisphere & recommendations for treatment of cholera." Current Trends. *MMWR*, Aug 16, 1981; 40(32): 562–565

"Update: cholera outbreak—Peru, Ecuador & Colombia." [reprint from *Wkly Epidemiol Record*, WHO & CDC ed'al note] *MMWR*, Apr 5, 1991; 40(13): 225–227

"Update: *Vibrio cholerae* 01—Western Hemisphere, 1991–1994 & *V. cholerae* 0139—Asia, 1994." *MMWR*, Mar 24, 1995; 44(11): 215–219

Vugia, DL et al, "Surveillance for epidemic cholera in the Americas: an assessment." *MMWR*, 1992; 41(SS-1): 27–34

Wilber, JA et al, "Importation of cholera from Peru." Epidemiol Notes Repts. *MMWR*, Apr 19, 1991; 40(15): 258–259

Wilson, MM, "Cholera is walking south." Letter from Buenos Aires. *JAMA*, Oc 19, 1994; 272(15): 1226–1227

Vibrio parahaemolyticus

Adler, K, "*Vibrio parahaemolyticus* risk assessment methodology endorsed by micro committee." *Fd Chem News*, Oct 4, 1999, 9–13

Altman, LK, "Diarrhea outbreak on 2 ships linked to contaminated seafood." *NY Times*, Apr 3, 1975

Balter, S et al, "*Vibrio parahaemolyticus* infections associated with consumption of raw shellfish—three states, 2006." *MMWR*, Aug 11, 2006; 55(31): 854–856

Briley, J, "Multi-state *Vibrio parahaemolyticus* outbreak sparks recall of all Galveston Bay oysters." *Fd Chem News*, July 6, 1998, 21

—— "Texas oyster sites will be cleared if FDA finds no more evidence of *Vibrio*." *Fd Chem News*, Sept 14, 1998, 25–26

—— "*V. parahaemolyticus* strikes again, this time in New York region, high water temperature & oxygen depletion suspected." *Fd Chem News*, Sept 21, 1998, 3, 23–24

Butler, ME, "*Vibrio parahaemolyticus* risk assessment released." *Fd Chem News*, Jan 22, 2001: 8–9

—— "*Vibrio parahaemolyticus* levels reduced through postharvest treatment." *Fd Chem News*, Jan 29, 2001: 7–9

Byron, J, "*V. parahaemolyticus* control plan approved by ISSC [Interstate Shellfish Sanitation Conference] *Fd Chem News*, Aug 3, 1998, 28–29

Daniels, NA et al, "Emergence of a new *Vibrio parahaemolyticus* serotype in raw oysters; a prevention quandary." Original Contribut. *JAMA*, Sept 27, 2000; 284(12): 1541–1545

Dern, A, "New York shellfish areas reopened after being found free of *V. parahaemolyticus*." *Fd Chem New*, Nov 2, 1998: 5

—— "Levels of *Vibrio* in raw oysters sold at retail being studied by CFSAN." [Center for Food Safety & Nutrition] *Fd Chem News*, Nov 23, 1998: 10–11

Doyle, MP, "Foodborne illness, pathogenic *Escherichia coli, Yersinia enterocolitica, & Vibrio parahaemolyticus." Lancet,* Nov 3, 1990; 336: 1114–1115

Fyle, M, "Outbreak of *Vibrio parahaemolyticus* infections associated with eating raw oysters—Pacific Northwest, 1997." *MMWR,* July 12, 1987; 47(22): 457–462

Gonzalez-Escalona, M et al, "*Vibrio parahaemolyticus* diarrhea, Chile, 1998 & 2004." Dispatches. *Emerg Infect Dis,* Jan 2005; 11(1): 129–131

Martinez-Urtaza, J et al, "Pandemic *Vibrio parahaemolyticus* 03:K6, Europe." Lett. *Emerg Infect Dis,* Aug 2005; 11(8): 1319–1320

"More information may be needed for reliable *Vibrio parahaemolyticus* risk assessment, FDA staffer says." *Fd Chem News,* June 7, 1999: 13–16

Murphy, J, "Texas law spurs debate on sampling waters for *Vibrio parahaemolyticus." FDA. Fd Chem News,* May 24, 1999: 4–5

—— "ISSC approves controversial *Vibrio parahaemolyticus* control plan drawing ire from Gulf lawmaker." ISSC Conference. [Interstate Shellfish Sanitation Conference] *Fd Chem News,* Aug 2, 1999: 24–25

Oliver, JF and SM Ostroff, "Preventing *Vibrio parahaemolyticus* infection." Lett. *JAMA,* Jan 3, 2001; 285(1): 42–43

Quillici, ML et al, "Pandemic *Vibrio parahaemolyticus* 03:K6 spread, France." Lett. *Emerg Infect Dis,* July 2005; 11(7): 1148–1149

"*Vibrio parahaemolyticus* foodborne outbreak—Louisiana." *MMWR* Sept 15, 1978; 27: 345–346

"Washington State closes three oyster harvest areas due to *Vibrio parahaemolyticus." Fd Chem News,* Sept 8, 1997: 13

Wechsler, E et al, "Outbreak of *Vibrio parahaemolyticus* infection associated with eating raw oysters & clams harvested from Long Island Sound—Connecticut, New Jersey, & New York, 1998." *MMWR,* Jan 29, 1999; 48(3): 48–51

Winter, G, "Doubts cast on U.S. effort for the safety of shellfish." *NY Times,* July 19, 2001: C7

Vibrio vulnificus

Bisharat, N et al, "Hybrid *Vibrio vulnificus." Res. Emerg Infect Dis,* Jan 2005; 11(1): 30–35

Butler, ME, "ISSC evaluating *Vibrio vulnificus* illness-reduction strategy." *Fd Chem New,* Jan 29, 2001, 6–7

—— "ISSC asking states to implement *Vibrio* illness reduction steps." FDA. *Fd Chem News,* Feb 5, 2001, 13

Chung, PH et al, "Cutaneous injury & *Vibrio vulnificus* infection." Lett. *Emerg Infect Dis,* Aug 2006; 12(8): 1302–1303

"Concern continues about *Vibrio vulnificus." FDA Drug Bull,* Apr 1988, 3

Davis, C, "Viral gastroenteritis associated with consumption of raw oysters—Florida, 1983." Epidemiol Notes Repts. *MMWR,* June 24, 1994; 43(24): 446–449

"Death in California blamed on *V. vulnificus* in Gulf oysters." *Fd Chem News,* Sept 26, 1994: 33–36

"Educating public about raw oyster problem." Update. *FDA Consumer,* Nov 1994: 4

"FDA official highly critical of oyster tracing record." *Fd Chem News,* June 27, 1994: 40–42

"FDA shellfish consumption warnings arouse ISSC." *Fd Chem News,* July 20, 1992: 44–47

"Florida agencies planning to meet on oyster safety issues." *Fd Chem News,* Feb 1, 1993: 21–22

"Florida issues raw-oyster health advisory after 7 people die." *Fd Chem News,* Dec 14, 1991: 39

"Florida researchers using depuration, chilling on shellfish." *Fd Chem News,* Aug 22, 1994: 48

Glaros, T, "Oyster blues, scientists are warning rare seafood lovers of new hazards." Rest. Notebk. Capitol Comment. *Rest Hospitality,* Aug 1985: 28

"Good sanitation could stem glow-in-the-dark seafood, FDA-er." *Fd Chem News,* July 29, 1991: 16–17

Hlady, WG et al, "*Vibrio vulnificus* infections associated with raw oyster consumption—Florida, 1981–1992." Epidemiol Notes Repts. *MMWR,* June 4, 1993; 42(21): 405–407

Hlady, WG and KC Klontz, "The epidemiology of *Vibrio* infections in Florida, 1981–1993." *J Infect Dis,* May 1996; 173: 1176–1183

Hsuch, Po-Ren et al, "*Vibrio vulnificus* in Taiwan." *Emerg Infect Dis,* Aug 2004; 10(8): 1363–1368

Johnson, JM et al, "*Vibrio vulnificus,* man & the sea." *JAMA,* May 17, 1985; 253(19): 2850–2853

Kizer, KW, "*Vibrio vulnificus* hazards in patients with liver disease." Lett. *Conn Med,* Aug 1994, 480

Lash, S, "Shellfish industry calls for 60% *Vibrio vulnificus* reduction." FDA. *Fd Chem News,* Aug 6, 2001; 1: 17

"Low heat, cold storage said to reduce *Vibrio* in raw oysters." *Fd Chem News,* Jan 18, 1993: 40–42

Mascola, L, "*Vibrio vulnificus* infections associated with eating raw oysters—Los Angeles, 1996." *MMWR;* 45: 621–624, from CDC Leads from *MMWR. JAMA,* Sept 25, 1996; 276(12): 937–938

Miller, RW, "Fewer months 'R' safe for eating raw Gulf oysters." *FDA Consumer,* June 1988: 22–25

Mouzin, E et al, "Prevention of *Vibrio vulnificus* infections, assessment of regulatory educational strategies." Brief Rept. *JAMA* Aug 20, 1997; 278(7): 576–578

Murphy, J, "ISSC rejects proposal to set performance standard for *Vibrio vulnificus* in raw shellfish." ISSC Conference [Interstate Shellfish Sanitation Commission] *Fd Chem News,* Aug 2, 1999: 25–26

Osvath, R, "Florida adopts voluntary plan to battle Vv in oysters." *Fd Chem News,* Mar 12, 2001: 13

—— "Gulf oyster industry seeks $1 million for *Vibrio* education." *Fd Chem News,* Feb 4, 2002: 16

—— "Oyster-related illnesses prompt FDA health advisory." *Fd Chem News,* Nov 29, 1993: 40–41

—— "Oyster related infections can occur any time, study finds." *Fd Chem News,* Dec 13, 1993: 7

"Plan to reduce Vibrio infections." Update. *FDA Consumer,* Dec 1993: 4–5

Pollak, SJ et al, "*Vibrio vulnificus* septicemia, isolation of organism from stool & demonstration of antibodies by indirect immunofluorescence." *Arch Intern Med,* Apr 1983; 143: 837–838

Proceedings of the 1994 Vibrio vulnificus Workshop. USDHHS, US Dept Commerce Interstate Shellfish Sanitation Conference. Wash, D.C. June 15–26, 1994

"Raw shellfish warning viewed as last resort by FDA's Billy." *Fd Chem News,* Sept 23, 1991: 11–12

"Seafood safety warnings posted in California restaurants." *Pub Voice Fd Hlth Advocate.* Update. Feb 1991; 10(2): 2

Sun, Y and JD Oliver, "Hot sauce: no elimination of *Vibrio vulnificus* in oysters." *J Fd Protect,* Apr 1995; 58: 441–442

"To eat or not to eat (raw shellfish). Part I, *Vibrio vulnificus* infections in California—a ten year review." *Cal Morbidity,* Aug 13, 1993; 31(32): 1; Part II "*Vibrio vulnificus* & other infections— is the risk unacceptable?" *Cal Morbidity,* Aug 27, 1993; 33(34): 1

"Vibrio infections: high risk patients should avoid raw shellfish." *FDA Med Bull,* Mar 1993: 6

"Vibrio reported 80 times worse for adults with liver disease." *Fd Chem News,* June 7, 1993: 31

"*Vibrio vulnificus* & patients with liver disease." *FDA Drug Bull,* Apr 1985; 15(1): 6

"V. *vulnificus* nonculturable cells called health threat." *Fd Chem News,* June 8, 1992: 19

Wright, A, "Nondetectable performance standard for *Vibrio* in raw oysters supported by public health & consumer groups." FDA. *Fd Chem News,* May 10, 1999: 8–10

—— "New Zealand Agriculture Ministry supports 'nondetectable' standard for *Vibrio* in oysters." FDA. *Fd Chem News,* June 7, 1999: 21–22

Chapter 12

Amin, MK and FA Draughon, "Infection of shell eggs with *Yersinia enterocolitica.*" *J Fd Protect,* Oct 1990; 53(10): 826–830

Anderson, DM and O Schneewind, "A mRNA signal for the type III secretion of Yop proteins by *Yersinia enterocolitica.*" Repts. *Sci,* Nov 7, 1997; 278: 1140–1143

Badon, SJ and RG Cable, "*Yersinia enterocolitica* contamination of blood products." *Conn Med,* June 1992; 56(6): 287–289

Bhaduri, S, "Test detects, recovers harmful foodborne bacterium." *Sci Res News,* USDA, Feb 1991: 1–2

Bhaduri, S and S Palumbo, "Effect of enrichment procedures on the stability of the virulent plasmid & virulence-associated characteristics in *Yersinia enterocolitica.*" Paper. 81E-3, annual meeting. *Instit Fd Technol,* 1995

Black, RE et al, "Epidemic *Yersinia enterocolitica* infection due to contaminated chocolate milk." *N Engl J Med*, 1978; 298: 76–79

Bondarev, LS et al, "Variant manifestations of generalized form of yersiniosis." *Vrach Delo* (Kiev, Ukraine) 1991; 5: 96–98, from abstract. *JAMA*, June 13, 1992, 2980

"Brief Notes." *Fd Chem News*, Feb 20, 1995: 14; June 30, 1997: 44

Delmas, CL et al, "Isolation of *Yersinia enterocolitica* & related species from foods in France." *Appl Environ Microbiol*, Oct 1985; 50(4): 767–771

Doyle, MP, "Foodborne illness, pathogenic *Escherichia coli, Yersinia enterocolitica*, and *Vibrio parahaemolyticus*." *Lancet*, Nov 3, 1990; 336: 1111–1115

"Food poisoning detection tests patented." USDA Res. *Fd Review*, Apr–June 1991; 14(2): 54

Francis, DW et al, "Enterotoxin production & thermal resistance of *Yersinia* in milk." *Appl Environ Microbiol*, 1980; 40: 174–176

Fukushima, H and M Gomyoda, "Inhibition of *Yersinia enterocolitica* serotype 0:3 by natural microflora of pork." *Appl Environ Microbiol*, May 1986; 51(5): 990–994

Gaul, GM, "Intestinal infection affects blood supply safety, recent deaths following transfusions alarm medical community." Pub Hlth. *Wash Post Hlth*, Feb 19, 1991: 9

Granhek-Ogden, D et al, "Outbreak of *Yersinia enterocolitica* serogroup 0:9 infection & processed pork, Norway." Dispatches. *Emerg Infect Dis*, May 2007; 13(5): 754–756

Guan, K and JE Dixon, "Protein tyrosine phosphatase activity of an essential virulent determinant in *Yersinia*." Repts. *Sci*, Aug 3, 1990; 249: 553–556

Halpin, TJ et al, "Red blood cell transfusions contaminated with *Yersinia enterocolitica*— United States, 1991–1996, & initiation of a national study to detect bacteria-associated transfusion reactions." *MMWR*, June 20, 1997; 46(24): 553–555

Hanna, MO et al, "Development of *Yersinia enterocolitica* on raw beef & cooked beef & pork at different temperatures." *J Fd Protect*, 1977; 42: 1180–1184

Hunter, BT, "Yersinia Infection." *Consumers' Research Mag*, Sept 1993: 8–9

Isberg, RR, "Discrimination between intracellular uptake & surface adhesion of bacterial pathogens." Articles. *Sci*, May 17, 1991; 252: 934–938

Jones, RC et al, "*Yersinia enterocolitica* gastroenteritis among infants exposed to chitterlings—Chicago, Illinois, 2002." *MMWR*, Oct 10, 2003; 52(40): 956–958

Jones, TP et al, "From pig to pacifier: chitterling-associated yersiniosis outbreak among black children." Dispatches. *Emerg Infect Dis*, Aug 2003; 9(8): 1007–1009

Kuehnert, MJ et al, "Platelet transfusion reaction due to *Yersinia enterocolitica*. " Lett. *JAMA*, Aug 20, 1997; 278(7): 550

Lee, LA et al, "*Yersinia enterocolitica* 0:3 infections in infants & children associated with the household preparation of chitterlings." Brief Rept. *N Engl J Med*, Apr 5, 1990; 322(14): 984–987

Lofgren, JP et al, "Multi-state outbreak of yersiniosis." Epidemiol Notes Repts. *MMWR*, Sept 24, 1982; 31(37): 505–506

Monroe, MW, "*Yersinia enterocolitica* infections during the holidays in black families— Georgia." Topics Minority Hlth, *MMWR*, Nov 16, 1999; 39(44): 819–821

Nesbakken, T et al, "Comparative study of a DNA hybridization method & two isolation procedures for detection of *Yersinia enterocolitica* 0:3 in naturally contaminated pork products." *Appl Environ Microbiol,* Feb 1991; 57(2): 389–394

Nightingale, SL, "Possibility of *Yersinia enterocolitica* bacteremia due to transfusion." From FDA. *JAMA,* July 10, 1991; 266(2): 190

Orth, K et al, "Inhibition of the mitogen-activated protein kinase kinase superfamily by a *Yersinia* effector. Repts. *Sci,* Sept 17, 1999; 285: 1920–1923

Ostroff, SM et al, "Sources of sporadic *Yersinia enterocolitica* in Norway: a prospective case-control study." *Epidemiol Infect,* Feb 1994; 112(1): 133–141

"Outbreak of *Yersinia enterocolitica*—Washington State." Epidemiol Notes Repts. *MMWR,* Oct 22, 1982; 31(41): 562–564

"Pathogenic *Yersinia enterocolitica* found in half of swine herds in baseline study." *Fd Chem News,* Nov 27, 1995: 14

Pritchard TJ et al, "Environmental surveillance of dairy processing plants for the presence of *Yersinia* species." *Journal of Food Protection,* Apr 1995; 58(4): 395–397

"Research supports FDA advice on *Yersinia* in dairy plant coolers." *Fd Chem News,* Oct 9, 1995, 40–41

Richards, C et al, "Autologous transfusion-transmitted *Yersinia enterocolitica*." Lett. *JAMA,* Sept 23–30, 1992; 268(12): 1541–1542

"Six *Yersinia enterocolitica* cases in NH, VT are of concern but not unusual, NH heart official says." *Fd Chem News,* Nov 27, 1995: 9

Stanley, D, "Arthritis from foodborne bacteria?" *Agric Res,* Oct 1996: 16

Stolk-Engelaar, V and J Koegkamp-Korstanje, "Clinical presentation & diagnosis of gastrointestinal infections by *Yersinia enterocolitica* in 261 Dutch patients." *Scand J Infect Dis,* 1996; 28: 571–575

Tacket, CO et al, "A multistate outbreak of infections caused by *Yersinia enterocolitica* transmitted by pasteurized milk." Original Contribut. *JAMA,* Jan 27, 1984; 251(4): 483–486

Tauxe, RV et al, "*Yersinia enterolitica* infections & pork: the missing link." *Lancet,* 1987: 1129–1132

Ternhag, A et al, "Short- and long-term effects of bacterial gastrointestinal infections." Res. *Emerg Infect Dis,* Jan 2008; 14(1): 143–148

Vidon, DJ and CL Delmas, "Incidence of *Yersinia enterocolitica* in raw milk in eastern France." *Appl Environ Microbiol,* 1981; 41: 335–359

Woernle, CH et al, "*Yersinia enterocolitica* bacteremia & endotoxin shock associated with red blood cell transfusions—United States, 1991." *MMWR,* 1999; 40: 176–178. From CDC. Leads from *MMWR. JAMA,* May 1, 1991; 265(17): 2174–2175

"*Yersinia enterocolitica* gastrointestinal outbreak—Montreal." *Canada Dis Wkly Rept.* 1976; 2: 41–44

"*Yersinia* in market swine." *Fd Chem News,* Jan 11, 1999: 19

Chapter 13

"Advice for travelers." *Conn Med,* May 1998; 62(5): 279–281

Bader, TF et al, "Hepatitis E in a U.S. traveler to Mexico." Lett. *N Engl J Med*, Dec 5, 1991; 325(23): 1659

Beers, A, "Company is forced to pay for the removal of tainted berries." *Fd Chem News*, Sept 22, 1997: 30–31

"Brief Notes." *Fd Chem News*, Feb 10, 1997, 52–53; Apr 15, 1997, 37; May 12, 1997, 39–40; May 19, 1997, 41; May 26, 1997, 32, 35; June 16, 1997, 35; Oct 13, 1997, 30; Nov 17, 1997, 33–34; Apr 15, 1999, 35; Aug 2, 1999, 35; May 8, 2000, 21

"Briefs." *Fd Chem News*, Sept 8, 1997, 29–30; Sept 21, 1997, 39

Burros, M, "Food-borne illness from produce on the rise." *NY Times*, Nov 23, 2003: 23

Calvin, L et al, "The economics of food safety: the case of green onions & hepatitis A outbreaks." *Outlook Report from ERS, USDA*, Dec 2004

Chodick, G, "Declining incidence of hepatitis A." Lett. *JAMA*, Jan 18, 2006; 295(3): 282

Cliver, DO, "Virus transmission via food." *IFT Scientific Status Summary. Expert Panel Food Safety & Nutrition*. [revision from Oct, 1988] *Fd Tech*, Apr 1999, 51(4): 71–77

—— "Hepatitis A from strawberries: who's to blame?" Back Page. *Fd Tech*, June 1997: 132

Cromeans, TL, "Understanding & preventing viral transmission via foods." *Fd Tech*, Apr, 1997; 51(4): 20

Dagon, R et al, "Incidence of hepatitis A in Israel following universal immunization of toddlers." *JAMA*, 2005; 292: 202–210

Dato, V et al, "Hepatitis A outbreak associated with green onions at a restaurant—Monaca, Pennsylvania, 2003." *MMWR*, Nov 28, 2003; 52(47): 1155–1157

Desorbo, MA. "Tough luck for Puck." News Notes. *Fd Qual*, Apr–May, 2007:14

"Don't drink—or rinse with?—the water." *Fd Qual*. Nov–Dec 2003: 7

"Epitope dumps A&W over bad berries." *Nature Biotechnol*, June, 1997; 15(6): 491

Fackelmann, K, "The hepatitis G enigma, researchers corner new viruses associated with hepatitis." *Sci News*, Apr 13, 1996: 238–239

"FDA approval for a continued hepatitis A & B vaccine." *MMWR*, Sept 21, 2001; 50(7): 806–607

"FDA reports recalls of strawberry products processed from lots associated with Michigan hepatitis A outbreak." Enforcement. *Fd Chem News*, May 26, 1997: 15

Frank, C et al, "Major outbreaks of hepatitis A associated with orange juice among tourists, Egypt, 2004." Dispatches. *Emerg Infect Dis*, Jan 2007; 13(1): 156–158

"Fruits linked with hepatitis A outbreak in Michigan recalled." Enforcement. *Fd Chem News*, Apr 28, 1997: 24

Gordenker, A, "Illnesses in more states linked to 1997 frozen strawberry outbreak." *Fd Chem News*, Mar 1, 1999: 28–29

Grady, D, "Produce items are vulnerable to biological contamination." [sidebar]. *NY Times*, Nov 18, 2003: A20

"Green onions associated with hepatitis A outbreaks." Updates. *FDA Consumer*, Jan–Feb 2004: 5

"Hepatitis A associated with consumption of frozen strawberries—Michigan, Mar, 1997." *MMWR*, Apr 4, 1997; 46(13): 288, 295

"Hepatitis A-contaminated strawberries blamed on NAFTA by Bonier." *Fd Chem News*, May 5, 1997: 42

"Hepatitis A control discussed by CDC." *Fd Chem News*, Feb 24, 1997: 5–6

"Hepatitis A outbreak energizes effort to label foreign produce." *Fd Qual*, Apr 1997: 10

"Hepatitis A outbreak in a day-care center—Inyo County, Dec 1993." *Cal Morbidity*, Mar 25, 1994; 11(12)

"Hepatitis E, *Arcobacter butzleri* involvement in foodborne disease reported." *Fd Chem News*, Sept 8, 1997: 8–9

"Hepatitis E in U.S. patients; infection linked to travel." *Am Med News*, Feb 1, 1993: 34

Herrera, JL et al, "Hepatitis E among U.S. travelers, 1989–1992." *MMWR*, 1993; 42: 1–4. From CDC, *JAMA*, Feb 17, 1993; 269(7): 845–846

"House subcommittee wants more inspections of school lunch commodities." *Fd Chem News*, June 21, 1997: 19–21

Hughes, James M, ed. *Prevention of Hepatitis A through Active or Passive Immunization: Recommendations of the Advisory Committee on Immunization Practices (ACIP)*. Atlanta, GA: CDC, *MMWR*, Oct 1, 1999; RR-12 [Recommendation & Reports]

Hunter, BT, "Food-borne transmission of hepatitis A." *Consumers' Research Mag;* Jan 1995: 8–9

Lebois, V "Hepatitis A—the food sector risk," *Internatl Fd Hyg*, 1997; 7(7): 5–6

Lett, SM et al, "Update: prevention of hepatitis A after exposure to hepatitis A virus & in international travelers. Updated recommendations of the Advisory Committee on Immunization practices (ACIP)." *MMWR*, Oct 19, 2007; 56(41): 1080–1084

Mattock, C and B Brace, "New hepatitis viruses." *J Royal Soc Med*, Jan 1992; 85(1): 50–53

O'Connor, A, "Experts seek new effort to control hepatitis A." *NY Times*, Dec 30, 2003: F7

Otto, Pam Erickson, "Tainted berries prompt legislative & regulatory action." News. *Fd Prod Design*, June, 1997, 16–17;19

Pebody, RG et al, "Foodborne outbreaks of hepatitis A in a low endemic country: an emerging problem?" *Epidemiol Infect*, Feb, 1998, Vol 120, No 1, 55–59

Phibbs, P, "Hepatitis A outbreak linked to Mexican strawberries illegally introduced into school food program." *Fd Chem News*, Apr 7, 1997: 35–37

Polgreen, L, "Hepatitis inquiry moves deliberately from farm to plate." *NY Times*, Nov 11, 2003: A20

"Possible hep[atitis] A contamination results in donut recall." Enforcement. *Fd Chem News*, Apr 21, 1997: 13

"Potential hepatitis A exposure among interstate 95 travelers—North Carolina, 1999." PH Dispatch. *MMWR*, Aug 20, 1999; 48(32): 717

"Prevention of hepatitis A by vaccine & immune globulin." *Cal PH Update;* 2001(1): 1–4

"Processors charged with mislabeling strawberries tied to outbreak of hepatitis A virus." Enforcement. *Fd Chem News*, June 16, 1997: 5–6

Scharschmidt, BF, "Hepatitis E: a virus in waiting." *Lancet*, Aug 26, 1995; 346(8974): 519–520

"School lunch program scrutinized by Congress following outbreak." *Fd Chem News*, Apr 14, 1997: 24–25

Shoyer, E et al, "Ascertainment of secondary cases of hepatitis A—Kansas, 1996–1997." *MMWR*, July 23, 1999; 48(28): 608–610, 619

Thayer, A, "Biotech firm tries to rid itself of tainted berry distributor." *Chem Engineer News*, Apr 14, 1997: 6–7

Tumey, B, "Customers of Georgia deli sue chain, claiming work practices spread hepatitis A." Litigation. *Fd Safety Rept;* May 19, 1999: 487–488

Wasley, A et al, "Incidence of hepatitis A in the United States in the era of vaccination." *JAMA*, 2005; 294: 194–201

Welty, T et al, "Hepatitis A vaccination programs in communities with high rates of hepatitis A." *MMWR*, July 4, 1997; 46(26): 600–603

"What about those scallions?" News Notes. *Fd Qual*, Feb–Mar 2004: 9–10

Williams, I et al, "Hepatitis A vaccination coverage among children aged 24–35 months—United States, 2004–2005." *MMWR*, July 13, 2007; 56(27): 678–68

Chapter 14

Alfano-Sobsey, EM et al, "Human challenge pilot study with Cyclospora cayetanensis." Dispatches. *Emerg Infect Dis*, Apr 2004; 10(4): 726–728

Ashford, R et al, "Human infection with cyanobacterium-like bodies." *Lancet*, Apr 17, 1993; 341(8851): 1034

Binkley, A, "Toronto health officials want to continue ban on Guatemalan berries." *Fd Chem News*, Apr 10, 2000: 19–20

"Brief Notes." *Fd Chem News*, June 30, 1997, 44; July 7, 1997, 33; Feb 9, 1998, 27; Dec 1, 1998, 26; Feb 1, 1999, 26; May 3, 1999, 37; May 24, 1999, 34; July 5, 1999, 34; July 26, 1999, 36–37; Nov 8, 1999, 33; Dec 20, 1999, 33; Jan 17, 2000, 29; Apr 3, 2000, 38

"Briefs." *Fd Chem News*, Aug 16, 1999, 40; Dec 6, 1999, 41

Briley, J, "Health investigators again confounded by *Cyclospora* outbreak, this time in basil." *Fd Chem News*, July 28, 1997: 25–26

—— "Florida *Cyclospora* outbreak traced to mesclun greens." *Fd Chem News*, Feb 23, 1998: 6

Briley, J & A Gordenker, "Guatemala plans September raspberry exports to U.S. after FDA finds farms in compliance." *Fd Chem News*, July 13, 1998: 30–32

Carroll, M, "Source of parasite remains a mystery." *Chow Line*. [news release] Wooster, OH: Ohio State U/Ohio Agric Res Devel Center, July 4, 1996: 1

"Cause of *Cyclospora* outbreak continues to elude FDA & CDC." *Fd Chem News*, July 15, 1996: 35–36

"CDC: water in pest spray likely source of *Cyclospora* in outbreak." *Fd Chem News*, Feb 10, 1997: 24

Charaton, FB, "*Cyclospora* outbreak in US." *Br Med J*, July 13, 1996; 313(7049): 71

Clapp, S, "Central kitchen suspected in *Cyclospora* outbreak linked to basil." *Fd Chem News*, Sept 1, 1997: 19–20

Colley, DG, "Widespread foodborne cyclosporiasis outbreaks present major challenges." Lett. *Emerg Infect Dis*, Oct–Dec 1996; 2(4): 354–356

Connor, BA and DR Shim, "Foodborne transmission of *Cyclospora*." Lett. *Lancet*, Dec 16, 1995; 346(8990): 1634

Connor, BA et al, "Reiter syndrome following protracted symptoms of *Cyclospora* infection." Dispatches. *Emerg Infect Dis*, May–June 2001; 7(3): 453–454

Crist, A, "Outbreak of cyclosporiasis associated with snow peas—Pennsylvania, 2004." *MMWR*, Sept 24, 2004; 53(37): 876–878

"*Cyclospora* outbreak can't be pinned to one fruit, FDA-er says." *Fd Chem New*, July 8, 1996: 21–22

"*Cyclospora* outbreaks in Toronto in May still under investigation." *Fd Chem News*, June 22, 1998: 4–5

"*Cyclospora* probes move away from strawberries." *Fd Chem News*, July 1, 1996: 46–48

"*Cyclospora* traced to imported berries." *Sci News*, Aug 17, 1996: 107

De Graw, E et al, "Update: Outbreak of cyclosporiasis—United States & Canada, 1997." *MMWR*, June 13, 1999; 48(23): 521–523

Dibbell, J, "Berry puzzling this summer's stomach bug is still on the lam." *Time*, July 15, 1996: 59

Döller, PC et al, "Cyclosporiasis outbreak in Germany associated with the consumption of salad." Dispatches. *Emerg Infect Dis*, Sept 2002; 8(9): 992–994

Eberhard, ML et al, "Laboratory diagnosis of *Cyclospora* infections." *Arch Pathol Lab Med*, 1997; 121: 792–797

"FDA inspectors to check raspberry production in Guatemala." *Fd Chem News*, Dec 29, 1997: 14

"FDA says 'no' to Guatemalan raspberries." *Fd Prod Design*, Feb 1998: 28

"FDA to cut back on *Cyclospora* testing of Guatemala berries." *Fd Chem News*, Nov 4, 1996: 29–30

Frankel, DH, "U.S. bad berries may be from below the border." *Lancet*, July 20, 1996; 348(9021): 185

Garcia-López, HL et al, "Identification of *Cyclospora* in poultry." Lett. *Emerg Infect Dis*, Oct–Dec 1996; 2(4): 356–357

Gordenker, A and J Briley, "*Cyclospora* outbreak investigations underway, but no sources identified." *Fd Chem News*, May 26, 1997: 20–22

Gordenker, A, "Imported raspberries implicated in *Cyclospora* investigations as likely source of illness." *Fd Chem News*, June 2, 1997: 20–22

——— "FDA to convene *Cyclospora* meeting July 23 in Washington." *Fd Chem News*, June 16, 1997: 22–24

——— "Guatemalan berry growers accuse US authorities of bias." *Fd Chem News*, Sept 6, 1997: 14

—— "Canada bans fall import of Guatemala raspberries pending audit of new food safety program." *Fd Chem News,* Sept 30, 1998: 18–19

Gorman, C, "The strawberry sickness, a mysterious intestinal infection is striking the US & Canada. Is unwashed fruit the source?" *Time,* July 1, 1996: 59

Graczyk, TK et al, "Recovery of waterborne oocysts of *Cyclospora cayetanensis* by Asian freshwater clams (*Corbicula fluminea*)." *Am J Trop Med Hyg,* 1998; 59: 928–932

"Guatemalan berry safety program, formed with FDA & CDC help, to take effect April 21, risk assessment criteria set for farms." *Fd Chem News,* Apr 14, 1997: 12–13

Herwaldt, BL et al, "An outbreak in 1996 of cyclosporiasis associated with imported raspberries." *N Engl J Med,* May 29, 1997; 336(22): 1548–1556

Ho, AY et al, "Outbreak of cyclosporiasis associated with imported raspberries, Philadelphia, Pennsylvania, 2000." Research. *Emerg Infect Dis,* Aug 2002; 8(8): 783–788

Hoge, CW, "Epidemiology of diarrheal illness associated with coccidian-like organisms among travelers & foreign residents in Nepal." *Lancet,* May 8, 1993; 341(8854): 1175–1179

Huang, P et al, "The first reported outbreak of diarrheal illness associated with *Cyclospora* in the United States" *Ann Intern Med,* Sept 15, 1995; 123(6): 409–414

Hunter, BT, "*Cyclospora:* an emerging pathogen." Fd for Thought. *Consumers' Research Mag,* Aug 1996: 8–9

Jackson, GJ et al, "*Cyclospora*—still another new foodborne pathogen." *Fd Tech* Back Page. *Fd Tech,* Jan 1997; 51(1): 120

Jacquette, G et al, "Update: Outbreaks of cyclosporiasis—United States, 1997." *MMWR,* May 31, 1997; 46(21): 461–462

Letendre, LJ, "Outbreaks of *Cyclospora cayetanensis* infection: United States & Canada, 1996." *J Assoc Fd Drug Officials,* Mar 1997; 61(1): 13–17

"Long history of pathogen detection. *Cyclospora* discussed by FDA-ers." *Fd Chem News,* Dec 16, 1996: 8

Morton, E, "CDC official predicts 'outbreaks' of *Cyclospora,* a diagnosis." *FdChem News,* May 19, 1997: 35–36

Murphy, J, "*Cyclospora* research & other pathogens work among 23 FDA research priorities in three-year plan." *Fd Chem News,* June 8, 1998, 3; 21–23

—— "Guatemala says berries largely unaffected by heavy rains from Hurricane Mitch." *Fd Chem News,* Nov 9, 1998: 15

—— "FDA braces for backlash if Guatemalan berries are tied to Florida outbreak." *Fd Chem News,* Aug 9, 1999: 35, 36

—— "FDA still trying to find out which fruit items may have caused a *Cyclospora* outbreak." *Fd Chem News,* Aug 23, 1999: 20–21

—— "FDA scientists report breakthrough in detecting *Cyclospora* in foods." *Fd Chem News,* Oct 25, 1999: 18–19

Ortega, YR et al, "*Cyclospora* species—a new protozoan pathogens of humans." *N Engl J Med,* May 6, 1993; 328(18): 1308–1312

—— "Isolation of *Cryptosporidium parvum* & *Cyclospora cayetanensis* from vegetables collected in markets of an endemic region in Peru." *Am J Trop Med Hyg*, 1997; 57: 683–686

Osterholm, MT, "Cyclosporiasis & raspberries—lessons for the future." Ed'al. *N Engl J Med*, May 29, 1997; 336(22): 1597–1599

"Outbreak of cyclosporiasis—Ontario, Canada, May 1998." *MMWR*, Oct 2, 1998; 47(38): 806–809

"Outbreaks of cyclosporiasis, United States 1997." *MMWR*, May 23, 1997: 451–452

Pargas, N, "*Cyclospora* outbreaks go beyond Guatamala raspberries, CDC official reminds IAMFES [Internat'l Assoc Milk, Fd & Environ Sanitarians]." *Fd Chem News*, Aug 31, 1998: 8–9

—— "*Cyclospora* may be becoming endemic in US." *Fd Chem News*, Sept 28, 1998: 8–9

Pieniazek, NJ et al, "PCR [polymerase chain reaction] confirmation of infection with *Cyclospora cayetanensis*." Lett. *Emerg Infect Dis*, Oct–Dec 1996; 2(4): 357–358

"Possible presence of parasite on strawberries leads to warning to consumers." Enforcement. *Fd Chem News*, June 24, 1996: 23

"Possible sources(s) of *Cyclospora*-linked illnesses under investigation by federal, state health officials." *Fd Chem News*, June 24, 1996: 29–30

Prichett, R et al, "Outbreak of cyclosporiasis—Northern Virginia–Washington DC–Baltimore, Maryland, metropolitan area, 1997." *MMWR*, Aug 1, 1997; 46(30): 689–691

Shelton, DL, "*Cyclospora* outbreak difficult to track, prevent." Media Rounds. Health. *Am Med News*, Aug 5, 1996: 19–20

"Skimpy knowledge base on *Cyclospora* aided by 1995 outbreak." *Fd Chem News*, July 15, 1996: 25–27

Steinberg, S, "Sleuths probe mystery of parasitic infection." *Sci News*, July 6, 1996: 7

Sterling, CR, "Outbreaks of pseudo-infection with *Cyclospora* & *Cryptosporidium*—Florida & New York City, 1995." *MMWR*, Apr 25, 1997; 46(16): 354–358

—— & YR Ortega, "*Cyclospora*: an enigma worth unraveling." Synopses. *Emerg Infect Dis*, Jan–Feb 1999; 5(1): 48–53

Chapter 15

Addiss, DG et al, "Assessing the public health threat associated with waterborne cryptosporidiosis: Report of a workshop." *MMWR*, June 16, 1995; 44(RR6) [Recommendations and Rept]: 1–16

Akhter, MN et al, "Assessment of inadequately filtered public drinking water—Washington, DC, Dec 1993." *MMWR*, Sept 16, 1994; 43(36): 661–663

Alden, NB et al, "Cryptosporidiosis outbreaks associated with recreational water use—five States, 2006." *MMWR*, July 27, 2007; 56(29): 729–732

"An enhanced laboratory-based surveillance system for *Cryptosporidium* infection." *Cal Morbidity*, Oct 1998: 1–3

ARS, APHIS [Animal & Plant Health Inspection Service] find bovine cryptosporidiosis widespread." *Fd Chem News*, Dec 20, 1993: 28–30

Awad-El-Kariem et al, "Is human cryptosporidiosis a zoonotic disease?" Corresp. *Lancet*, June 12, 1993; 341: 1535

Aziz, M & B Loftus, "Cryptosporidiosis: a cause of gastroenteritis in children." *J Irish Coll Physicians Surgeons*, July 1993; 22(3); 193–194

Beers, A, "Green onions likely source of outbreak." *Fd Chem News*, July 20, 1998: 26

Bell, A et al, "A swimming pool-associated outbreak of cryptosporidiosis in British Columbia." *Can J PH*, Sept–Oct 1993; 84(5); 334–337

Besser-Wiek, JW et al, "Foodborne outbreak of diarrheal illness associated with *Cryptosporidium parvum*—Minnesota 1995." *MMWR*, Sept 13, 1996; 45(36): 783–784

Blackburn, BG et al, "Cryptosporidiosis associated with ozonated apple cider." Dispatches. *Emerg Infect Dis*, Apr 2006; 12(4): 684–686

Blair, K, "*Cryptosporidium* & public health." *Health Environ Digest*, 1994; 8: 61–67

Blanshard, C et al, "*Cryptosporidium* in HIV-seropositive patients." *Quarterly J Med*, 1992; 85(307–308): 813–823

Boyce, N, "Why Uncle Sam feels under the weather." *New Scientist*, Mar 21, 1998; 157(2126): 12

Bridgman, SA et al, "Outbreak of cryptosporidiosis associated with a disinfected groundwater supply." *Epidemiol Infect*, Dec 1995; 115: 555–566

Briley, J, "*Cryptosporidium* found in Chesapeake Bay oysters; no human illness link established." *Fd Chem News*, Oct 27, 1997: 14

Cacciò, S et al, "Human infection with *Cryptosporidium felis:* case report & literature review." Dispatches. *Emerg Infec Dis*, Jan 2002; 8(1): 85–86

Cama, V et al, "Mixed *Cryptosporidium* infections & HIV." *Emerg Infect Dis*, June 2006; 12(6): 1025–1028

Colford, Jr, JM et al, "Participant blending & gastrointestinal illness in a randomized, controlled trial of an in-home drinking water intervention." Research. *Emerg Infect Dis*, Jan 2002; 8(1): 29–36

Conrad, L, "The tedious hunt for *Cryptosporidium*." *Today's Chem at Work*, Mar 1998: 24–27

Cordell, RL et al, "Impact of a massive waterborne cryptosporidiosis outbreak in child care facilities in Metropolitan Milwaukee, Wisconsin." *Pediat Infect Dis J*, July 1997; 16(7): 639–644

Corso, PS et al, "Cost of illness in the 1993 waterborne *Cryptosporidium* outbreak, Milwaukee, Wisconsin." Research. *Emerg Infect Dis*, Apr 2003; 9(4): 426–431

"*C. parvum* found threat to some, not all food uses of tap water." *Fd Chem News*, July 11, 1994: 28

"Crypto bigger problem in water than in food, expert says." *Fd Chem News*, June 26, 1995: 1–6

"Cryptosporidiosis—a growing public health concern." *Cal Morbidity*, May 5, 1995; (17–18): 1–2

"Cryptosporidiosis linked to tap water." *Lancet*, Mar 2, 1996; 347(9001): 605

"Cryptosporidiosis outbreak in the U.K." *Lancet*, Mar 8, 1997; 349(9053): 705

"*Cryptosporidium* infections associated with swimming pools—Dane County, Wisconsin, 1993." From the CDC, *MMWR*. *JAMA*, Sept 28, 1994; 272(12): 914–915

"*Cryptosporidium* seen as food industry problem." *Fd Chem News,* Feb 11, 1991: 14

Deneen, VC, "Outbreak of cryptosporidiosis associated with a water sprinkler fountain—Minnesota, 1997." *MMWR,* Oct 16, 1998; 47(40): 856–860

Dern, A, "Green onions cited as likely source of 1997 outbreak of cryptosporidiosis." *Fd Chem News,* Sept 21, 1998: 6–7

Du Pont, HL et al, "The infectivity of *Cryptosporidium parvum* in healthy volunteers." *N Engl J Med,* Mar 30, 1995; 332(13): 855–859

Durham, S, "*Cryptosporidium* clarified in U.S. cattle." *Agric Res,* May 2005: 22

Dworkin, MS, "Cryptosporidiosis in Washington State: an outbreak associated with well water." Concise Communications. *J Infect Dis,* Dec 1996; 174(6): 1372–1376

Emmerson, AM, "Emerging waterborne infections in health-care settings." Special Issue. *Emerg Infect Dis,* Mar–Apr 2001; 7(2): 272–276

Fayer, R & BLP Ungar, "*Cryptosporidium spp* & cryptosporidiosis." *Microbiol Reviews,* Dec 1986; 50(4): 458–483

Fayer, R, ed, *Cryptosporidium & Cryptosporidiosis.* Boca Raton, FL: CRC Press, 1997

—— "*Cryptosporidium parvum* in oysters from commercial harvesting sites in the Chesapeake Bay." Dispatches. *Emerg Infect Dis,* Sept–Oct 1999; 5(5): 706–710

"Foodborne, waterborne diseases to be addressed by CDC strategy." *Fd Chem News,* May 2, 1994: 33–35

Fox, LM et al, "Emergency survey methods in acute cryptosporidiosis outbreak." *Emerg Infect Dis,* May 2005; 11(5): 729–731

Gelletlie, R et al, "Cryptosporidiosis associated with school milk." *Lancet,* Oct 4, 1997; 350(9083): 1005–1006

Glaberman, S et al, "Three drinking-water-associated cryptosporidiosis outbreaks, Northern Ireland." Dispatches. *Emerg Infect Dis,* June 2002; 8(6): 631–633

Goh, S et al, "Sporadic cryptosporidiosis, North Cumbria, England, 1996–2000." *Emerg Infect Dis,* June 2004; 10(6): 1007–1015

—— "Sporadic cryptosporidiosis decline after membrane filtration of public water supplies, England, 1996–2002." *Emerg Infect Dis,* Feb 2005; 11(2): 251–259

Gorman, J, "Summertime, when people & parasites head for the water." Side Effects, *NY Times,* June 8, 2005: D5

Graham, DR, "Hot tub associated mycobacterial infections in immunosuppressed persons." Lett. *Emerg Infect Dis,* July 2002; 8(7): 750

Guerrant, D et al, "Association of early childhood diarrhea & cryptosporidiosis with impaired physical fitness & cognitive function four-seven years later in a poor urban community in northeast Brazil." *Am J Trop Med Hyg,* 1999; 61: 707–713

Guerrant, RL, "Cryptosporidiosis, an emerging, highly infectious threat." Synopses. *Emerg Infect Dis,* Jan–Mar 1997; 3(1): 51–57

Hashmey, R et al, "Cryptosporidiosis in Houston, Texas, a report of 95 cases." *Med;* 76(2): 118–139

Hayes, EB et al, "Large community outbreak of cryptosporidiosis due to contamination of a filtered public water supply." *N Engl J Med,* May 25, 1999; 320(21): 1372–1376

Healey, MC, "Better treatment for a 'new' disease." *Utah Sci,* Spring 1993: 13–14, 23

Hlavsa, MiC et al, "Cryptosporidiosis surveillance—United States, 1999–2002." *MMWR,* Surveillance Summaries. Jan 28, 2005; 54(SS1): 1–8

Hoskin, JC & RE Wright, "*Cryptosporidium:* an emerging concern for the food industry." *J Fd Protect,* Jan 1991; 54(1): 53–57

Howe, AD et al, "*Cryptosporidium* oocysts in a water supply associated with a cryptosporidiosis outbreak." Research. *Emerg Infect Dis,* June 2002; 8(6): 619–624

Hunter, BT, "*Cryptosporidium:* an emerging human health hazard." *Consumers' Research Mag,* Mar 1993: 8–9

Hunter, PR et al, "Waterborne diseases." Conference Panel Summaries. *Emerg Infect Dis,* June 2001, Supplement; 7(3): 544–545

—— "Subtypes of *Cryptosporidium parvum* in humans & disease risk." Research. *Emerg Infect Dis,* Jan 2007; 13(1): 82–88

Knott, M, "Fatal dose for water parasite." *New Scientist,* Apr 27, 1996; 150(2037): 23

Lake, IR et al, "Cryptosporidiosis decline after regulation, England & Wales, 1989–2005." *Emerg Infect Dis,* Apr 2007; 13(4): 623–625

Liorente, MT, "*Cryptosporidium felis* infection, Spain." Lett. *Emerg Infect Dis,* Sept 2006; 12(9): 1471–1472

MacKensie, WR et al, "A massive outbreak in Milwaukee of *Cryptosporidium* infection transmitted through the public water supply." *N Engl J Med,* July 21, 1994; 331(3): 161–167

—— "An outbreak of cryptosporidiosis associated with a resort swimming pool." *Epidemiol Infect,* Dec 1995; 115(3): 545–553

McAnulty, JM et al, "A community-wide outbreak of cryptosporidiosis associated with swimming at a wave pool." *JAMA* Nov 23–30, 1994; 272(20): 1597–1600

McCarthy, M, "USA: cryptosporidiosis outbreak." *Lancet,* Apr 24, 1993; 341(8852): 1084

McClain, J et al, "Assessing parents' perception of childrens' risk for recreational water illness." Research. *Emerg Infect Dis,* May 2005; 11(5): 670–676

Mercado, R et al, "*Cryptosporidium hominis* infection of the human respiratory tract." Dispatches. *Emerg Infect Dis,* Mar 2007; 13(3): 462–464

Millard, PS et al, "An outbreak of cryptosporidiosis from fresh-pressed apple cider." *JAMA,* Nov 23–30, 1994; 272(20): 1592–1596

Minshew, P et al, "Outbreak of gastroenteritis associated with an interactive water fountain at a beachside park—Florida, 1999." *MMWR,* June 30, 2000; 49(25): 565–568

Mølback, K, "Risk factors for *Cryptosporidium* diarrhea in early childhood: a case control study from Guinea-Bissau, West Africa." *Am J Epidemiol,* 1994; 139: 734–740

Morris, RD, "Temporal variation in drinking water turbidity & diagnosed gastroenteritis in Milwaukee." *AJPH,* Feb 1996; 86(2): 237–239

Mshar, PA et al, "Outbreaks of *Escherichia coli 0157: H7* infection & cryptosporidiosis associated with drinking unpasteurized apple cider—Connecticut & New York, Oct, 1996." *MMWR,* Jan 10, 1997; 46(1): 4–8

Murphy, J, "New study shows *Cryptosporidium* can survive in seawaters, infect oysters." *Fd Chem News,* Mar 30, 1996: 6

—— "*Cryptosporidium*-tainted oysters prompt new warnings from CDC." *Fd Chem News,* Sept 6, 1999: 8–9

Nash, JM et al, "The waterworks flu, a tiny parasite gets the blame for making thousands of Milwaukeeans miserable." Pollution. *Time,* Apr 19, 1993: 41

Naumova, EN et al, "The elderly & waterborne *Cryptosporidium* infections: gastroenteritis hopitalization before & during the 1993 Milwaukee outbreak." Research. *Emerg Infect Dis,* Apr 2003; 9(4): 418–425

Navin, TR, "Detecting cryptosporidiosis as a cause of diarrheal illness: implications for clinicians." Lett. *JAMA,* May 7, 1997; 277(17): 1355–1356

"New drug for parasitic infections in children." Update. *FDA Consumer,* May–June 2001: 4

Newman, A, "Final drinking water monitoring rule set for June." *Environ Sci Tech,* Jan 1995; 29(1): 20A

"Normal chlorination processes won't kill *Cryptosporidium.*" *Fd Chem News,* July 18, 1994: 45–46

Okun, DA, "We need watershed protection & filtration." *NY Times,* May 28, 1994: A18

Olson, BH, "The safety of our drinking water, reason for concern but not alarm." Ed'al. *N Engl J Med,* May 25, 1989; 320(21): 1413–1414

Ong, C et al, "Novel *Cryptosporidium* genotypes in sporadic cryptosporidiosis case: first report of human infection with a cervine genotype." Research. *Emerg Infect Dis,* Mar 2002; 8(3): 263–268

Patten, KJ & JB Rose,"Viability of *Cryptosporidium parvum* oocysts in beverages." *Paper.* Annual Meeting, Inst Fd Tech, 1994

"Physicians try unusual drugs to fight *Cryptosporidium* in AIDS patients. Health. *Am Med News,* Oct 7, 1996: 21

"Prevalence of parasites in fecal material from chlorinated swimming pools—United States, 1999." *MMWR,* May 25, 2001; 50(20): 410–412

Proctor, ME et al, "Surveillance data for waterborne illness detection: an assessment following a massive waterborne outbreak of *Cryptosporidium* infection." *Epidemiol Infect,* Feb 1998; 120(1): 43–54

"Products recalled due to *Cryptosporidium.*" *Fd Chem News,* June 14, 1993: 65

Quinn, K, "Foodborne outbreak of cryptosporidiosis-Spokane, Washington, 1997." *MMWR,* July 17, 1998; 47(27): 565–567

"Responding to fecal accidents in disinfected swimming venues." Notice to Readers. *MMWR,* May 25, 2001; 50(20): 416–417

Robertson, LJ et al, "Survival of *Cryptosporidium parvum* oocysts under various environmental pressures." *Appl Environ Microbiol,* Nov 1992; 58(11): 3494–3500

Rose, JB et al, "Survey of potable water supplies for *Cryptosporidium & Giardia.*" *Environ Sci Tech,* Aug 1991; 25(8): 1393–1400

Segal, M, "Parasitic invaders & the reluctant human host." *FDA Consumer,* July–Aug 1993, 7–13

Sorville, FJ et al, "Swimming-associated cryptosporidiosis—Los Angeles County." Epidemiol Notes Repts. *MMWR,* May 25, 1990; 39(20): 343–345

Stoeckie, M & RG Douglas, Jr., "Infectious diseases." Contemp 1995, *JAMA,* June 7, 1995; 273(21): 1686–1688

Tzipori, S, "Cryptosporidiosis in animals & humans." *Microbiol Reviews,* Mar 1983; 47(1): 84–96

Veverka, F et al, "Protracted outbreaks of cryptosporidiosis associated with swimming pool use—Ohio & Nebraska, 2000." *MMWR,* May 25, 2001; 50(20): 406–410

Vugia, DJ et al, "Mycobacteria in nail salon, whirlpool footbath, California." Dispatches. *Emerg Infect Dis,* Apr 2005; 11(4): 616–618

"Waterborne *Cryptosporidium* is killed by ozone in soft drinks." *Fd Chem News* Mar 20, 1995: 6

"Waterborne illness prevention measures recommended by CDC 'optimal filtration' seen needed for *Cryptosporidium*." *Fd Chem New,* Aug 23, 1993: 22–23

Whitman, D, "The sickening sewer crisis." *US News & World Rept,* June 12, 2000: 16–18

Chapter 16

Becker, H, "Reinventing systematics. Tracking trichinosis carriers." *Agric Res,* May 1995: 5–6

"Education, control measures to stem trichinosis urged by CDC." *Fd Chem News,* Feb 10, 1992: 72

CDC."Summary of Notifiable Diseases, United States." *MMWR* 2006 55(53); 2005 54(53); 2004 53(53); 2003 52(53); 2002 51(53); 2001 50(53); 2000 49(53); 1999 48(53); 1998 47(53); 1997 46(54); 1996 45(53)

Federal Register. "Trichinae certification program: final rule." APHIS, USDA 9FR, Parts 149, 160, 161, Oct 2008

Frongillo, RF et al, "Report of an outbreak of trichinellosis in Central Italy." *Eur J Epidemiol,* Mar 2002; 8: 282–288

"FSIS defines pork products to be treated for trichinae," *Fd Chem News,* May 10, 1993: 40–41

Greenbloom, SL et al, "Outbreak of trichinosis in Ontario secondary to the ingestion of wild boar meat." *Can J PH,* Jan–Feb 1997; 88(1): 52–56

Hall, KN, "Trichinosis from commercial pork: a review." *Fd Safety Notebk,* July–Aug 1992; 3(7–8): 76–77

Landry, SM et al, "Trichinosis: common source outbreak related to commercial pork." *South Med J,* Apr 1992; 85(4): 428–429

Mazzola, V, "Real-world research: it's pigs & chickens." *Agric Res,* July 1990: 10–12

McAuley, JB et al, "Trichinosis surveillance, United States, 1987–1990." *MMWR,* Dec 1991; 40(SS3): 35–42

—— "Trichinosis surveillance, United States, 1987–1990." *MMWR,* Feb 7, 1992; 41(5): 87

McBride, J, "Giving pork a new image." *Agric Res,* Aug 2000: 18–19

Murrell, KD, "Parasites: the problems persist." Forum. *Agric Res*, Dec 1996: 3

Newman, A, "In pursuit of autoimmune worm cure." Health & Fitness. *NY Times*, Aug 31, 1999: D5

Phabmixey, V et al, "*Trichinella spiralis* infections—United States, 1990." Epidemiol Notes. Repts. *MMWR*, Feb 1, 1991; 40(4): 57–60

Ranque, S et al, "*Trichinella pseudospiralis* outbreak in France." Dispatches. *Emerg Infect Dis.* Sept–Oct 2000; 6(5): 543–547

Rehmet, S et al, "Trichinellosis outbreaks—Northrhine—Westfalia, Germany, 1998–1999." *MMWR*, June 18, 1999: 488–492

Roy, SL et al, "Trichinellosis surveillance—United States, 1997–2001." Surveillance Summaries. *MMWR*, July 25, 2003; 52(SS–6): 1–8

Smith, P, "Trichinellosis associated with bear meat—New York & Tennessee, 2003." *MMWR*, July 16, 2004; 53(27): 606–610

"Specifies trichinae treatment for poultry products containing pork." *Fd Tech*, Aug 1992: 70

Stack, PS, "Trichinosis still a public health threat." *Postgrad Med*, June 1995; 97(6): 137–144

"*Trichinella spiralis* Infections—United States, 1990." *MMWR*, Feb 1, 1991; 40(4): 57–60

"Trichinosis outbreak prompts French ban on U.S. horsemeat." *Fd Chem News*, Apr 1, 1991: 50–51

"Trichinosis outbreaks." Updates. *FDA Consumer*, May 1991: 4–5

"USDA trichinae proposal warns firms on pathogen control." *Fd Chem News*, Jan 14, 1991: 14–15

Vollbrecht, A et al, "Outbreak of trichinellosis associated with eating cougar jerky—Idaho, 1995." *MMWR*, Mar 15, 1996; 45(10): 205–206

"Wisconsin trichinosis outbreak called largest in decade." *Fd Chem News*, Apr 8, 1991: 30

Woodwossen A et al, "Seroprevalence of *Trichinella, Toxoplasma,* and *Salmonella* in antimicrobial-free and conventional swine production systems." *Foodborne Pathogens and Disease,* April 2008; 5(2): 199–203

Zimmerman WJ, "Evaluation of microwave cooking procedures and ovens for devitalizing *Trichinae* in pork roasts." *Journal of Food Science* 1983; 48(3): 856

Chapter 17

Altman, LK, "Botulinum toxin's promise as drug may rival its potential as weapon." Health. *NY Times*, Mar 10, 1998: C7

Anderson, I, "End of the line for deadly stowaway?" *New Scientist*, Oct 24, 1992; 36(1844): 12–13

Andres, C, "Acidulants: flavor, preserve, texturize & leaven foods." *Fd Process*, July 1985: 52–54

Anonsen, C, "Botulinum toxin for treatment of spastic dysphonia." Lett. *Conn Med*, Aug 1989; 53(8): 464–465

Baird, B, "Sous vide: What's all the excitement about?" *Fd Tech* Nov 1990; 44(11): 92; 94; 96

Bell, E et al, "Botulism associated with commercially distributed kapchunka—New York City." *MMWR*, Sept 6, 1985; 34(35): 546–547

Blatherwick, FJ et al, "Update: International outbreak of restaurant-associated botulism—Vancouver, British Columbia, Canada." *MMWR*, Oct 18, 1985; 34(41): 643

Blumenthal, D, "The canning process, old preservation technique goes modern." *FDA Consumer*, Sept 1990: 14–18

"Botulin & commercial pot pie—California." *MMWR*, Jan 28, 1983; 32(3): 39–40, 45

"Botulinum toxin." *Consensus Statement*, NIH, Nov 1990; 8(8): 1–20

"Botulinum toxin relaxes stiffness of cerebral palsy." *Med Trib*, Mar 12, 1992: B10

"Botulism & vacuum-packaged foods at issue in FSIS letter." *Fd Chem News*, Mar 13, 1995: 10

"Botulism from fresh foods—California." Epidemiol Notes & Repts. *MMWR*, Mar 22, 1985; 34(11): 156–159

"Botulism from home-canned bamboo shoots—Nan Province, Thailand, Mar 2006." *MMWR*, Apr 14, 2006; 55(14): 389–395

"Botulism guilty of fowl play." Constance Holden, ed. Random Samples. *Sci*, Nov 7, 1997: 1019

"Botulism toxin effective against excessive sweating." News. *Am Med News*, Mar 23–30, 1998: 36

"Brief report: foodborne botulism from home-prepared fermented tofu—California, 2006." *JAMA*, Mar 28, 2007; 297(12): 1311–1312

Burros, Marian, "Trying to solve the botulism mystery." *NY Times*, Apr 28, 1982: C1

Byron, J, "Botulism a possible threat to packaged products, IFPA [International Fresh-cut Produce Association] warned." *Fd Chem News*, Dec 15, 1997: 9–10

Calderon, M & Rivka BG, eds. *Food Preservation by Modified Atmospheres*. Boca Raton, FL, CRC Press, 1990

Cawthorne, A et al, "Botulism & preserved green olives." Lett. *Emerg Infect Dis*, May 2005; 11(5): 781–782

Chen, I, "Toxin to the rescue: tapping a deadly botulinum protein to treat neuromuscular disorders." *Sci News*, Jan 19, 1991: 42–43

"Controlled atmosphere extends meat shelf life." Pkging News & Trends. *Pkging*, Aug 1984: 8

Corlett, Jr, DA, "Refrigerated foods & use of hazard analysis & critical control point principles." *Fd Tech*, Feb 1989: 91–94

Corwin, E, "A food poisoning whodunit." *FDA Consumer*, Nov 1980: 4–7

D'Argenio, P et al, "Type B botulism associated with roasted eggplant in oil—Italy 1993." *MMWR*, Jan 20, 1995; 44(2): 33–36

Desorbo, MA, "The carbon monoxide conundrum." *Fd Qual*, Feb–Mar 2006: 12–13

Dickson, EC et al, "A study of the resistance of the spores of *Bacillus botulinus* to various sterilizing agencies which are commonly employed in the canning of fruits & vegetables." *Arch Intern Med*, 1919; 24: 581–589

Doughty, SC et al, "Foodborne botulism—Illinois." *MMWR*, Jan 20, 1984; 33(2): 22–23

Downing, DL, ed, "Refrigerated foods & emerging pathogens." *Special Rept*, Nov 1989, Geneva, NY: NY State Agr Exp Sta, No 64, Sept 1990

"Drug from botulism toxin." Updates. *FDA Consumer*, Mar 1990: 2

Ember, L, "Botox: neuromuscular modulator." *C&EN*, June 20, 2005: 50

Flieger, K et al, "Don't trifle with truffles." Investigators' Repts. *FDA Consumer*, July–Aug 1989: 36

Forcinio, H, "Extending freshness & shelf life." *Prep Fds*, Nov 1984: 87–88, 90

Franz, DR et al, "Clinical recognition & management of patients exposed to biological warfare agents." *JAMA*, Aug 6, 1997; 278(5): 407

French, G et al, "Outbreak of Type E botulism associated with an uneviscerated salt-cured fish product—New Jersey 1992." Epidemiol Notes & Repts. *MMWR*, July 24, 1992; 41(29): 521–522

"Garlic-oil preparation, 34 botulism cases linked." *Am Med News*, Nov 1, 1985: 42

"Get rid of the garlic, FDA says." Updates, *FDA Consumer*, June 1999: 2

Ginsberg, MM et al, "Botulism associated with commercially canned chili sauce—Texas & Indiana, July 2007." *MMWR*, Aug 3, 2007; 56(30): 767–769

Glass, KA & MP Doyle, "Relationship between water activity of fresh pasta & toxin production by proteolytic *Clostridium botulinum*." *J Fd Protect*, Mar 1991; 54(3): 162–165

Hall, T, "Pouches offer fresher foods, but FDA warns of risk." *NY Times*, Mar 23, 1988: C1, C8

Handy, B et al, "That deadpan look: if injections of a lethal toxin can eliminate unsightly wrinkles, who cares if it also paralyzes your face?" *Time*, July 13, 1998: 72

Hauschild, A, HW & KL Dodds, eds. *Clostridium Botulinum: Ecology & Control in Foods.* NY: Marcel Dekker, 1993

Hays, SM, "Innovations in foods: safety first." *Agric Res*, Jan 1989: 10–11

Hecht, A et al, "Acid test for tomatoes." Investigators' Repts, *FDA Consumer*, Apr 1986: 36

Higgin, KT, "Petition puts MAP for meat in spotlight." *Fd Engineer*, Apr 2006: 19

Hopkins, H, "The way of botulism." *FDA Consumer*, Oct 1984: 33

Horn, A et al, "Botulism outbreak associated with eating fermented food—Alaska, 2001." *MMWR*, Aug 17, 2001; 50(32): 680–682

Horvitz, E & J Mans, "Perdue's CAP pack powers new products." *Prep Fds*, June 1988: 76–78, 80, 82, 84

Huhtanen, CN et al, "Acid enhancement of *Clostridium botulinum* inhibition in ham & bacon prepared with potassium sorbate & sorbic acid." *J Fd Protect*, Sept 1983; 46(9): 807–810

Hunter, BT, "Packaging Food," Fd for Thought. *Consumers'Research Mag*, Feb 1985: 8–9

—— "Preventing botulism." Food for Thought. *Consumer's Research Mag*, July 1986: 8–9

—— "The pros & cons of aseptic packaging: is it environmentally correct?" *Consumers' Research Mag*, Aug 1991: 15–17

—— "Food recalls: how well do they work? Could they be better?" *Consumers' Research Mag*, Aug 2002: 10–14, 25

"Is carbon monoxide a good gas or a bad gas?" *Fd Qual Mag*, Apr–May 2006: 19

Katz, F, "Formulating for increased shelf life." *Fd Process*, Mar 2006: 34–35, 37–38

Kershaw, P et al, "Fish botulism—Hawaii 1990." Epidemiol Notes. *MMWR*, June 23, 1991; 40(24): 442–444

Knubley, W et al, "Foodborne botulism—Oklahoma 1994." *MMWR* Mar 24, 1995; 44(11): 200–202

Kotev, S et al, "International outbreak of Type E botulism associated with ungutted, salted whitefish." *MMWR*, Dec 18, 1987; 36(49): 812–813

Lambert, AD et al, "Continued effect of modified atmosphere packaging & low-dose irradiation on toxin produced by *Clostridium botulinum* in fresh pork." *J Fd Protect*, Feb 1991; 54: 94–101

Lang, SS, "'Microatmosphere packaging' preserves unrefrigerated fruit for months." *News Summary*, Ithaca, NY: Cornell U, Oct 11, 1983

Liston, J, "Microbial hazards of seafood consumption." *Fd Tech*, Dec 1990; 44(12): 56, 58–62

Lombardi, S & J Knight, "Armour beef stew recalled nationwide." Press Release No 0787 93, USDA, Sept 16, 1993

Ludlow, CL, "Treatment of speech & voice disorders with botulinum toxin." Grand Rounds at the Clinical Center of the NIH. *JAMA*, Nov 28, 1990; 264(20): 2671–2675

MacDonald, KL et al, "Type A botulism from sautéed onions." *JAMA*, Mar 1, 1985; 253(9): 1275–1278

Mann, JM. "Economic impact of a botulism outbreak: importance of the legal component in food-borne disease." *JAMA*, Mar 11, 1983; 249(10): 1299–1301

"MAP/polyester boosts meat shelf life to 40 days." *Pkging Digest*, Oct 1997: 4, 10

McLaughlin, JB. "Botulism Type E outbreak associated with eating a beached whale, Alaska." *Emerg Infect Dis*, Sept 2004; 10(9): 1685–1687

McLean, HE et al, "Restaurant-associated botulism from mushrooms bottled-in-house—Vancouver, British Columbia, Canada." *MMWR*, Feb 27, 1987; 36(7): 103

Miller, RW, "How onions & a baked potato became sources of botulism poisoning." *FDA Consumer*, Oct 1984: 711–712

Morris, CE. "Vac-pack, MAP focus FDA concern on botulism toxicity can occur before spoilage in chilled food packaged under modified atmosphere or vacuum." Fd Pkging. *Fd Engineer*, Oct 1989: 64–65

Morse, DL, "Garlic-in-oil associated botulism: episode leads to product modification." *AJPH*, Nov 1990; 80(11): 1372–1373

Murphy, J, "Milk products scrutinized after California dairy cows die from botulism." *Fd Chem News*, June 7, 1999: 24

"New packaging machine improves shelf life of fresh meats." *Fd Engineer*, Apr 1990, 31

Notermans, S et al, "Botulism risk of refrigerated, processed foods of extended durability."*J Fd Prot*, Dec 1990; 53(12): 1020–1024

Ogoma, K et al, "Infant botulism due to *Clostridium botulinum* Type C toxin." Lett. *Lancet*, Dec 8, 1990; 336(8728): 1449–1450

Patel, T, "Botulism wipes out French wildfowl." *New Scientist*, Nov 25, 1995; 148(2005): 6

Paul, TO, "Botulinum toxin for the treatment of blepharospasm & strabismus." Lett. *Conn Med*, Dec 1990; 54(12): 664–665

"Potatoes wrapped in aluminum foil, baked & held at room temperature can cause botulism." Brief Notes. *Fd Chem News*, July 6, 1998: 33

Poulson, J, "Shouting from the rooftop—looking under the table." *Utah Sci*, Fall 1990: 97–99

Reddy, D et al, "Nitrite inhibition of *Clostridium botulinum*: electron spin resonance detection of iron-nitric acid complexes." *Sci*, Aug 19, 1983; 221: 769–770

"Restaurant-associated botulism—Vancouver, British Columbia." Epidemiol Notes & Repts. *MMWR*, Sept 20, 1985; 34(37): 571

"Retail vacuum packaging of meat: a hazard." *Utah Sci*, Fall 1990: 99

Rhodehamel, EJ, "FDA's concerns with sous vide processing." *Fd Tech*, Sept 1992: 73–76

Rifkin, G et al, "Foodborne botulism from eating home-pickled eggs—Illinois 1997." *MMWR*, Sept 1, 2000; 49(34): 778–780

Robbins, J, "Outbreaks of a rare botulism strain stymie scientists." *NY Times*, Oct 22, 2002: F3

Seals, JE, el al, "Restaurant-associated Type A botulism: transmission by potato salad." *Am J Epidemiol*, 1981; 113: 436–444

Segal, M, "Fish 'delicacy' causes botulism & death." Investigators' Repts. *FDA Consumer*, May 1988: 33

—— "Native food preparation fosters botulism, Alaskan dilemma." *FDA Consumer*, Jan–Feb 1992: 23–27

Shapiro, RL et al, "Botulism surveillance & emergency response: a public health strategy for a global challenge." *JAMA*, Aug 6, 1997; 278(5): 433–435

Shuler, C et al, "Botulism associated with commercial carrot juice—Georgia & Florida, Sept 2006." *MMWR*, Oct 13, 2006; 55(40): 1098–1099

Sobel, J et al, "Foodborne botulism in the United States, 1990–2000." Research. *Emerg Infect Dis*, Sept 2004; 10: 1606–1611

Solomon, HM et al, "Outgrowth of *Clostridium botulinum* in shredded cabbage at room temperature under a modified atmosphere." *J Fd Protect*, Oct 1990; 53(10): 831–833

Sterba, JP, "The history of botulism." *NY Times*, Apr 28, 1982: C6

"Sulfite masks C. bot growth in vacuum-packed potatoes, FDA-er." *Fd Chem News*, July 26, 1993: 48–49

"Toxic gas & meat—perfect together?" *Fd Qual*, Dec 2005–Jan 2006: 17

Uldrich, J, "Nanotechnology: The next small thing in food." Culinary Vistas. *Culinology,* Dec 2007: 15–16, 18–19

"Vacuum-packed shredded lettuce stays fresh for 12 full days." Reprint. *Fd Engineer,* Apr 1977 [unpaginated]

Vangelova, L, "Botulinum toxin: a poison that can heal." *FDA Consumer,* Dec 1995: 16–19

Varma, JK, "Foodborne botulism in the Republic of Georgia." *Emerg Infect Dis,* Sept 2004; 10(9): 1601–1604

Villar, RG et al, "Outbreak of Type A botulism & development of a botulism surveillance & antitoxin release system in Argentina." Lett from Buenos Aires. *JAMA,* Apr 14, 1999; 281(14): 1334–1340

"Warning letter hits uneviscerated fish." *Fd Chem News,* June 8, 1992: 32

Weiss, R, "FDA is urged to ban carbon-monoxide-treated meat." *Wash Post* Feb 20, 2006: A01

Wongwatcharapaiboon, P et al, "Foodborne botulism associated with home-canned bamboo shoots—Thailand, 1998." *MMWR,* June 4, 1999; 48(21): 437–439

Zilinskas, RA, "Iraq's biological weapons." *JAMA,* Aug 6, 1997; 278(5): 421

Chapter 18

Bar-Dayan, Y, "Food-borne outbreak of streptococcal pharyngitis in an Israel airforce base." *Scand J Infect Dis,* 1966; 28: 563–566

Cary, WE et al, "An institutional outbreak of food poisoning possibly due to a *Streptococcus.*" *Proc Soc Exp Biol Med,* 1931; 29: 214–215

CDC: Foodborne Disease Surveillance. *Annual Summary,* June 1983, HHS Pub No (CDC) 83–8185; 16: 38

Cohen, AD et al, "Foodborne epidemic of streptococcal pharyngitis at an Israeli military training base." *Military Med, 1982;* 147: 318–319

Decker, MD et al, "Food-borne streptococcal pharyngitis in a hospital pediatric clinic." Brief Repts. *JAMA,* Feb 1, 1985; 253(5): 679–681

DeCunto, CL et al, "Prognosis of children with poststreptococcal reactive arthritis." *Pediat Infect Dis J,* 1988; 7: 683–686

Dirks, T et al, "A foodborne outbreak of streptococcal pharyngitis—Portland, Oregon." *MMWR,* Jan 22, 1982; 31(1 & 2): 3–5

Elsea, WR et al, "An epidemic of food-associated pharyngitis & diarrhea." *Arch Environ Hlth,* 1971; 23: 48–56

Espinosa, FH et al, "Group C streptococcal infections associated with eating homemade cheese—New Mexico." Epidemiol Notes Repts. *MMWR,* Oct 7, 1983; 32(39): 510, 515–516

Fackelmann, KA, "Does strep trigger movement disorders?" *Sci News,* July 17, 1993: 39

Farber, RE & FA Korff, "Foodborne epidemic of group A beta-hemolytic *Streptococcus.*" *Pub Hlth Rept,* 1958; 73: 203–209

Farley, TA et al, "Direct inoculation of food as the cause of an outbreak of group A strepto-coccal pharyngitis." *J Infect Dis*, May 1993; 167(5): 1232–1235

Flanagan, K et al, "Group A, B [beta-] hemolytic *Streptococcus* skin infections in a meat-packing plant—Oregon." Epidemiol Notes Repts. *MMWR*, Oct 10, 1986; 35(40): 629–630

"Foodborne group A strep pharyngitis." *Infect Dis*, Mar 1978: 8–9

Gallo, G et al, "An outbreak of group A food-borne streptococcal pharyngitis." *Europ J Epi-demiol*, Mar 1992; 8(2): 292–297

Getting, VA et al, "A food-borne *Streptococcus* outbreak." *Am J Pub Hlth*, 1943; 33: 1217–1223

Groseclose, SL et al, *Summary of Notifiable Diseases—United States, 2000.* pub. June 14, 2002 for 2000. *MMWR*; 49(53): xix–xx, 66–67

—— *Summary of Notifiable Diseases—United States, 2001.* pub. May 2, 2003 for 2001. *MMWR*; 50(53); xxi–xxii, 106

"Group A streptococcal infections." *Natl Inst Allerg Infect Dis, NIH*, Dec 1997

Hill, HR et al, "Food-borne epidemics of streptococcal pharyngitis at the United States Air Force Academy." *N Engl J Med*, 1969; 280: 917–921

Jordan, WS, "Commission on Acute Respiratory Diseases," in The History of the Commis-sions (Section I), ed. TE Woodward. Washington, DC: Borden Institute, Office of the Sur-geon General Department of the Army, 1994

Lossos, IS et al, "Food-borne outbreak of group A beta-hemolytic streptococcal pharyngitis." *Arch Intern Med*, Apr 1992; 152(4): 853–855

Lynch, M et al, "Surveillance for foodborne-disease outbreaks—United States, 1998–2002." Surveill Summ. *MMWR*, Nov 10, 2006; 55(SS–10); 40

McCormick, JB et al, "Epidemic streptococcal sore throat following a community picnic." *JAMA*, 1976; 236: 1039–1041

Nowak, R, "Flesh-eating bacteria: not new, but still worrisome." Bacteriol. *Sci*, June 17, 1994; 264: 1665

Olsen, SJ et al, "Surveillance for foodborne disease outbreaks—United States, 1993–1997." CDC Surveill Summ. *MMWR*, Mar 17, 2000; 49(SS–1): 58

"Outbreak of foodborne streptococcal disease—Florida." *MMWR*, 1974; 23: 365–366

"Rice linked to pharyngitis outbreak." *Am Med News*, Feb 8, 1985: 50

Rigau, JG, "Streptococal foodborne outbreaks—Puerto Rico, Missouri." Epidemiol Notes Repts. *MMWR*, Nov 30, 1984(47): 669–672

Scamman, CL et al, "Scarlet fever outbreak due to infected food." *Am J Pub Hlth*, 1927; 17: 311–316

Seachrist, L, "The once & future scourge, could common anti-inflammatory drugs allow bacteria to take a deadly turn?" *Sci News*, Oct 7, 1995: 234–235

Stryker, WS et al, "Foodborne outbreak of group G streptococcal pharyngitis." *Am J Epi-demiol*, 1982; 116: 533–540

Weinstein, M et al, "Invasive infection with *Streptococcus iniae*—Ontario, 1995–1996." *MMWR*, Aug 2, 1996; 45(30): 650–653

—— "Invasive infections due to a fish pathogen, *Streptococcus iniae*." For the *S. iniae* Study Group. *N Engl J Med*, Aug 28, 1997; 337(9): 589–594

Chapter 19

Archer, G & JM Boslievac, "Signalling antibiotic resistance in staphylococci." Perspect Microbiol. *Sci*, Mar 9, 2001; 291: 1915–1916

Aubrey-Damon, H et al, "Antimicrobial resistance in commensal flora of pig farmers." Research. *Emerg Infect Dis*, May 2004; 10(5): 873–879

"Barrier teat dips fail to prevent *S. aureus* in milk." *Fd Chem News*, Jan 11, 1999: 17–18

Barstow, JA et al, "Staphylococcal food poisoning in Florida." *MMWR*, Apr 6, 1979: 153

Bell, KM et al, "Staphylococcal food poisoning—New York." Epidemiol Notes Repts. *MMWR*, Feb 2, 1979: 45

Brennan, M, "Plant may hold key to ultimate antibiotic." *Chem Engineer News*, Feb 21, 2000: 6–7

Campbell G et al, "Growth of lettuce & cauliflower tissues in vitro & their production of antimicrobial metabolites." *Can J Microbiol*, 1965; 11: 785–789

Chambers, HF, "The changing epidemiology of *Staphylococcus aureus*?" Special Issue, *Emerg Infect Dis*, Mar–Apr 2001; 7(2): 178–182

Chickamori, T, "Endocarditis from *Staphylococcus aureus*." Lett. *JAMA*, Dec 21, 2005; 294(23): 2972

"Chitin-containing canned foods may be prone to outbreaks." *Fd Chem News*, Aug 5, 1996: 11–12

Coglan, A, "Animal antibiotics threaten hospital epidemics." *New Scientist*, July 27, 1996; 15(2040): 7

Collingon, P et al, "*Staphylococcus aureus* bacteremia, Australia." Research. *Emerg Infect Dis*, Apr 2005; 11(4): 554–561

Collins, RK, "Multiple outbreaks of staphylococcal food poisoning caused by canned mushrooms." Epidemiol Notes Repts. *MMWR*, June 23, 1989; 38(24): 417–418

Conners, E et al, "Staphylococcal food poisoning—Delaware." Epidemiol Notes Repts. *MMWR*, Sept 21, 1979: 445–446

Cox, L et al, "Interstate common-source outbreaks of staphylococcal food poisoning—North Carolina, Pennsylvania." *MMWR*, Apr 15, 1983; 32(14): 183–184; 189

Day, N et al, "A link between virulence & ecological abundance in natural populations of *Staphylococcus aureus*." Repts. *Sci*, Apr 6, 2001; 292: 114–116

Enserink, M, "Resistant staph finds new niches." Infect Dis. *Sci*, Mar 14, 2003; 299: 1639–1641

Foodborne Disease Surveillance. Annual Summary 1982. HHS Pub No (CDC) 85, 8185, Sept 1985: 14

Fowler, VG, "Endocarditis from *Staphylococcus aureus*." Lett. *JAMA*, Dec 21, 2005; 294(23): 2973

Francis, BJ, "Presumed staphylococcal food poisoning associated with whipped butter." Epidemiol Notes Repts. *MMWR*, Aug 12, 1977; 26: 268

"Gastroenteritis from contaminated milkshakes." *Infect Dis*, June 1974: 25

Gravet, A et al, "*Staphylococcus aureus* isolated in cases of impetigo produces both epidermolysin A or B & LukE-LukD in 78% of 131 retrospective & prospective cases." *J Clin Microbiol*, 2001; 39: 4349–4356

Hageman, JC et al, "Severe community-acquired pneumoniae due to *Stapylococcus aureus*, 2003–2004 influenza season." Research. *Emerg Infect Dis*, June 2006; 12(6): 894–899

Hart-English, P et al, "Staphylococcal food poisoning outbreaks caused by canned mushrooms from China." *Fd Tech*, Dec 1990, 74: 76–77

Hiramatsu, K et al, "Reduced susceptibility of *Staphylococcus aureus* to vancomycin—Japan, 1996." *MMWR*, July 1997; 46(27): 624–626

Holmberg, SD & PA Blake, "Staphylococcal food poisoning in the United States—new facts & old misconceptions." *JAMA*, Jan 27, 1984; 251(4): 487–499

Levine, WC et al, "Foodborne disease outbreaks in nursing homes, 1975 through 1987." *JAMA*, Oct 16, 1991; 266(15): 2105–2109

Lorber, M, "Endocarditis from *Staphylococcus aureus*." Lett. *JAMA*, Dec 21, 2005; 294(23): 2972

Marrack, P & J Kappler, "The staphylococcal enterotoxins & their relatives." Articles. *Sci*, May 11, 1990; 248: 705–711

Martin, R et al, "*Staphylococcus aureus* with reduced susceptibility to vancomycin—United States, 1997." *MMWR*, Aug 22, 1997; 46(33): 765–766

—— "Update: *Staphylococcus aureus* with reduced susceptibility to vancomycin—United States, 1997." *MMWR*, Sept 5, 1997; 46(35): 813–815

Mazmanian, SK et al, "*Staphylococcus aureus* sortase, an enzyme that anchors surface proteins to the cell wall." Rept. *Sci*, July 30, 1999; 285: 760–763

Mount, JR et al, "Effect of temperature & CO_2 concentration on growth of *Staphylococcus aureus* in fresh pasta." *Presentation*. 59-C-21, Inst Fd Tech, annual meeting, 1994

Munoz, R, "Staphylococcal food poisoning from turkey at a country club buffet—New Mexico." Epidemiol Notes Repts. *MMWR*, Nov 21, 1986; 35(46): 715–722

"NIH: measles deaths linked to *S. aureus*." *Med Trib*, Nov 28, 1991: 24

Nishina, A et al, "2,6-Dimethoxy-p-benzoquinone as an antibacterial substance in the bark of *Phyllostachys heterocycla var. pubescens*, a species of thick-stemmed bamboo." *Journal of Agricultural and Food Chemistry*, Feb 1991; 39(2): 266–269

"Over 7,000 sickened by Snow Brand milk in Japan." *Prep Fds*, July 2000: 33

"Overwrapping found to promote pathogen growth in packaged fresh mushrooms." *Fd Chem News*, Oct 14, 1996: 4–5

Palumbo, SS & JL Smith, "Repair of heat-injured *Staphylococcus aureus* 196E on food substrates & additives & at different temperatures." *J Fd Prot*, Apr 1982; 45(5): 455–461

"Pork pathogen survey conducted." Fd Safety Consortium. *FSIS Fd Safety Rev*, Summer 1992: 2(2): 20–22

Rasmussen, N, "Tales of a wonder drug." Bks et al, Pharmacol. *Sci*, Aug 24, 2007; 317: 1037–1038

Røder, BL et al, "Clinical features of *Staphylococcus aureus* endocarditis: a 10-year experience in Denmark." *Arch Intern Med*, 1999; 159: 462–469

Schneewind, O et al, "Structure of the cell wall anchor of surface proteins in *Staphylococcus aureus*." Rept. *Sci*, Apr 7, 1995; 268: 103–106

Segal, M, "Problem pasta pulled from market." Investigators' Repts. *FDA Consumer*, Sept 1994: 33–34

Siam, AR & M Hammoudeh, "*Staphylococcus aureus* triggered reactive arthritis." *Ann Rheum*, 1995; 54, 131–133

Sievert, DM et al, "*Staphylococcus aureus* resistant to vancomycin—United States, 2002." *MMWR*, July 5, 2002; 51(25): 565–567

Slack, R et al, "Staphylococcal food poisoning—West Virginia." Epidemiol Notes Repts. *MMWR*, Aug 1, 1980, 367–368

Smith, T et al, "Methicillin-resistant *Staphylococcus aureus* (MRSA) strain ST398 is present in midwestern U.S. swine and swine workers." PLoS ONE 4(1): e4258. doi:10.1371/journal. pone.0004258

Sokari, TG & SO Anozie, "Occurrence of enterotoxin producing strains of *Staphylococcus aureus* in meat & related samples from traditional markets in Nigeria." *J Fd Prot*, Dec 1990; 53(12): 1069–1070

"Staphylococcal food poisoning associated with Genoa & hard salami—United States." Epidemiol Notes Repts. *MMWR*, Apr 20, 1979: 179–180

"Staphylococcal food poisoning on a cruise ship." *MMWR*, June 10, 1983; 32(22): 294–295

"Staphylococcal infections." *Natl Inst Allerg Infect Dis*, NIH, Spring 1995

Stermitz, FR et al, "Synergy in a medicinal plant: antimicrobial action of berberine potentiated by 5'-methoxyhydnocarpin, a multidrug pump inhibitor." *Proceedings of the National Academy of Sciences*, 2000; 97(4): 1433–1437

"Sticky treatment for staph infections." Antibiotic Resistance. *Sci News*, June 9, 2007: 366

Strauss, E, "A possible new approach to combating staph infections." Microbiol. *Sci*, Apr 17, 1998; 280: 379

Surveillance for Food-borne Disease Outbreaks—United States, 1993–1997, CDC Surveill Summ. *MMWR*, Mar 17, 2000; 49(SS–1): 58

Tranter, HS, "Foodborne staphylococcal illness." Fdborne Ill. *Lancet*, Oct 27, 1990; 336: 1044–1046

van Duijkeren, E et al, "Methicillin-resistant *Staphylococcus aureus* in pigs with exudative epidermitis." Dispatches. *Emerg Infect Dis*, Sept 2007; 13(9): 1408–1410

Ward, K et al, "Outbreak of staphylococcal food poisoning associated with precooked ham—Florida, 1997." *MMWR*; 46(50): 1189–1191

Watanakunakorn, C, " *Staphylococcus aureus* endocarditis at a community teaching hospital, 1980 to 1991: an analysis of 106 cases." *Arch Intern Med*, 1994; 154: 2330–2335

Chapter 20

Alper, J, "Ulcers as an infectious disease." *Sci*, Apr 9, 1993; 260(5105): 1559–1560

—— "New bind for ulcer bacterium." *Sci*, Dec 17, 1993; 262: 1817

Altman, LK, "Lymphomas are on the rise in U.S., and no one knows why." Med Sci, Doctor's World, *NY Times*, May 24, 1994: B7

—— "Two win Nobel Prize for discovering bacterium tied to stomach ailments." Health & Fitness, *NY Times*, Oct 4, 2005: F5

—— "Nobel came after years of battling the system." Doctor's World, *NY Times*, Oct 11, 2005: F5, F8

—— "A scientist gazing toward Stockholm, ponders 'what if?' " Doctor's World, *NY Times*, Dec 6, 2005: F5, F8

"Antibiotics help fight stomach cancer." *Sci News*. Sept 1, 1993: 189

Armuzzi, A et al, "Effect of *Lactobacillus GG* supplementation in antibiotic-associated gastrointestinal side effects during *Helicobacter pylori* eradication therapy: A pilot study." *Digestion*, 2001; 63: 1–7

Bankhead, CD, "Office test for *H. pylori* at hand." *Med World News*, June 1991: 58

Bishop, JE, "Bacterium causes most peptic ulcers." Tech & Health, *Wall St J*, Feb 10, 1994: B6

Blaser, MJ, "Not all *Helicobacter pylori* strains are created equal; should all be eliminated?" *Lancet*, Apr 5, 1997; 349(9057): 1020–1022

—— "Where does *Helicobacter pylori* come from and why is it going away?" *JAMA*, Dec 15, 1999; 282(23): 2260–2262

Borén, T et al, "Attachment of *Helicobacter pylori* to human gastric epithelium mediated by blood group antigens." *Sci*, Dec 17, 1993; 262: 1892–1894

Bosch, JA et al, "Salivary MUC5B-mediated adherence (ex vivo) of *Helicobacter pylori* during stress." *Psychosom Med*, Jan–Feb 2000; 62(1): 40–49

Castelvecchi, D, "Ulcer bug linked to stroke." Biomed. *Sci News*, Aug 10, 2002: 94

Carlson, S et al, "Progression of gastritis to monoclonal B cell lymphoma with resolution recurrence following eradication of *Helicobacter pylori*." Clin Invest, *JAMA*, Mar 27, 1996; 275(12): 937–939

Carmel, R et al, "*Helicobacter pylori* infection and food-cobalamin malabsorption." *Digest Dis Sci*, Feb 1944; 39(2): 300–314

Christiensen, D, "Is your stomach bugging you? The rise and fall of the bacterium *H. pylori*." *Sci News*, Oct 9, 1999: 234–236

Correa, P, "Is gastric carcinoma an infectious disease?" Ed'al. *N Engl J Med*, Oct 17, 1991: 1170–1171

—— et al, "Chemoprevention of gastric dysplasia: randomized trial of antioxidant supplements & anti-*Helicobacter pylori* therapy." *J NCI*, 2000; 92: 1881–1888

Corvaglia, L, "Accuracy of serology and 13C-urea breath test for detection of *Helicobacter pylori* in children." *Pediat Infect Dis J*, 1999; 18: 976–979

DeGerome, JH, "*Helicobacter pylori* & mucosa-associated lymphoid tissue lymphoma." Lett. *JAMA* Oct 2, 1996; 275(13): 1034

Desai, HG et al, "Dental plaque: A permanent reservoir of *Helicobacter pylori*?" *Scand J Gastroenterol*, 1991; 26(11): 1205–1208

DiMarino, Jr, AJ, "*Helicobacter pylori* & peptic ulcer disease: an interview with Barry J. Marshall, M.D." *Intern Med World Rept,* Sept 1–14, 1993; 8(15): 14, 16, 28

Dimario, P et al, "Use of lactoferrin for *Helicobacter pylori* eradication: preliminary results." *J Clin Gastroenterol*, 2003; 36: 396–398

Dominici, P et al, "Familial clustering of *Helicobacter pylori* infection: population-based study." *Br Med J*, 1999; 119: 537–541

Dubois, A, "Spiral bacteria in the human stomach: the gastric *Helicobacters*." Synopses. *Emerg Infect Dis*, July–Sept 1995; 1(3): 79–85

"Easy way to find ulcers: Breathe." Tech. *NY Times,* Apr 10, 2003: F6

Ebell, MH, "Peptic ulcer disease." Practical Therapeutics. *Am Family Phy,* July1992; 46(1): 218–219

Forman, D et al, "EUROGAST Study Group: An international association between *Helicobacter pylori* infection & gastric cancer. *Lancet,* May 29, 1993; 341(8857): 1359–1362

Fox, JG et al, "Hepatic *Helicobacter* species identified in bile & gallbladder tissue from Chileans with chronic cholecystitis." *Gastroenterol*, 1998; 114: 755–763

Frigo, P et al, "*Hyperemesis gravidarum* associated with *Helicobacter pylori* seropositivity." *Obstetrics and Gynecology,* Apr 1998; 91: 615–617

Gilvarry, J et al, "Eradication of *Helicobacter pylori* affects symptoms in non-ulcer dyspepsia." *Scand J Gastroenterol*, 1997; 12: 535–540

Giordano, N et al, "*Helicobacter pylori* infection & primary Sjögren's syndrome: a possible association & new therapeutic approach." *Curr Ther Res,* 1995; 56: 1265–1269

Giovannucci, E, "Tomatoes, tomato-based products, lycopene, & cancer: review of the epidemiologic literature." *J NCI,* 1999; 91, 317–331

Goodman, KJ et al, "*Helicobacter pylori* infection in the Colombian Andes: a population-based study of transmission pathways." *Am J Epidemiol,* Aug 1996; 144(3): 290–299

Goodwin, CS et al, "*Helicobacter pylori* infection." Seminar. *Lancet,* Jan 25, 1997; 349(9047): 265–269

Gunn, M et al, "Significant association of cagA positive *Helicobacter pylori* strains with risk of premature myocardial infarction." *Heart,* 2000; 84: 267–271

"*Helicobacter,* diet linked to development of stomach cancer." *Fd Chem News,* July 10, 1995, 41–42

"*Helicobacter pylori* in peptic ulcer disease." *NIH Consensus Statement,* Feb 7–9, 1994; 12(1)

"Heroics for humble broccoli." In the Lab. *NY Times,* May 28, 2002: F6

"*H. pylori* infections preceded non-Hodgkin's stomach lymphomas." *Fd Chem News,* May 9, 1994: 7–8

Jarosz, M et al, "Effects of high dose vitamin C treatment on *Helicobacter pylori* infection and total vitamin C concentration in gastric juice." *Eur J Cancer Prev*, 1998; 7: 449–454

Johnson-Henry, KC et al, "Probiotics reduce bacterial colonization & gastric inflammation in *Helicobacter pylori*-infected mice." *Digest Dis Sci*, Aug 2004; 49(7–8): 1095–1102

Kawakubo, M et al, "Natural antibiotic function of a human gastric mucin against *Helicobacter pylori* infection." *Sci*, Aug 11, 2003; 105: 1003–1006

Kennedy, J, "Vitamin C seen protective against ulcer, stomach cancer." *Fd Chem News*, Nov 24, 1997: 9

Kockar, C et al, "*Helicobacter pylori* eradication with beta-carotene, ascorbic acid, and allicin." *Acta Medica*, 2001; 44: 97–100

Kolibasova, K et al, "Eradication of *Helicobacter pylori* as the only successful treatment in rosacea." *Arch Dermatol*, 1996; 132(11): 1393

Kountouras, J et al, "Eradication of *Helicobacter pylori* may be beneficial in the management of chronic open-angle glaucoma." *Arch Intern Med*, 2002; 162, 1237–1244

Kuelin, BM, "Nobels honor research on ulcer microbe." "Green" Drug Production Method, *JAMA*, Nov 9, 2005; 294(18): 2289–2290

Kumar, N et al, "Do chillies influence healing of duodenal ulcer?" Clin Res. *Br Med J*, 1984; 288: 1803–1804

Laino, C, "*H. pylori* implicated in allergies. *Med Trib*, Mar 24, 1994: 1

Lambert, JR et al, "High prevalence of *Helicobacter pylori* antibodies in an institutionalized population: Evidence of person-to-person transmission." *Am J Gastroenterol*, 1995; 90: 2167–2171

Leung, WK et al, "Does the use of chopsticks for eating transmit *Helicobacter pylori*?" *Lancet*, July 5, 1997; 350(9070): 31

"Link with heart disease." The World in Med. *JAMA*, June 10, 1998: 1771

Mahdavi, J et al, "*Helicobacter pylori* SabA adhesin in persistent infection & chronic inflammation. *Sci*, July 26, 2002; 297: 573–578

Marcus, H & MA Mendall, "*Helicobacter pylori* infection: A risk factor for ischaemic cerebrovascular disease and carotid atheroma." *J Neurol Neurosurg Psychiat*, 1998; 64: 104–107

Markle, HV, "Coronary artery disease associated with *Helicobacter pylori* infection is at least partially due to inadequate folate status. *Med Hypoth*, Oct 1997; 49( ): 4, 289–292

Marshall, BJ et al, "Attempt to fulfill Koch's postulates for pyloric *Campylobacter*." *Med J Austral*, Apr 15, 1985; 142: 439

—— et al, "Pyloric *Campylobacter* infection gastroduodenal disease." *Med J Austral*, Apr 15, 1985; 142: 439

—— "*Helicobacter pylori*: the etiologic agent for peptic ulcer." The 1995 Albert Lasker Med Res Awards. *JAMA*, Oct 4, 1995; 274(14): 1064–1066

Marwick, C, "*Helicobacter*: New name, new hypothesis involving type of gastric cancer." *JAMA*, Dec 5, 1990; 264(21): 2724–2727

Mendall, MA et al, "Relation of *Helicobacter pylori* infection and coronary heart disease." *British Heart Journal*, 1994, 71(5): 437–439

Mlot, C, "Can houseflies spread the ulcer bacterium?" *Sci News*, June 7, 1997: 350

Nalin, DR, "Cholera & severe toxigenic diarrhoeas." Lead Article. *Gut,* Feb 1994; 15(2): 145–149

"New views on *H. pylori.*" Quick Uptakes. *JAMA,* June 25, 1997; 277(24): 1926

Nomura, A et al, "*Helicobacter pylori* infection & gastric carcinoma among Japanese Americans in Hawaii." *N Engl J Med,* Oct 17, 1991; 325(16): 1132–1136

Odenbreit, S et al, "Translocation of *Helicobacter pylori* CagA into gastric epithelial cells by type IV secretion." *Sci,* Feb 25, 2000; 287: 1497–1500

Parsonnet, J et al, "*Helicobacter pylori* infection & the rise of gastric carcinoma." *N Engl J Med,* Oct 17, 1991; 325(16): 1127–1136

—— "Gastric adenocarcinoma & *Helicobacter pylori* infection." Lett. *Conn Med,* Aug 1994; 58(8): 474–475

—— et al, "Fecal & oral shedding of *Helicobacter pylori* from healthy infected adults." *JAMA,* Dec 15, 1999; 282(23): 2240–2245

Pattison, CP & BJ Marshall, "Proposed link between *Helicobacter pylori* and sudden infant death syndrome." *Med Hypoth,* Nov 1997; 49(5): 365–369

Peach, HG et al, "*Helicobacter pylori* infection in an Australian regional city: Prevalence & risk factors." *Med J Austral,* Sept 15, 1997; 167(6): 310–313

Perry, S et al, "Gastroenteritis & transmission of *Helicobacter pylori* infection in households." *Emerg Infect Dis,* Nov 2006; 12(11): 1701–1708

Phillips, P, "Bacterium-ulcer link is clinched." Chronic Care. Gastroenterol. *Med World News,* Oct 1990: 17

"Plants active against *Helicobacter.*" *Townsend Lett Doctors,* Feb–Mar 2000: 170

Plummer, M et al, "*Helicobacter pylori* cytotoxin-associated genotype and gastric precancerous lesions." *Journal of the National Cancer Institute,* Sept 5, 2007; 99(17): 1328–1334

Pocecco, M et al, "High risk of *Helicobacter pylori* infection associated with cow's milk antibodies in young diabetics." *Acta Pediat,* July 1997; 86(7): 700–703

Podolsky, D, "Kill the bug & you kill the ulcer." *US News & World Rept,* May 13, 1991: 94

Ponzetta, A, "*Helicobacter pylori* seroprevalence in cirrhotic patients with hepatitis B virus infection." *Nether J Med,* 2000; 56: 206–210

Portnoi, VA, "*Helicobacter pylori* infection & anorexia of aging." *Arch Intern Med,* Feb 10, 1997; 157(31): 269–272

"Raw poultry may be vector for *Helicobacter pylori* infection." *Fd Chem News,* Aug 2, 1993: 28

Rice, JM, "*Helicobacter hepaticus:* A recently recognized bacterial pathogen, associated with chronic hepatitis hepatocellular neoplasia in laboratory mice." Dispatches. *Emerg Infect Dis,* Oct–Dec 1995; 1(4): 129–131

Rosioru, C et al, "Esophagitis & *Helicobacter pylori* in children: incidence & therapeutic implication." *Am J Gastroenterol,* 1993; 13(4): 510–513

Ruiz, B et al, "Vitamin C concentration in gastric juice before & after anti-*Helicobacter pylori* treatment." *Am J Gastroenterol,* 1995; 89: 533–539

Saijo, Y et al, "Relationship of *Helicobacter pylori* infection to arterial stiffness in Japanese subjects." *Hypertension Research,* 2005; 28(4): 283–292

Sakurane, M et al, "Therapeutic effects of antibacterial treatment for intractable skin diseases in *Helicobacter pylori*-positive Japanese patients." *Journal of Dermatology,* 2002; 29(11): 22–27

Sarraf-Zadegar, N et al, "*Helicobacter pylori* relation to acute myocardial infarction in an Iranian sample." *Coronary Health Care,* 2001; 5: 202–207

Seppa, N, "Did colonization spread ulcers?" Biomed. *Sci News,* June 17, 2000: 195

—— "Bad bug: microbe raises stomach cancer risk." *Sci News,* Sept 1, 2007: 134

"Sharing chopsticks transmits *Helicobacter pylori.* Fd Chem News, July 7, 1997: 34

Shigeto, N et al, "Eradication of *Helicobacter pylori* for idiopathic thrombocytopenic purpura." *Nippon Shokakibyo Gakkai Zasshi,* 2004; 101(6): 598–608

Shiotani, A et al, "Beneficial effect of *Helicobacter pylori* eradication in dermatologic diseases." *Helicobacter,* 2001; 6(1): 60–65

Singh, RK et al, "Prospective analysis of the association of infection with CagA bearing strains of *Helicobacter pylori* and coronary heart disease." *Heart,* 2002; 88: 43–46

Sivam, GP et al, "*Helicobacter pylori:* In vitro susceptibility to garlic (*Allium sativum* extract)." Brief Comm. *Nutr & Cancer,* 1997; 27(2): 118–121

Tabak, M et al, "In vitro inhibition of *Helicobacter pylori* by extracts of thyme." *J Appl Bacteriol,* 1996; 80(6): 667–672

Thomas, JE et al, "Protection by human milk IgA against *Helicobacter pylori* infection in infancy." Lett, *Lancet,* July 10, 1993; 142: 121

"Ulcer-causing bacteria found in water." *Sci News,* June 10, 1995: 367

Utas, S et al, "*Helicobacter pylori* eradication treatment reduces the severity of rosacea." *Journal of the American Academy of Dermatology,* Mar 1999; 40: 433–435

Voelker, R, "Where did *H. pylori* come from?" *JAMA,* June 14, 2000; 283(22): 2923

Wainwright, RB, "The U.S. Arctic Investigations Program: infectious disease prevention & control research in Alaska." *Lancet,* Feb 14, 1996; 147(9000): 517–520

Weeks, DL et al, "A H+Gated urea channel: The link between *Helicobacter pylori* urease & gastric colonization." *Sci,* Jan 21, 2000; 287: 482–485

Wood, H & M Feldman, "*Helicobacter pylori* & iron deficiency." Ed'al. *JAMA,* Apr 9, 1997; 277(14): 1166–1167

Yang, M, "Advances in TCM research and treatment of gastropathies associated with *Helicobacter pylorum.*" *Journal of Traditional Chinese Medicine,* 2000; 20(2): 152–157

Yip, R et al, "Pervasive occult gastrointestinal bleeding in an Alaskan native population with prevalent iron deficiency: role of *Helicobacter pylori* gastritis." *JAMA,* Apr 9, 1997; 277(14): 1135–1139

Zoler, Mitchel L, "*H. pylori* links to cancer unfolds." *Med World News,* Feb 1991: 20

—— "Fast tests face a slow demand." *Med World News,* Dec 1991: 38

Zullo, A et al, "Ascorbic acid & intestinal metaplasia in the stomach: a prospective random-ized study." *Aliment Pharmacol Therapeut*, 2000; 14: 1301–1309

Chapter 21

Gloves

Abin, MS et al, "Anatomy of a defective barrier sequential glove leak detection in a surgical and dental environment." *Crit Care Med*, 1992; 20(2): 170–184

Adler, K, "Recommendations on bare-hand contact with ready-to-eat foods finalized by micro committee." Micro Comm Meeting. *Fd Chem News*, Oct 4, 1999: 9

Bernstein, FA, "Latex, vinyl, or soap?" *NY Times*, Mar 14, 2007: 1, 6

Butler, ME, "AFDO [Association of Food & Drug Officials] asking for model variances for barehanded contact." FDA. *Fd Chem News*, Mar 20, 2000: 16–17

Denman, S et al, "Handwashing & glove use in a long-term care facility—Maryland, 1992." Epidemiol Notes Repts. *MMWR*, Sept 10, 1993; 42(35): 672–675

Dodd, RD et al, "Self protection in surgery in the use of double gloves." *Br J Surg*, 1990; 77(2): 219–220

"Effects of gloves on bacterial cross contamination between hands & food." *J Pub Hlth*, June 2001

"Foodborne illness often handborne, sanitarians reminded." *Fd Chem News*, Aug 5, 1991: 13–14

"Gloved one, The" *Fd Creations*, May 2005: 9

Larson, E et al, "Effect of antibacterial home cleaning and handwashing products on infec-tious disease symptoms: a randomized, double-blind trial." *Annals of Internal Medicine*, 2004 Mar 2; 140(5): 321–329

"Leaky gloves have become infection control nightmare." *Med Post*, Jan 13, 1998: 34

Michaels, B, "Are gloves the answer?" *Dairy Fd Environ Sanitation*, 2001; 21(6): 489–492

——"Understanding the glove risk paradigm: clean operations." *Fd Safety Mag*, (Part 1) June–July 2004: 24, 26, 30; (Part 2) July–Sept 2004: 32, 34, 37, 69

—— "There's more to it at hand." Gloves. Fd Serv Retail. *Fd Qual*, Feb–Mar 2005: 71–76

Murphy, J, "Bare-hand contact ban for ready-to-eat foods debated by micro committee." *Fd Chem News*, Sept 27, 1999: 17–18

Olsen, RJ, "Examination gloves as barriers to hand contamination in clinical practice." *JAMA*, July 21, 1993; 270(3): 350–353

Handwashing

Auerswald, BA, "Good sanitation is in your hands." *Fd Qual*, Apr 1999: 22–26

Green, JD, "The five w's of handwashing." Sanitation. *Fd Safety Mag*, June–July 2007: 12, 14–16, 65

"Guidelines for hand hygiene in health-care settings." Recomm Repts. *MMWR*, Oct 25, 2002; 51(RR–16): 1–45

Hovey, L, "One in three caterers don't wash hands after using lavoratory (UK) survey shows." *Fd Protect Trends*, 2003: 23, 53–54

Larson, EL, "APIC [Association for Professionals in Infection Control & Epidemiology] Guidelines for handwashing and hand antisepsis in health-care settings." *Am J Infect Control*, 1995; 23: 251–269

Lin, CM et al, "Influence of fingernail length and type on removing *E. coli* from the nail regions using different handwashing interventions." *J Fd Protect*, 2002; 65: 117

Mann, J, "Handwashing: 5 steps to a best-practice payoff." Sanitation. *Fd Safety Mag*, Oct–Nov 2005: 26, 28, 30–31, 67–68

Michaels, B, "Handwashing: an effective tool in the food safety arsenal." Sanitation Tech. *Fd Qual*, Sept–Oct 2002: 45–46, 48–53

Nuland, SB, *"The Doctor's Plague: Germs, Childbed Fever & the Strange Story of Ignác Semmelweis.* NY: Norton/Atlas Bks, 2003

Pittet, D, "Improving adherence to hand hygiene practice: a multidisciplinary approach." Special Issue. *Emerg Infect Dis*, Mar–Apr 2001; 7(2): 234–240

Powitz, RW, "A practical perspective on handwashing." Sanitarian's File. *Fd Safety Mag*, June–July 2003: 16–17

Shelton, DL, "Physicians get an AMA reminder: wash your hands." Annual Meet News. *Am Med News*, July 17, 1995: 26

Starobin, A, "Cleanliness is next to effectiveness; handwashing compliance can lead to improved food safety." Safety Sanitation. Handwashing. *Fd Qual*, Oct–Nov 2006: 60, 62

Monitoring Hygiene

"Automated hand & glove washing systems." Sanitation Tech. *Fd Qual*, May 1998: 82

"Clean hand, clean buns: automated handwashing meets HACCP [Hazard Analysis Critical Control Point] compliance & FDA regulations." Field Repts. *Fd Engineer*, June 2007: 94

"Did you wash your hands?" Sanitation Tech. *Fd Qual*, Mar 1997: 52–53

"FDA should adopt HACCP [Hazard Analysis Critical Control Point] requirements for handwashing compliance in food service, company says." *Fd Chem News*, June 7, 1999: 20–21

Frederick, T, "The do's & don'ts of food plant personal hygiene practices." Sanitation. *Fd Safety Mag*, Dec 2004–Jan 2005; 18: 20–23, 74–75

"Giving hygiene a hand." *Fd Prod Design*, Oct 1992: 68

"Hands-free soap dispenser." *Prep Fds*, Feb 1999: 82

"Handwash training kit." *Fd Tech*, Nov 1998: 89

"Innovative hand and glove washing system." *Fd Qual*, Nov–Dec 1999: 90

Lehrman, Dion, "Handwashing: more than an SSOP [Sanitation Standard Operating Procedures] Sanitation Tech. *Fd Qual*, Mar–Apr 2001: 52, 54–55

"Mandatory use of hands-free taps in food processing facilities." Brief Notes. *Fd Chem News*, Sept 20, 1999: 37

Milliorn, M, "Inspection: employee hygiene monitoring." *Fd Qual,* Apr–May 2004: 66, 68, 70

—— "Monitoring hygiene: keeping a watchful eye on employees' hygiene will bolster food safety & minimize the chance of illness." *Fd Qual,* Dec 2004–Jan 2005: 81–82

"No-touch hand drying." Sanitation Tech. *Fd Qual,* Mar 1998: 60

O'Harrow, Jr, R, "Did you remember to wash your hands? A high-tech bathroom watchdog system has privacy advocates up in arms." Natl Wkly Add. *Wash Post,* Sept 8, 1997: 1–2

Pargas, N, "Hand contact with foods at the foodservice level is a global concern, McDonald's official says." *Fd Chem News,* Mar 1, 1999: 19

"Touch-free hygiene." What's New for You. Prods Systems. *Fd Qual,* May–June 2001: 68

Soaps & Alcohol Sanitizers

"From cuticles to countertops: alcohol sanitizers aid hygiene." Fd Safety Insiders. Sanitation Systems Solutions. *Fd Safety Mag,* Feb–Mar 2003: 30

Zaragoza, M, "Handwashing with soap or alcoholic solution? A randomized clinical trial of its effectiveness." *Am J Infect Control,* 1999; 27: 258–261

Triclosan

Aiello, AE et al, "Antibacterial cleaning products & drug resistance." Research. *Emerg Infect Dis,* Oct 2005; 11(10): 1565–1570

Boyce, JM, "Antiseptic technology: access, affordability, & acceptance." Special Issue. *Emerg Infect Dis,* Mar–Apr 2001; 7(2): 231–234

Boyce, JM & D Pittet, "Guidelines for hand hygiene in health-care settings: recommendations for the Healthcare Infection Control Practices Advisory Committee & the HICPAC/SHEA/APIC/IDSA Hand Hygiene Task Force." Recomm Rept. *MMWR,* 2002; 51(RR–16): 1–45

Cunningham, A, "Tainted by cleanser, antimicrobial agent persists in sludge." Sci News This Wk. *Sci News,* May 6, 2006: 275

Davidson, PM & MA Harrison, "Resistance and adaptation to food antimicrobials, sanitizers, & other process controls." IFT [Institute of Food Technologists] Sci Status Summ. *Fd Tech,* Nov 2002: 69–78

Larson, EL, "Hygiene of the skin: when is clean too clean?" Special Issue. *Emerg Infect Dis,* Mar–Apr 2001; 7(2): 225–230

Lesney, MS, "Home-use antibacterials: high risk, low benefit." *Intern Med News,* Dec 1, 2005; 38(23): 48

Levy, SB, "Antibacterial household products: cause for concern." Conference Presentations. Supp. *Emerg Infect Dis,* June 2001; 7(3 Supp): 512–521

Reynolds, SA et al, "Hand sanitizer alert." Lett. *Emerg Infect Dis,* Mar 2006; 12(3): 527–528

Sofos, JN, "Stress-adapted, cross-protected resistant: a concern?" News Anal. Sci Comm Govt Relations. *Fd Tech,* Nov 2002: 22

Suszkiw, J, "New test to detect triclosan in water." *Agric Res,* Jan 2009: 13

Tan, L et al, "Use of antimicrobial agents in consumer products." *Arch Dermatol*, 2002; 138: 1082–1086

Veldhoen, N et al, "The bacterial agent triclosan modulates thyroid hormone-associated gene expression and disrupts postembryonic anuran development." *Aquatic Toxicology*, Dec 1, 2006; 80(3): 217–227

Weber, DJ et al, "Efficacy of selected hand hygiene agents used to remove *Bacillus atrophaeus* (a surrogate of *Bacillus anthracis*) from contaminated hands." Brief Rept. *JAMA*, Mar 12, 2003 289(10): 1274–1277

Chapter 22

Ak, NO et al, "Cutting boards of plastic & wood contaminated experimentally with bacteria." *J Fd Protect*, 1994; 57: 16–22

—— "Decontamination of plastic & wood cutting boards for kitchen use." *J Fd Protect*, 1994; 57: 23–30

Altekruse, SF et al, "Consumer knowledge of foodborne microbial hazards & food-handling practices." *J Fd Protect*, 1996; 59: 287–294

Anderson, JB et al, "A camera's view of consumer food-handling behaviors." Current Res. *J Am Diet Assoc*, Feb 2004; 104: 186–191

Brody, JE, "Clean cutting boards are not enough: new lessons in food safety." Personal Hlth. *NY Times* Jan 30, 2001: D5

"Can openers teem with bacteria." *Med Wrld News*, Nov 12, 1971: 56

Cogan, TA et al, "Achieving hygiene in the domestic kitchen: the effectiveness of commonly used cleaning procedures." *J Appl Microbiol*, 2002; 92: 885–892

Daniels, RW, "Home food safety." *Fd Tech*, Feb 1998: 54–56

Dawson, P et al, "Residence time and food contact time effects on transfer of *Salmonella Typhimurium* from tile, wood and carpet: testing the five-second rule." *Journal of Applied Microbiology*, Apr 2007; 102(4): 945–953

Filipic, M, "Mild bleach solution good for sanitizing." *Chow Line*. News Media Relations. Ohio State U, Wooster, Ohio, Sept 17, 2006

"Focus on cutting board safety." *FSIS, USDA,* 1997

Gerba, C, "On germ patrol, at the kitchen sink." Hlth Fitness. *NY Times*, Feb 23, 1999: D6

Heenan, J, "Can your kitchen pass the food storage test?" *FDA Consumer*, Mar 1974: 20–25

Hesser, A, "A cutting board with the right stuff." Test Kitchen. *NY Times*, Aug 4, 1999: D3

Hunter, BT, "Safe microwave oven use." *Consumers' Research Mag*, Dec 1988: 8–9

—— "Overlooked threats of foodborne illness, don't let your guard down." *Consumers' Research Mag*, Oct 1995: 14–18

—— "Simple ways to prevent foodborne illness; good habits to develop." *Consumers' Research Mag*, Aug 1997: 25–28

—— "Cutting boards (wood or plastic?)" *Consumers' Research Mag*, Mar 1998: 8–9

Kiernan, V, "Dishing the dirt on dishcloths." *New Scientist*, Sept 2, 1995; 147: 8

Knabel, SJ, *Scientific Status Summary: Foodborne Illness: Role of Home Food Handling Practices.* Fd Tech, Apr 1995: 119–131

Marston, W, "On germ patrol, at the kitchen sink." Scientist at Work. Charles Gerba. Hlth Fitness. *NY Times*, Feb 23, 1999: D6

Medieros, LC et al, "Food safety education: what should we be teaching consumers?" *J Nutr Ed*, Mar–Apr 2001

—— "Identification & classification of consumer food-handling behaviors for food safety educators." Res. *J Am Diet Assoc*, Nov 2001; 101(11): 1326–1332, 1337–1339

Murphy, J, "Bleach-based cleaning products superior in home-based food handling study." General. *Fd Chem News*, Nov 6, 2000: 7–8

Parnell, TL & LJ Harris, "Reducing *Salmonella* on apples with wash practices commonly used by consumers." *J Fd Protect*, May 2003; 66: 741–747

Powitz, RW, "Creating a great cutting boards & wipe rag program." Sanitarian File. *Fd Safety Mag*, Aug–Sept 2007: 20–25

Raloff, J, "Wood wins, plastic trashed for cutting meats." *Sci News* Feb 6, 1993: 84–85

—— "Sponges & sinks & rags, oh, my! Where microbes lurk & how to rout them." *Sci News*, Sept 14, 1996: 172–173

Redmond, EC et al, "Consumer food handling in the house: a review of food safety studies." *J Fd Protect*, 2003; 66: 130–161

Reese, KM, "Remarks on cutting boards . . ." Newscripts. *Chem Engineer News*, Apr 6, 1993: 88

—— "Wooden cutting boards safer than plastic ones." Newscripts. *Chem Engineer News*, Mar 1, 1993: 136

Swientex, B, "Home unsafe home." Ed'al. *Prep Fds*, Aug 1999: 11

"Washing vegetables is no small potatoes." Sanitarian Tech. *Fd Qual*, 1997: 51–52

Williamson, DM et al, "Correlating food safety knowledge with home-food preparation practices." *Fd Tech*, May 1992: 94–100

Wolf, ID, "Food handling, a timely Scientific Status Summary." *Fd Tech*, Apr 1995: 28

"World Health Organization's golden rules for safe food preparation." *Cal Morbidity*, May 7, 1993; 17(18): 1

Zang, S et al, "Multistate surveillance for food-handling, preparation & consumption behaviors associated with foodborne diseases, 1995 & 1996 BRFSS [Behavioral Risk; Factor Surveillance Systems] food-safety operations." Surveill Summ. *MMWR*, Sept 11, 1998; 47(SS4): 33–57

Index

About the Author

Beatrice Trum Hunter has written more than thirty books on food issues, including *Probiotic Foods for Good Health* (Basic Health, 2008), *The Sweetener Trap & How to Avoid It* (Basic Health, 2008), *A Whole Foods Primer* (Basic Health, 2007), *Food & Your Health* (Basic Health, 2003), *The Mirage of Safety: Food Additives and Public Policy* (Charles Scribner's Sons, 1975), and *Consumer Beware: Your Food & What's Been Done to It!* (Simon & Schuster, 1971). As food editor for more than twenty years at *Consumers' Research Magazine*, her monthly columns and feature articles brought cutting-edge issues to the public before general recognition.

Hunter has received many awards and recognitions for her work. The International Academy of Preventive Medicine made her an Honorary Fellow. Other honorary memberships include the American Academy of Environmental Medicine, the Price-Pottenger Nutrition Foundation, the Weston A. Price Foundation, and the Nutrition for Optimal Health Association. She received the prestigious Jonathan Forman Award for outstanding contributions to the field of environmental medicine, was honored by the International College of Applied Nutrition, and was recipient of the President's Award for the National Nutritional Foods Association.